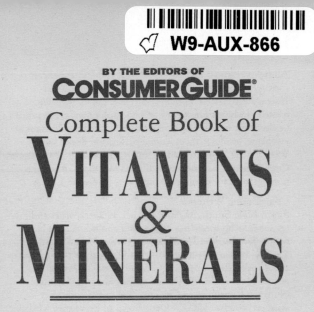

BY THE EDITORS OF
CONSUMER GUIDE®

Complete Book of

VITAMINS
&
MINERALS

SUSAN MALE SMITH, M.A., R.D.
ARLINE MCDONALD, PH.D.
ANNETTE NATOW, PH.D., R.D.
JO-ANN HESLIN, M.A., R.D.

PUBLICATIONS INTERNATIONAL, LTD.

Contributing Writers:
Susan Male Smith, M.A., R.D., is a freelance writer and consultant who specializes in nutrition and health. She has written for *American Health, Family Circle, McCall's,* and *Redbook* and has co-authored the books *Foods for Better Health* and *All-New Family Medical Guide to Health & Prevention.*
Arline McDonald, Ph.D., is a nutritionist with Scientific Nutrition Consulting in Chicago. She serves as adjunct assistant professor with the Department of Preventive Medicine at Northwestern University Medical School in Chicago and the Department of Human Nutrition and Dietetics at the University of Illinois, Chicago. **Annette Natow, Ph.D., R.D.,** is professor emeritus at the Adelphi University School of Nursing and is the editor of *The Journal of Nutrition for the Elderly.* **Jo-Ann Heslin, M.A., R.D.,** is the associate editor of *The Journal of Nutrition for the Elderly* and has written extensively on nutrition for numerous health publications.

Illustrations: Leonid Mysakov

Cover photo: Sacco Productions Limited, Chicago

Acknowledgments:

Vitamin and Mineral Counter (version 22) information provided by the Nutrition Coordinating Center at the University of Minnesota.

Nutritional analysis of recipes provided by Linda Yoakam, M.S., R.D., Naperville Nutrition Network.

The publishers would like to thank the following organizations for the use of their recipes in this publication: Almond Board of California; American Celery Council; American Lamb Council; California Apricot Advisory Board; California Cling Peach Advisory Board; California Tree Fruit Agreement; Canned Food Information Council; Florida Department of Citrus; Minnesota Cultivated Wild Rice Council; National Broiler Council; National Live Stock & Meat Board; National Pasta Association; National Turkey Federation; The Sugar Association, Inc.; Walnut Marketing Board; Washington Apple Commission; Western New York Apple Growers; and Wisconsin Milk Marketing Board.

Contents

Introduction

The year is 1700. It's almost dawn. At last count, 25 more sailors aboard His Majesty's ship have taken ill. The journey has been long and treacherous. Many months have passed since the crew of hale and hearty men set sail across the high seas. Now, as the captain looks around him, his men are slowly dying, one by one. Mysterious, irregular patches of red and purple skin cover their weakened bodies. Their gums are swollen and bleeding, and their teeth are falling out.

This scene was all too common on sailing ships of the time. In fact, the mysterious condition had plagued many since the time of Hippocrates, in 400 B.C. Yet it wasn't until 1747 that a British doctor, James Lind, began to solve the puzzle of this elusive killer by recognizing that men who were at sea for extended periods of time were deprived of certain foods, particularly fresh fruits. And not until 1795 did the British remedy the situation by issuing lime juice to the sailors aboard their naval vessels, earning them the nickname "limeys." Miraculously, it seemed, the elusive killer disappeared.

Why? What had this doctor discovered? What possible role could lime juice play in warding off a centuries-old killer? We know now that the men on those long ocean voyages were suffering from a deficiency of vitamin C—the dreaded killer was *scurvy*.

Throughout most of history, no one knew vitamins or minerals existed—at least, not by name. People knew only the *results* of not having certain foods in their diets.

Deciding what to eat back then was relatively simple. You ate whatever food was around. If you were lucky, nutrients balanced themselves in the available food, keeping you and your neighbors healthy. But at times, inevitably, the diet lacked various essential nutrients, and the entire population suffered the consequences. By trial and error, people improved their diets, recognizing in some elementary way the connection between good food and good health.

Today, of course, we have a wealth of knowledge about essential nutrients. We know what each nutrient does for us in normal amounts, as well as effects they may have when taken in large doses. Now, we have a new problem—too much information. For example, which report do we believe? The one that says megadoses of vitamin A can cure cancer, or the other that says the same nutrient can be toxic and is dangerous for pregnant women?

Some of the claims you see in vitamin and mineral advertisements, books, newspaper articles, and magazine stories may tempt you. Take a little of this mineral or a large dose of that vitamin, they say, and you'll be able to grow hair, smooth wrinkles, avoid cancer, and stop the aging process. Being seduced by such promises is easy.

But stop and think. If it were really that easy—if all these claims were true—then no one would ever go bald, develop wrinkles, get cancer, or look a day over 25. As we all know, this is hardly the case. Such fantastic claims are often anecdotal—the "it worked for me, so you try it" type of advice. The testing of such claims is rare, so there's no way to know if coincidence was responsible for the outcome. If it was just a fluke, you could actually endanger your health, and you'll most certainly waste your money.

Scientific evidence, not hearsay, is the type of advice you can use and trust—evidence that's supported by repeated studies, tests, and long, hard hours of research. The confusing part is that more and more of this kind of hard evidence supports what we used to think was simply hearsay. So, where do you turn to separate the good advice from the bad?

Right here. CONSUMER GUIDE® and a team of recognized experts in the field of nutrition provide you with a thorough, medically sound, up-to-date source book. We've cut through the confusion and have come up with a clear explanation of the function, value, and possible dangers of deficiency and overdose for each nutrient.

In the *Complete Book of Vitamins & Minerals* you can find answers to such questions as:

- Which nutrients do I need?
- How much of each should I take?
- What foods are rich sources?
- What about supplements?
- Will large doses help prevent or cure diseases?
- Are there any dangers?
- What's the latest research?

We'll first explain how the challenge of eating right is up to you. Then, we'll tell you everything you need to know about vitamins and minerals. Finally, we'll tackle everything you should know about over-the-counter supplements, in case your doctor determines you need them. We emphasize throughout that you should meet recommended nutrient intakes by eating a balanced diet. It's our hope that the information in this book will compel you to select foods that will contribute to a healthier life.

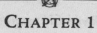
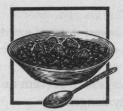

CHAPTER 1

Eating Right
Is Up to You

Studying only vitamins and minerals in the school of nutrition is like studying only verbs and nouns in an English class—they're only part of the overall picture. We must also understand what other elements food contains, why we need it, and how it's used in our bodies. Once we understand the intricate workings of essential nutrients, we'll have the knowledge to eat better and live a healthier life.

HISTORY

Human beings have walked the face of the earth for at least 250,000 years. For most of that time, our ancestors were hunters and gatherers, scrounging for food from among the plants and animals available in the immediate area. When the local food sources became scarce, tribes and individuals either moved on to greener pastures or perished.

About 10,000 years ago, people developed agriculture. They began to farm and domesticate animals, thereby working with the environment to take care of themselves. From ignorance evolved curiosity about how food sustains life. With the dawning of the scientific age, people began to ask even more questions: What happens to food when it's eaten? How does food generate energy? What foods are important for growth and the maintenance of health? These and other questions remained unanswered until chemistry, biochemistry, physiology, and other related sciences advanced.

In the late 1700s, the Frenchman Antoine Lavoisier, considered by many to be the "Father of Nutrition," investigated the relationship between respiration and energy production. His studies showed that our bodies use the oxygen we inhale to produce body heat and energy. He also observed that, in the process, we create and exhale carbon dioxide. Lavoisier concluded that the food we eat acts as fuel, which the body oxidizes, or burns, to release energy.

In a coal furnace, for example, coal burns in the presence of oxygen, releasing carbon dioxide and energy as heat. The oxidation of food is similar: In the presence of oxygen, the food we eat is burned to release carbon dioxide and energy. Lavoisier's work was the first step to uncovering how food sustains life. But the oxidation of food is only a part of a complex series of reactions that occur in the body—reactions we refer to as *metabolism*.

METABOLISM AND ENERGY

Metabolism encompasses all the chemical reactions that take place in the body's trillions of cells. Every minute of every day our cells are busy breaking down the molecules of some substances and building up the molecules of others. These chemical reactions are necessary to produce proteins, hormones, enzymes, fats, and stored forms of sugar that are vital to life. The reactions produce chemical waste products that the body must eliminate. And, of course, all-important energy is either stored or released.

What is energy? Energy is simply the ability to do work. We get energy from burning food as fuel, and we can determine how much energy a certain food supplies. We talk about the energy value of foods by comparing the number of calories foods provide. A *calorie* is the unit of heat energy. The energy value of individual foods depends on the amount of carbohydrates, fats, and proteins present. Carbohydrates and proteins supply four calories per gram, while fats yield nine calories per gram. (One gram is about equal to the mass of a paper clip. For comparison to more meaningful measures: There are 28.3 grams in an ounce and 453 grams in a pound. A milligram (mg) is 1/1,000 of a gram; a microgram (µg) is 1/1,000,000 of a gram, or 1/1,000 of a milligram.)

Different types of energy are interchangeable. For example, the chemical energy of carbohydrate converts into heat energy to help maintain a constant body temperature. It can also change to kinetic energy necessary for muscle action, or it can be trapped as chemical energy and stored in other body compounds.

THE ESSENTIAL NUTRIENTS

As the science of chemistry developed in the 18th and 19th centuries, so did procedures to analyze what we eat. Scientists soon discovered the great variety of chemically distinct compounds in foods. Their experiments determined parts of foods best suited for growth and health.

In 1827, the English physician William Prout was probably among the first to define an "adequate diet." He described the three "staminal principles" of foods necessary to support life:

• The oily
• The saccharin
• The albuminous

Today, we recognize these three basic components as fats, carbohydrates, and proteins.

By this time, the study of food chemistry had caught up to the theory and was becoming increasingly sophisticated. Researchers also began to use animals in their investigations. By the latter part of the 19th century, they expanded the definition of the "adequate diet" proposed by Prout to include inorganic elements, known as *minerals*. Today, we recognize about 17 minerals as essential nutrients for humans, and the list is growing. In the future, some 20 or 30 other minerals in foods may prove to be essential.

But something was still missing. By the dawn of the 20th century, scientists found that experimental animals perished when fed diets containing only highly purified preparations of fats, carbohydrates, proteins, and the known minerals. The missing vital nutrients turned out to be *vitamins*, the fifth class of nutrients discovered. (Previous researchers had failed to recognize the existence of vitamins because the diets prepared for experimental animals were not sufficiently "pure"—they were "contaminated" with vitamins.)

CLASSES OF ESSENTIAL NUTRIENTS

Carbohydrates (Starches; sugars): Used primarily to supply energy; carbohydrates furnish four calories per gram.

Fats and Oils (Essential fatty acids): Also called *lipids;* used to supply energy; fats furnish nine calories per gram. Dietary fat supplies the "essential fatty acids," which the body cannot make itself. A layer of fat under the skin insulates the body. Fat around internal organs cushions and protects them. Accumulation of too much fat leads to overweight and obesity.

Proteins (Essential amino acids): Used primarily in the growth and maintenance of lean body tissues—muscle. If necessary, our bodies use proteins for energy, furnishing four calories per gram. Proteins comprise smaller units—called *amino acids*—nine of which are essential and must come from food.

Vitamins: Regulators of metabolism necessary for normal formation and breakdown of body carbohydrates, fats, and proteins. Many vitamins play roles as coenzymes, helping to trigger important reactions.

Inorganic Elements (Minerals; water): Used for various functions. Some elements—like calcium and phosphorus—contribute to body structure as an important part of bones. Iron is a part of hemoglobin, the red pigment in blood that transports oxygen from the lungs to body tissues. Some inorganic elements are essential for how well nerves and muscles respond to stimuli. Others are essential for normal enzyme action. The elements in body fluids help maintain acid–base balance and water balance. Water is a component of every cell in the body, accounting for 60 percent of body weight. Blood, a water solution, carries nutrients to cells and waste products away from them.

RECOMMENDED DIETARY ALLOWANCES

The Food and Nutrition Board of the National Research Council—an arm of the National Academy of Sciences—establishes and periodically updates the Recommended Dietary Allowances (RDAs). The first RDA table was an outgrowth of the need to determine the food and nutrition status in the United States to ensure national defense during World War II. The productivity of the American people depended on good health, and good health depended on good nutrition.

The RDAs are estimates, based on available scientific knowledge, of the amount of nutrients that people need to maintain good health over a period of time. The RDAs are useful when planning menus for groups of people, such as those in schools, hospitals, or nursing homes. The government also uses them to evaluate food programs at the federal, state, and local levels.

Evaluating an *individual's* food intake was never the intention of the RDAs, though their use for that is not uncommon. It is important to remember they are not daily goals. Your intake of a nutrient is probably sufficient if your *average* intake of that nutrient equals two thirds of the RDA over a reasonable length of time. When evaluating intakes for groups of individuals, such as school-children or nursing-home patients, it's best to average five to ten days' worth of intakes.

RDAs are also not *minimum* dietary requirements. They represent amounts of nutrients that meet the needs of most healthy people. Except for calories, the RDAs contain a sizable margin of safety. Officials deliberately set them at levels higher than what's needed for the average person. This allows room for the occasional anomalous individual requirement and for those infrequent but inevitable stress situations of life that boost our nutrient requirements. The RDA also takes into account differences in the absorption level of nutrients from various sources. They are not, however, intended to meet the needs of seriously ill people or of those with genetic or metabolic disorders that cause profound changes in nutrient needs.

The very first RDAs, established in 1943, recommended intakes for 6 vitamins, 2 minerals, calories, and protein. The most current RDAs—the 10th edition, issued in 1989—gives an RDA for 11 vitamins, 7 minerals, calories, and protein, divided into 18 different age and sex categories (see Table 1, pages 18–19).

In addition, it gives "Estimated Safe and Adequate Daily Dietary Intakes of Additional Selected Vitamins and Minerals" for seven more vitamins and minerals (see Table 2, page 21). Less information is available about the nutrients in this table; therefore, there are no definite allowances made. The RDAs give estimations, as ranges, instead.

The same is true for the three minerals listed in "Estimated Sodium, Chloride, and Potassium Minimum Requirements of Healthy Persons" (see Table 3, page 21).

Rounding out the RDAs are "Median Heights and Weights and Recommended Energy Intake," provided for 15 different age and sex categories (see Table 4, pages 22–23). Also included in this table are additional allowances for pregnant women during each trimester and for lactating women during the first and second six-month periods after giving birth.

The 10th edition of the RDA published in 1989 differs from previous editions in several ways. It uses actual height and weight measures of American adults of different ages, taken from the most recent National Health and Nutrition Examination Survey (NHANES II), as the basis for the requirement for energy. Previous editions of the RDAs used arbitrary weight-for-height standards.

For the first time, the current edition features RDAs for vitamin K and selenium, reflecting the availability of better research. Another first: Smokers now have an additional allowance for vitamin C to reflect their higher needs (see Chapter 5 on antioxidants). And breast-feeding mothers now have two sets of requirements to differentiate needs specific to the first six months after delivery versus the second six-month period.

Table 1
FOOD AND NUTRITION BOARD, NATIONAL ACADEMY OF SCIENCES–NATIONAL RESEARCH COUNCIL
RECOMMENDED DIETARY ALLOWANCES,[a] Revised 1989

Designed for the maintenance of good nutrition of practically all healthy people in the United States.

Category	Age (years) or Condition	Weight[b] (kg)	(lb)	Height[b] (cm)	(in)	Protein (g)	Calcium (mg)	Phosphorus (mg)	Magnesium (mg)	Iron (mg)	Zinc (mg)	Iodine (µg)	Selenium (µg)
Infants	0.0-0.5	6	13	60	24	13	400	300	40	6	5	40	10
	0.5-1.0	9	20	71	28	14	600	500	60	10	5	50	15
Children	1-3	13	29	90	35	16	800	800	80	10	10	70	20
	4-6	20	44	112	44	24	800	800	120	10	10	90	20
	7-10	28	62	132	52	28	800	800	170	10	10	120	30
Males	11-14	45	99	157	62	45	1,200	1,200	270	12	15	150	40
	15-18	66	145	176	69	59	1,200	1,200	400	12	15	150	50
	19-24	72	160	177	70	58	1,200	1,200	350	10	150	150	70
	25-50	79	174	176	70	63	800	800	350	10	15	150	70
	51-	77	170	173	68	63	800	800	350	10	15	150	70
Females	11-14	46	101	157	62	46	1,200	1,200	280	15	12	150	45
	15-18	55	120	163	64	44	1,200	1,200	300	15	12	150	50
	19-24	58	128	164	65	46	1,200	1,200	280	15	12	150	55
	25-50	63	138	163	64	50	800	800	280	15	12	150	55
	51-	65	143	160	63	50	800	800	280	10	12	150	55
Pregnant						60	1,200	1,200	320	30	15	175	65
Lactating	1st 6 months					65	1,200	1,200	355	15	19	200	75
	2nd 6 months					62	1,200	1,200	340	15	16	200	75

[a] The allowances, expressed as daily intakes over time, are intended to provide for individual variations among most normal persons as they live in the United States under usual environmental stresses. Diets should be based on a variety of common foods in order to provide other nutrients for which human requirements have been less well defined.

[b] Weights and heights of reference adults are actual medians for the U.S. population of the designated age, as reported by NHANES II. The median weights and heights of those under 19 years of age were taken from Hamill et al (1979). The use of these figures does not imply that the height-to-weight ratios are ideal.

Tables 1-4 reprinted with permission from Recommended Dietary Allowances, 10th Edition, ©1989, by the National Academy of Sciences, National Academy Press, Washington, D.C.

Table 1 (cont.)

FOOD AND NUTRITION BOARD, NATIONAL ACADEMY OF SCIENCES—NATIONAL RESEARCH COUNCIL
RECOMMENDED DIETARY ALLOWANCES,[a] Revised 1989

Designed for the maintenance of good nutrition of practically all healthy people in the United States.

Category	Age (years) or Condition	Fat-Soluble Vitamins				Water-Soluble Vitamins						
		Vitamin A (µg RE)[b]	Vitamin D (µg)[c]	Vitamin E (mg α-TE)[d]	Vitamin K (µg)	Vitamin C (mg)	Thiamin (mg)	Riboflavin (mg)	Niacin (mg NE)[e]	Vitamin B6 (mg)	Folate (µg)	Vitamin B12 (µg)
Infants	0.0-0.5	375	7.5	3	5	30	0.3	0.4	5	0.3	25	0.3
	0.5-1.0	375	10	4	10	35	0.4	0.5	6	0.6	35	0.5
Children	1-3	400	10	6	15	40	0.7	0.8	9	1.0	50	0.7
	4-6	500	10	7	20	45	0.9	1.1	12	1.1	75	1.0
	7-10	700	10	7	30	45	1.0	1.2	13	1.4	100	1.4
Males	11-14	1,000	10	10	45	50	1.3	1.5	17	1.7	150	2.0
	15-18	1,000	10	10	65	60	1.5	1.8	20	2.0	200	2.0
	19-24	1,000	10	10	70	60	1.5	1.7	19	2.0	200	2.0
	25-50	1,000	5	10	80	60	1.5	1.7	19	2.0	200	2.0
	51-	1,000	5	10	80	60	1.2	1.4	15	2.0	200	2.0
Females	11-14	800	10	8	45	50	1.1	1.3	15	1.4	150	2.0
	15-18	800	10	8	55	60	1.1	1.3	15	1.5	180	2.0
	19-24	800	10	8	60	60	1.1	1.3	15	1.6	180	2.0
	25-50	800	5	8	65	60	1.1	1.3	15	1.6	180	2.0
	51-	800	5	8	65	60	1.0	1.2	13	1.6	180	2.0
Pregnant		800	10	10	65	70	1.5	1.6	17	2.2	400	2.2
Lactating	1st 6 months	1,300	10	12	65	95	1.6	1.8	20	2.1	280	2.6
	2nd 6 months	1,200	10	11	65	90	1.6	1.7	20	2.1	260	2.6

[a] Retinol equivalents. 1 retinol equivalent = 1 µg retinol or 6 µg beta-carotene. To calculate IU: for fruits and vegetables, multiply the RE value by 10; for foods from animal sources, multiply the RE value by 3.3.
[b] As cholecalciferol. 10 µg cholecalciferol = 400 IU of vitamin D.
[c] α-Tocopherol equivalents. 1 mg d-α tocopherol = 1 α-TE.
[d] NE (niacin equivalent) is equal to 1 mg of niacin or 60 mg of dietary tryptophan.
Tables 1-4 reprinted with permission from Recommended Dietary Allowances, 10th Edition, ©1989, by the National Academy of Sciences, National Academy Press, Washington, D.C.

The latest RDAs also signaled changes for seven nutrients—one value was raised; six were lowered. The RDA for calcium increased from 800 mg to 1,200 mg for women aged 22 to 24 years—expanding the years for peak bone growth. The RDAs decreased for vitamin B_6, folate, vitamin B_{12}, magnesium, iron, and zinc. In addition, the low ends of the ranges for the Estimated Safe and Adequate Daily Dietary Intake fell even lower for four additional nutrients—biotin, manganese, copper, and molybdenum.

Some experts in nutrition have expressed concern that the most recent edition lowered so many RDAs. Clearly, the RDAs' focus is on preventing deficiency diseases more than protecting against chronic diseases of current importance to public health. Our need for some vitamins and minerals certainly would be greater than current recommendations if the stated goal was to prevent disease. This growing belief has led to some outspoken criticism about the usefulness of the current RDAs.

In particular, the requirements for folate in women of child-bearing age, and for vitamin B_{12} and zinc in the elderly, are under discussion. The National Academy of Sciences convened a special session of the Food and Nutrition Board to consider the merit of these criticisms.

The 1989 10th Edition of the RDA is on pages 18–19 of this chapter. Individual vitamin and min-

Table 2
Estimated Safe and Adequate Daily Dietary Intakes of Additional Selected Vitamins and Minerals[a]

Category	Age (years)	Vitamins	
		Biotin μg	Pantothenic Acid
Infants	0-0.5	10	2
	0.5-1	15	3
Children and adolescents	1-3	20	3
	4-6	25	3-4
	7-10	30	4-5
	11+	30-100	4-7
Adults		30-100	4-7

Category	Age (years)	Trace Elements[b]				
		Copper (mg)	Manganese (mg)	Fluoride (mg)	Chromium (μg)	Molybdenum (μg)
Infants	0-0.5	0.4-0.6	0.3-0.6	0.1-0.5	10-40	15-30
	0.5-1	0.6-0.7	0.6-1.0	0.2-1.0	20-60	20-40
Children and adolescents	1-3	0.7-1.0	1.0-1.5	0.5-1.5	20-80	25-50
	4-6	1.0-1.5	1.5-2.0	1.0-2.5	30-120	50-150
	7-10	1.0-2.0	2.0-3.0	1.5-2.5	50-200	75-250
	11+	1.5-2.5	2.0-5.0	1.5-2.5	50-200	75-250
Adults		1.5-3.0	2.0-5.0	1.5-4.0	50-200	75-250

[a] Because there is less information on which to base allowances, these figures are not given in the main table of RDA and are provided here in the form of ranges of recommended intakes.

[b] Since the toxic levels for many trace elements may be only several times usual intakes, the upper levels for the trace elements given in this table should not be habitually exceeded.

Table 3
Estimated Sodium, Chloride, and Potassium Minimum Requirements of Healthy Persons[a]

Age	Weight		Sodium (mg)[a,b]	Chloride (mg)[a,b]	Potassium (mg)[c]
	(lb)[d]	(kg)[d]			
Months					
0-5	9.9	4.5	120	180	500
6-11	19.6	8.9	200	300	700
Years					
1	24.2	11.0	225	350	1,000
2-5	35.2	16.0	300	500	1,400
6-9	55.0	25.0	400	600	1,600
10-18	110.0	50.0	500	750	2,000
>18[d]	154.0	70.0	500	750	2,000

[a] No allowance has been included for large, prolonged losses from the skin through sweat.

[b] There is no evidence that higher intakes confer any health benefit.

[c] Desirable intakes of potassium may considerably exceed these values (~3,500 mg for adults).

[d] No allowance included for growth. Values for those below 18 years assume a growth rate at the 50th percentile reported by the National Center for Health Statistics (Hamill et al., 1979) and averaged for males and females.

Table 4

Median Heights and Weights

Age (years), Gender, or Condition	Weight (kg)	Weight (lb)	Height (cm)	Height (in)
Infants				
0.0–0.5	6	13	60	24
0.5–1.0	9	20	71	28
Children				
1–3	13	29	90	35
4–6	20	44	112	44
7–10	28	62	132	52
Males				
11–14	45	99	157	62
15–18	66	145	176	69
19–24	72	160	177	70
25–50	79	174	176	70
51+	77	170	173	68
Females				
11–14	46	101	157	62
15–18	55	120	163	64
19–24	58	128	164	65
25–50	63	138	163	64
51+	65	143	160	63
Pregnant				
1st trimester				
2nd trimester				
3rd trimester				
Lactating				
1st 6 months				
2nd 6 months				

[a]Calculation based on FAO equations, then rounded.
[b]In the range of light to moderate activity, the coefficient of variation is ± 20%.

Table 4 (cont.)

Recommended Energy Intake

REE[ad] (kcal/day)	Average Energy Allowance (kcal)[b]		
	Multiples of REE[d]	Per kg	Per day[c]
320		108	650
500		98	850
740		102	1,300
950		90	1,800
1,130		70	2,000
1,440	1.70	55	2,500
1,760	1.67	45	3,000
1,780	1.67	40	2,900
1,800	1.60	37	2,900
1,530	1.50	30	2,300
1,310	1.67	47	2,200
1,370	1.60	10	2,200
1,350	1.60	38	2,200
1,380	1.55	36	2,200
1,280	1.50	30	1,900
			+0
			+300
			+300
			+500
			+500

[c]Figure is rounded.
[d]REE = Resting Energy Expenditure; Multiples of REE = Adjustment for activity (light to moderate).

eral profiles appear in Chapters 7 and 11, with discussions of allowances for adults. For information about allowances for infants, children, teenagers, young adults, and women who are pregnant or breast-feeding, refer back to the complete tables in this chapter.

THE FOOD GUIDE PYRAMID

After World War II, officials developed the Basic Four Food Groups because of a concern that people were not getting enough protein, vitamins, and minerals in their diets. Meat, milk, and eggs anchored diets of that time. Little attention was paid to nutrients we try to eat less of today—fat, sugar, and calories.

To help people plan and evaluate their diets for adequate nutrition, the United States Department of Agriculture (USDA) developed the "Food Guide Pyramid" (see page 28) in 1992. This food guide is an updated version of the familiar Basic Four Food Groups, or Daily Food Guide of the 1950s, except that the number of food groups is now five instead of four. The new Pyramid also reflects a concern for moderation in intakes of fats, oils, and sweets.

Grouping by Nutrient

The Pyramid no longer lumps fruits and vegetables into one group, as in the past. By creating two distinct groups, the USDA is emphasizing the specific contributions each brings to the table.

Fruit provides some vitamins and minerals in amounts not necessarily found in vegetables, and vice versa. For example, without citrus fruit, it would be difficult to get enough vitamin C. Likewise, without a serving of a yellow-orange or dark-green, leafy vegetable, it might be difficult to get enough beta-carotene in the diet.

Moreover, citrus fruits are richer than vegetables in soluble fiber—the fiber that may lower blood cholesterol. But vegetables have more of insoluble fiber—the kind that may protect the colon from cancer.

Other than separating fruits from vegetables, the food groups in the Pyramid are identical to those in the Basic Four. As before, the nutrients they share are what determines the grouping of foods. The vegetable group provides potassium, magnesium, folate, vitamin E, vitamin K, and sometimes calcium, in addition to vitamin A and fiber, depending on your choice of vegetable. Fruits offer potassium as well as vitamin C and fiber.

The milk group includes yogurt and cheese—all good sources of calcium, phosphorus, vitamin D, and riboflavin (vitamin B_2), as well as protein. Grains include breads, cereals, rice, and pasta—important sources of B vitamins and fiber, along with such minerals as iron, potassium, zinc, copper, and selenium.

Most eclectic is the meat group, which includes poultry, fish, eggs, dried beans, and nuts as concentrated sources of protein. By placing dried beans and nuts with meat, it emphasizes that both are good alternative protein sources—for anyone, not just vegetarians. Dried beans, like meat, are also a source of iron and zinc. In addition, they provide folate, calcium, and fiber. Nuts also furnish magnesium and vitamin E.

Grouping foods according to the nutrients they provide allows you to choose from a variety of different foods. Just remember to include items from each of the food groups. This offers an easy way to plan a healthful diet with a balanced intake of nutrients, while avoiding the rigid approach and monotony of fixed menus.

By balancing foods from each of the food groups, the Pyramid eating plan also ensures adequate amounts of vitamins and minerals in the diet, with a few exceptions. Teenage girls and women in their child-bearing years may have difficulty getting enough iron unless they make an effort to include extra servings of iron-rich such foods as whole-grain or enriched breads and cereals in their diets.

These women, as well as postmenopausal women, also have special requirements for calcium. The recommended number of servings from the milk group may not completely meet their needs, nor will extra servings of other calcium sources such as dried beans and broccoli. Such instances might call for the use of dietary supplements.

Eating from the Bottom Up

The Pyramid's triangular shape better represents the relative proportion of foods in your diet than the old square Basic Four, which implied equality among the groups. However, you should not interpret the position of the food groups on the Pyramid to mean that one group is paramount over another. The groups on top are not more *important* than the lower ones. Each food group's placement on the Pyramid visually portrays its ideal *proportion* in the diet. You should eat more from the bottom of the Pyramid and less from the top. Yet selecting foods from each group is necessary to obtain a balanced diet with all the vitamins, minerals, and other nutrients you need.

The number of recommended servings from each group has changed to reflect the difference nutritionists place on the proportional value of the different groups. Furthermore, to take into account the differences in individuals' needs for calories, a range of servings replaces the single recommendations made in the past. (See "Examples of Single Servings" on page 31.)

The low end of the range given for number of servings is sufficient for older adults and inactive women who eat about 1,600 calories per day. The middle number meets the needs for most children, teenage girls, active adult women, and inactive adult men; it provides about 2,200 calories per day. Teenage boys, active adult men, and women who

Food Guide Pyramid
A Guide to Daily Food Choices

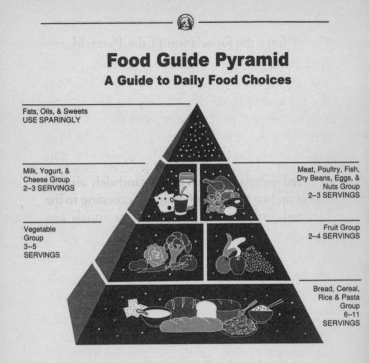

Fats, Oils, & Sweets
USE SPARINGLY

Milk, Yogurt, &
Cheese Group
2–3 SERVINGS

Meat, Poultry, Fish,
Dry Beans, Eggs, &
Nuts Group
2–3 SERVINGS

Vegetable
Group
3–5
SERVINGS

Fruit Group
2–4 SERVINGS

Bread, Cereal,
Rice & Pasta
Group
6–11
SERVINGS

KEY

● Fat (naturally occurring and added)

▼ Sugars (added)

These symbols show fats, oils, and
added sugars in foods.

are very active need about 2,800 calories daily and should aim for the highest number of servings listed. No one should eat fewer than the lowest number of servings listed for each food group. Small children who may need less than 1,600 calories should simply eat smaller portions.

Grains form the foundation of the Pyramid, emphasizing the role they should play as the base of your diet. This group shows the greatest change from the Basic Four in the number of servings recommended, increasing from the old 4 servings to the new 6 to 11 servings. This may seem like a lot more bread and pasta to eat, until you realize how little food is in one serving. Since one slice of bread equals one serving, a sandwich already makes up two servings of grains. According to the Pyramid, only one-half cup of pasta equals one serving, so an average plate of spaghetti easily translates into three or four Pyramid servings.

Take a step up from grains and you'll find the fruit and vegetable groups. They should be the next most plentiful foods in your diet. The Pyramid plan recommends three to five servings of vegetables plus two to four servings of fruits. This is more than double the Basic Four's recommendation, which called for only four servings from the combined group of fruits and vegetables. This reflects new research that shows fruits and vegetables can prevent chronic diseases, whether through their rich nutrient content or their contribution of phytochemicals—natural disease-fighting chemicals in plants (see Chapter 5).

Near the top of the Pyramid are the milk and meat groups, signaling their smaller roles relative to grains, fruits, and vegetables. They share a step because the proportions they contribute to the total diet should be about the same. The Pyramid plan recommends two to three servings from each group. This is unchanged from the Basic Four plan.

At the very top of the Pyramid are fats, oils, and sweets. These items are not a food group; their position on the Pyramid gives the message to use these items sparingly. Fat and sugar are also present in the other groups, of course, so you will need to take this into account when choosing specific foods.

The guidelines for fat limit your intake to 30 percent of calories. If you choose foods with the lowest fat contents from each group, the Pyramid eating plan will provide approximately half of the fat you need. You can then use the remainder of your fat allowance for cooking fats, spreads, and salad dressings.

The guidelines for sugar suggest limiting intake to 6 teaspoons for a 1,600-calorie diet, 12 teaspoons for a 2,200-calorie diet, and 18 teaspoons for a 2,800-calorie diet. This allowance includes any amount you might be getting from sweetened fruit juices, presweetened breakfast cereals, candy, and baked goods. Reading labels becomes essential (remember, four grams equals one teaspoon of sugar).

There are fat traps in almost all the groups. The meat group contains the most, because meats are more likely to be high in fat. But grain-based foods such as cookies, cakes, and pastries are also high in fat, and you shouldn't meet the recommenda-

EXAMPLES OF SINGLE SERVINGS

Food Group

Milk, Yogurt, and Cheese	1 cup of milk or yogurt 1½ ounces of natural cheese 2 ounces of processed cheese
Meat, Poultry, Fish, Dry Beans, Eggs, and Nuts	2–3 ounces of cooked lean meat, poultry, or fish ½ cup of cooked beans, 1 egg, or 2 tablespoons of peanut butter count as 1 ounce of lean meat
Vegetables	1 cup of raw leafy vegetables ½ cup of other vegetables, cooked or chopped raw ¾ cup of vegetable juice
Fruit	1 medium apple, banana, or orange ½ cup of chopped, cooked, or canned fruit ¾ cup of fruit juice
Bread, Cereal, Rice, and Pasta	1 slice of bread 1 ounce of ready-to-eat cereal ½ cup of cooked cereal, rice, or pasta

tions for grains by eating a lot of these foods. Fat in the milk group comes from whole-milk products, ice cream, and most cheeses. Vegetables can also be sources of fat if fried or eaten with cream sauces. Fruits can be sugar traps if you choose sweetened canned fruit, juice drinks, jellies, jams, or preserves.

These Pyramid recommendations mirror those promoted in the Dietary Guidelines for Americans, published jointly by the USDA and the Department of Health and Human Services, as well as in the U.S. Surgeon General's 1988 Report on Nutrition and Health. These dietary guidelines stress the need to lower our fat intake to protect against heart disease, cancer, and overweight.

Keep in mind that foods rich in fat and sugar are often devoid of vitamins and minerals. We should direct ourselves toward foods rich in the nutrients we need. These are the food choices most likely to supply the vitamins and minerals necessary for good health.

FOOD LABELING

The "Nutrition Facts" food label includes a measurement called Percent Daily Value, or %DV, which provides information about a food's nutrient content. The %DV reflects the RDA values for the age and sex group that has the greatest needs.

Nutrition Facts

Serving Size ¹/₂ cup (114g)
Servings per Container 4

Amount Per Serving

Calories 90	**Calories from Fat** 30

	% **Daily Value***
Total Fat 0g	5%
Saturated Fat 0g	0%
Cholesterol 0mg	0%
Sodium 300mg	13%
Total Carbohydrate 13g	4%
Dietary Fiber 3g	12%
Sugars 3g	
Protein 3g	

Vitamin A 80%	•	Vitamin C 60%
Calcium 4%	•	Iron 4%

*Percent Daily Values are based on a 2,000 calorie diet.
Your daily values may be higher or lower depending on your
calorie needs.

	Calories:	2,000	2,500
Total Fat	Less than	65g	80g
Sat Fat	Less than	20g	25g
Cholesterol	Less than	300mg	300mg
Sodium	Less than	2,400mg	2,400mg
Total Carbohydrate		300g	375g
Fiber		25g	30g

Calories per gram:

Fat 9   •   Carbohydrate 4   •   Protein 4

In 1990, Congress passed the Nutrition Labeling and Education Act to clear up confusion over food labels. All packaged foods and meat and poultry products must have nutrition information on their labels (see sample label, page 33). For unpackaged raw foods, such as fruits, vegetables, and raw fish, look for voluntary information provided by posters or pamphlets in the produce sections and at seafood counters.

There are strict definitions now about what claims manufacturers can make, governing words such as *lite* or *light*, *low*, *high*, *less*, *more*, *reduced*, *good source*, or *free*. A food has to meet strict guidelines to use these words. Even casual use of the word *fresh* is taboo. A food claiming to be a good source of vitamin E, for example, must provide ten percent of the recommended amount of vitamin E per serving. If a food claims to be cholesterol free, it cannot contain more than 2 mg per serving. But even a truly cholesterol-free food cannot make this claim if it is high in fat, because the message would be too confusing for consumers. The labeling on a food that naturally contains zero cholesterol, such as pinto beans, can make only general statements about being cholesterol-free.

To make comparisons easier, packages now express nutrition information exactly the same way from package to package, with only a few exceptions. Foods that contain insignificant amounts of many nutrients can use an abbreviated version of the chart. Foods that come in very small packages only have to provide a toll-free number where consumers can call for nutrition information.

Serving sizes are now standardized for similar types of foods. The size of a serving is based on details from food consumption surveys and is, thus, more realistic than the old serving sizes made up by the manufacturers. The label states the total number of calories per serving, along with the number of calories from fat in a serving.

Amounts of total fat, saturated fat, cholesterol, sodium, carbohydrate, dietary fiber, sugars, and protein are expressed in grams or milligrams per serving of the food. The relative amounts or percentages of vitamin A, vitamin C, calcium, and iron provided by one serving is also on the label. Other nutrients can also appear on the label as long as the Food and Drug Administration (FDA) has included them on its authorized list.

Preventing heart disease and cancer is a current health concern responsible for the shift in emphasis on the food label. The label relegates nutrients we might be underconsuming to lesser status, not mentioning some of them at all. At this time, evidence is not sufficient that vitamin and mineral deficiencies—except for deficiencies of vitamin A, vitamin C, calcium, and iron—are significant health problems. But as researchers complete more comprehensive studies on the health benefits of vitamins such as folate and vitamin E, or minerals such as selenium or chromium, this position could change. (See Chapters 6 and 10 for more information on the roles of vitamins and minerals in fighting diseases.)

Although the food label is now more informative about such nutrients as fat, sugar, and calories, it is less informative about vitamins and minerals. Now, the nutrient information just lists the 2 vitamins and 2 minerals a food is highest in, instead of the 11 vitamins and 3 or 4 minerals it did before. However, if a food claims to be high in a particular vitamin or mineral, then that nutrient must also appear on the label along with the required vitamins and minerals.

Despite these limitations, the label information is still useful in selecting foods to make up a healthful diet. A new term, *Daily Value* (DV), now appears on the label. The DV replaces the U.S. RDA. All nutrients on the label are expressed as a percentage of the DV (%DV) that one serving of the food contributes to a 2,000-calorie diet. If your daily caloric intake is more or less than 2,000 calories, the percentages applying to your diet will vary from the percentage listed. For diets of 2,000 and 2,500 calories, the actual %DV for some nutrients appear on the label. Because the DVs for vitamins and minerals do not change for different calorie intakes, only the %DVs appear on the label for these nutrients.

Some foods claim specific health benefits on their labels. If a food meets certain requirements, its label is allowed to state a relationship between particular foods and certain diseases, as long as it stresses the importance of the food as part of an overall healthful diet (see "Examples of Authorized Health Claims for Foods," page 38).

For example, labels can identify foods low in sodium (less than 140 mg per serving) as an important part of a diet aimed at lowering the risk of high blood pressure. Foods that are good sources of calcium or provide ten percent of the DV for this mineral (120 mg per serving) may carry a message about calcium's importance in the diets of young adult women, to help prevent osteoporosis.

Fruits and vegetables that provide ten percent of the DV for vitamin A, vitamin C, or dietary fiber may carry a statement saying they offer protection against cancer as part of a balanced diet that is low in fat.

Fruit, vegetable, and whole-grain products that are good sources of fiber and are also low in fat can make claims about cancer. Foods low in total fat, saturated fat, and cholesterol can make claims about heart disease. And foods that supply a critical amount of soluble fiber, such as oats, oranges, and peaches, can claim to have a benefit against heart disease.

As more clinical research accumulates, you may see additional claims on food labels to alert you to foods that may protect against disease. Although not yet approved, possible health claims on the horizon include:

- folate to protect against neural tube defects in pregnant women

- zinc to benefit immune system function in the elderly
- vitamin E to lower risk of heart disease
- calcium to combat high blood pressure

(For more information on these relationships, see Chapters 6 and 10.)

EXAMPLES OF AUTHORIZED HEALTH CLAIMS FOR FOODS

- Calcium and Osteoporosis
- Sodium and Hypertension
- Fat and Cancer
- Saturated Fat & Cholesterol and Coronary Heart Disease
- Fiber-containing Grain Products, Fruits & Vegetables and Cancer
- Fiber-containing Grain Products, Fruits & Vegetables and Coronary Heart Disease
- Fruits & Vegetables and Cancer

CHAPTER 2

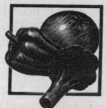

The Story of Vitamins

With all the talk about the importance of vitamins to good nutrition, it's time to ask, "What are vitamins?" Vitamins are organic substances that are necessary in very small amounts to maintain normal metabolism in the body.

In 1912, a Polish chemist by the name of Dr. Casimir Funk, working at the Lister Institute in London, coined the word *vitamine*. He derived it from *vita*, meaning "life," and *amine*, referring to a class of nitrogen-containing organic compounds. At the time, Dr. Funk was investigating thiamin—vitamin B_1—which is an amine. Later, scientists realized that not all vitamins are amines, so the final *e* in *vitamine* was dropped. The word *vitamin*, however, still reflects the vital life-giving importance of these substances.

The phrase "in very small amounts" included in the definition of vitamins sets them apart from the other classes of essential organic compounds. For example, proteins, fats, and carbohydrates are also organic substances, but we require them in considerably greater quantities. We measure vitamins in milligrams (mg) and micrograms (μg); in contrast, we measure proteins, fats, and carbohydrates in grams (g).

You may recall from the first chapter that a gram is about the mass of a paper clip. One milligram is 1/1,000 of a gram, and one microgram is 1/1,000,000 of a gram. Such extremely tiny amounts certainly sound insignificant. However, the British sailors who developed scurvy on long ocean voyages were deprived of mere milligrams of vitamin C and proved how absolutely vital these minute quantities are.

We've only known about the existence of vitamins since Dr. Funk's research in 1912. Since that time, scientists have identified 13 vitamins. The last to be isolated was vitamin B_{12} in the late 1940s. Upon its discovery, researchers assigned a letter designation to each vitamin in alphabetical order. It turned out, however, that some of the vitamins were actually several substances. The compound vitamin B, for example, turned out to be a group of compounds. So we now have vitamin B_1, vitamin B_2, vitamin B_6, and so forth. Although vitamins' alphabetical designations are still in common use, they also have chemical names. (The table on page 42 identifies the 13 vitamins and their chemical names.)

All vitamins are essential to life and must be supplied in the diet. As with any rule, though, there are exceptions. The body does produce small amounts of biotin, vitamin B_{12}, and vitamin K from intestinal bacteria, but in such negligible quantities that we still need more from the foods we eat.

Furthermore, if the body is supplied with the proper raw materials, it is capable of manufacturing certain other vitamins. For example, plant foods such as fruits and vegetables don't actually contain vitamin A but instead have vitamin A "activity." In other words, they are "precursors" to vitamin A, because they contain substances called *carotenes* that our bodies can convert to vitamin A. Carotenes, or carotinoids, are the yellow-orange pigments that give the characteristic color to vegetables and fruits such as carrots, squash, and cantaloupe. These precursors are sometimes called *provitamin A*. Carotenes may also function as antioxidants, giving them importance beyond their conversion to vitamin A (see Chapter 5).

We have a provitamin D in our skin. Sunlight triggers a chemical reaction in skin that begins the provitamin's complex conversion to vitamin D— a process that is later completed in the kidneys. This explains vitamin D's nickname, the "sunshine vitamin." Often, though, the amount pro-

Vitamins and Their Chemical Names

Vitamin	Chemical Name
A	carotenoids; beta-carotene; retinol; vitamin A acetate; vitamin A palmitate
B_1	thiamin; thiamin hydrochloride; thiamin mononitrate
B_2	riboflavin; riboflavin 5'-phosphate; sodium riboflavin phosphate; disodium riboflavin phosphate
B_3	niacin; nicotinic acid; nicotinamide; niacinamide
B_6	pyridoxine hydrochloride
B_{12}	cobalamin; cyanocobalamin; cyanocobalamin concentrate
C	ascorbic acid; sodium ascorbate; erythorbic acid (isoascorbic acid)
D	cholecalciferol; calciferol; ergocalciferol
E	tocopherol; alpha-tocopherol; alphatocopheryl acetate; alphatocopheryl acid succinate
K	naphthoquinone; menadione (K_3); phylloquinone (K_1, phytonadione) menaquinone (K_2)
Biotin	biotin
Folate	folic acid; folacin
Pantothenic acid	panthenol; calcium pantothenate

duced this way isn't enough to meet our bodies' needs, and we still need a dietary source. The body also meets some of its niacin needs by conversion from the amino acid, tryptophan. Because we must rely on diet to fulfill our requirements for these vitamins, they are all essential.

Another way to classify vitamins is by solubility. Fat-soluble vitamins—A, D, E, and K—require fat for absorption. Water-soluble vitamins include biotin, folate, niacin, pantothenic acid, vitamins B_1, B_2, B_6, B_{12}, and C. (Information about each of the 13 vitamins is provided in Chapter 7.)

SO MUCH FROM SO LITTLE

Many vitamins, especially those of the B complex, act as coenzymes, or small molecules attached to enzymes that help the enzymes do their job. An enzyme is an catalyst—a substance that regulates the speed of a chemical reaction without being used up or changed in that reaction. So our bodies can use enzymes over and over again to control specific reactions. The body can also repeatedly use vitamins that act as coenzymes.

However, the body still needs a regular supply of these and the other vitamins to replace those excreted in the urine or destroyed or changed by the body during certain metabolic processes.

SUBCLINICAL DEFICIENCY

Concern about vitamin deficiencies is rapidly being replaced with concern about the effects of marginally adequate vitamin intakes—amounts that may not cause a vitamin-deficiency disease but might interfere with normal body functions.

A *subclinical deficiency* can sneak up on you when the amount of a nutrient in your diet or your total "body pool" of a nutrient is only marginally adequate. Biochemical and metabolic changes can begin to take place, and then, you would be at risk for a vitamin deficiency.

Subclinical deficiencies can be deceptive. Outward signs are not apparent, but symptoms can develop rapidly if intake of the nutrient suddenly drops or if the person's nutrient requirement suddenly increases because of an illness or surgery. A person could appear to be the picture of health, even though the process leading to disease may already be set in motion. And once a disease is present, it isn't always possible to reverse the effects of a longtime inadequate vitamin intake.

Sometimes symptoms never develop or aren't recognized when they do. For example, a vitamin E deficiency does not have any clear symptoms to identify it. If you are subclinically deficient in vitamin E, your immune system suffers the effects of operating at less-than-optimal capacity and may be unable to protect you fully against infections or cancer.

Only laboratory tests can confirm subclinical vitamin deficiencies. Depending on the vitamin, these laboratory tests may measure the amount of the vitamin circulating in the blood or the amount of the vitamin's breakdown products excreted in the urine.

In some instances, they measure metabolic by-products of a vitamin. The amount of these compounds in the blood or urine often indicate the vitamin status of the individual. That's because certain compounds accumulate if the vitamin they need to function is in low supply.

It is also possible to measure the activity of certain enzymes that require vitamins as coenzymes. For example, the enzyme transketolase (present in red blood cells) exhibits below-normal activity when not enough thiamin, its coenzyme, is available.

Waiting to act on your nutrient needs until you have a clear deficiency or a disease is not a prudent approach. Fortunately, severe vitamin deficiencies are rare in the United States today, but they do still exist in developing areas of the world, where food shortages and malnutrition are more prevalent than we like to think.

One way to protect yourself from the dangers of undetectable subclinical deficiencies is to eat a wide variety of foods. If you do not eat enough calories, or if your eating habits are not as good as you would like, you may want to consider taking a multivitamin/mineral supplement. The supplement should balance what you are already getting from your diet.

TOXICITY

We know that large doses of vitamins can have harmful effects on the body. In fact, an overdose of a vitamin can be as serious as a vitamin deficiency. Overdoses are more likely to occur with fat-soluble vitamins, which are stored in body fat and the liver and used as needed. The more you take of fat-soluble vitamins, the more of them your body stores. If too much is stored, serious consequences result. Cases of toxicity from excesses of vitamins A and D are occasionally reported (see the profiles in Chapter 7).

Our bodies cannot store large amounts of water-soluble vitamins, so we need a more constant supply of them. Overdoses are unlikely, because we excrete any excess of these vitamins in urine if too much is consumed. Because of this, nutritionists used to believe you couldn't take in a dangerous amount of water-soluble vitamins. We now know, however, that large quantities of vitamin C and some of the B vitamins—particularly B_6—can trigger toxic effects.

Moreover, high doses of vitamins can create vitamin imbalances. That is, large amounts of one vitamin can cause a deficiency of another. For example, animal studies have shown that high doses of vitamin E may adversely affect a person's vitamin K status.

Hypervitaminosis is the clinical term for a vitamin overdose. The danger of this condition exists whenever you take large doses—megadoses—of vitamins. (For more information about megadoses, see Chapter 4.)

THERAPEUTIC USES: VITAMINS AS DRUGS

Many situations increase vitamin needs. For example, children from infancy to the end of puberty—a period of growth and development—often need extra vitamins. Since pregnant women are eating for two (or more), they usually require extra nutrients also. When people cannot consume a regular diet because of severe illness, surgery, or allergies, they may need vitamin supplements. Vitamin requirements are higher for those taking birth control pills, those who are on very restrictive diets, and those taking drugs that may interfere with vitamin function or absorption. In rare instances, a person may be born with an inherited disorder requiring higher vitamin intakes. A qualified physician should carefully evaluate and treat all these situations.

Currently popular is "megavitamin therapy" or "orthomolecular therapy," based on the premise that large doses of vitamins are useful for the treatment or cure of many diseases. It's true that large doses of certain vitamins can be medically useful. For example, nicotinic acid—a form of niacin—is often prescribed to reduce blood cholesterol levels. Unfortunately, most claims haven't been substantiated by carefully controlled studies.

Any druglike action of a vitamin is unrelated to its nutritional function. When taken in megadoses, a vitamin is no longer acting as a nutrient, because the amount far exceeds what's necessary to meet the body's nutritional requirements. Rather, the vitamin is acting as a drug. It is not yet clear whether moderately high doses of vitamins are active as nutrients or as drugs.

Caution: Self-treatment of real or suspected diseases with massive doses of vitamins is potentially hazardous. Not only does the danger of overdose exist, but self-diagnosis and self-treatment can only delay appropriate medical attention. Supplements that contain doses 500 to 1,000 times more than the amounts recommended by the RDA require proper medical supervision.

VITAMINS IN A PREVENTIVE ROLE

Any benefits of vitamin megadoses in the treatment of medical conditions remain largely unproved and cannot take the place of standard medical treatment. Nevertheless, interest has grown in the possibility that certain vitamins can *prevent* some diseases from developing in the first place. (For more about prevention, see Chapters 5 and 6.)

Prevention does not need to be as aggressive as treatment. Prevention is similar to buying an insurance policy to protect you from something that might happen. But because you are not sure it actually will happen, you do not want to risk any unwanted side effects. So before you consider consuming higher-than-recommended amounts of particular vitamins, you need to be sure that scientific evidence supports it.

Much of what we know about the role of vitamins in protecting against diseases comes from studying people who exhibit fewer diseases than other people, and comparing the foods they eat. One of the most striking differences in dietary habits is the abundance of fruits and vegetables eaten by groups with low rates of cancer and heart disease. Fruits and vegetables are the major sources of many vitamins and minerals—particularly antioxidants. This suggests a tentative link between these nutrients and protection from disease. But fruits and vegetables are also full of fiber and phytochemicals, so no one knows for sure if one component—or all of them together—is what's responsible.

The possibility that some vitamins may help prevent disease has raised questions about whether the current dietary recommendations are high enough. Since the RDAs recommend amounts sufficient only to prevent deficiency, they may be well below what is optimal to protect against disease. Some evidence points to levels even higher than what is in foods, especially for vitamin E. Some researchers believe we should simply eat more fruits and vegetables, as population studies support.

This debate revolves around the new roles recently identified for vitamins in the body. The RDAs are based on traditional vitamin-dependent functions, but recent discoveries are forcing us to reevaluate our vitamin needs in light of newly defined functions for vitamins. Most of these functions protect us against disease processes.

No matter which way the debate is resolved, we may need more of certain vitamins than previously thought if we want to protect ourselves against disease.

VITAMINLIKE SUBSTANCES

Certain substances, though not true vitamins, closely resemble vitamins in their activity. When these vitaminlike substances appear in vitamin preparations, a footnote on the label usually reads: "Need in human nutrition has not been established."

The nutritional status and biological role of vitaminlike substances are murky. At one time, choline, inositol, and para-aminobenzoic acid (PABA) were thought to be vitamins. It was later discovered that each of these could be synthesized in the body, and a lack of them did not cause deficiency symptoms. Therefore, they do not meet the definition of a vitamin.

Claims for these substances can be misleading. PABA is an ingredient in some sunscreens, but taking PABA internally will not prevent sunburn.

PABA also appears to prevent gray hair, because when it is lacking in some animals, their dark fur loses its pigment. However, PABA cannot reverse or prevent graying in humans. Once a person's hair has turned gray, nothing short of a bottle of dye will restore his or her natural color.

Other vitaminlike substances include: bioflavonoids (often sold in combination with vitamin C), carnitine (sometimes called *vitamin B-T*), coenzyme Q, and lipoic acid.

Current widespread promotion of vitaminlike supplements for the treatment or cure of serious diseases lacks sufficient scientific basis. Bioflavonoids have shown promise as phytochemicals, but research is only preliminary. Vitaminlike substances certainly are not essential for good health. Only the 13 vitamins discussed in the following chapters are essential in the human diet.

CHAPTER 3

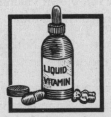

Vitamin Supplements

Confusion and misinformation surround the use of supplements. People hear stories about our food supply being robbed of its nutritional value and that it's impossible to get the required vitamins through food alone. Promoters of vitamin supplements encourage these stories with such expressions as "just to be sure you get all the vitamins you need." In addition, promotions abound for supplements—especially in massive doses—to prevent and cure diseases unrelated to known deficiencies.

The notion that vitamins are endowed with miraculous powers is a popular one. This idea, combined with a misunderstanding about how vitamins work, leads many to believe that daily supplements are essential for good health.

VITAMIN STATUS—USA

We seldom see full-blown vitamin deficiency diseases in the United States today. Most practicing doctors have never seen a case of scurvy, beriberi, pellagra, or rickets. Poverty, child neglect, ignorance about food selection, or adoption of bizarre eating habits account for most of the deficiencies that do occur. But just because vitamin deficiencies are rare doesn't mean that the vitamin status of the population is satisfactory. There is evidence that subclinical deficiencies are probably not uncommon in the United States.

From 1971 to 1974, the National Center for Health Statistics conducted its first Health and Nutrition Examination Survey (HANES) to evaluate the nutritional status of Americans. The more than 20,000 people surveyed represented a broad cross-section of the population, unlike previous surveys that concentrated on low-income populations. As in those surveys, the HANES survey uncovered nutrient deficiencies for vitamin A and iron, in addition to protein and calcium. Plus, a simple lack of calories could not explain it away, as in the low-income surveys.

In 1977, HANES II was conducted to see if the physical condition and laboratory test results of HANES II subjects correlated with the low nutrient intakes found in HANES I. Some of the participants did exhibit low laboratory values for such nutrients as protein, vitamin A, thiamin, riboflavin, and iron. Yet not everyone with a low intake of a nutrient had low laboratory values. Investigators determined that some of those with low intakes were probably at the very beginning stages of subclinical deficiency.

In 1977 and 1978, the U.S. Department of Agriculture (USDA) conducted a Nationwide Food Consumption Survey. Like earlier surveys, it found that dietary adequacy was related to income. But although Americans' weight had increased significantly (probably as a result of inactivity), calories had not. This meant that to keep weight from increasing, a person would have to reduce calories, thus reducing nutrient intake. Yet the survey indicated that for vitamins A, C, and B_6 and the minerals calcium, iron, and magnesium, about one third of the participants were already getting only 70 percent or less of the Recommended Dietary Allowance (RDA). Moreover, most of those surveyed were eating foods high in fat, sugar, and cholesterol.

A second Nationwide Food Consumption Survey was conducted in 1987 and 1988. It confirmed that most adults were not meeting the dietary guidelines. Those who ate fat-rich foods were most likely to have a low intake of vitamins and minerals. One third of the women were getting less than 67 percent of the RDA for vitamin A, vitamin E, vitamin B_6, folate, calcium, magnesium, iron, and zinc. For men, the problem nutrients were vitamin B_6, calcium, zinc, and magnesium.

Unfortunately, promotions for vitamin supplements often misuse findings from such nutrition surveys. Advertisements for vitamins may include statements like, "Surveys show that a large number of people in our country don't get all the vitamins they need." The implication is that these people need vitamin supplements. Statements of this sort ignore the fact that most people do not need 100 percent of the RDA for vitamins and minerals. And it presumes that supplements are the only answer. Yet most nutrition problems in the Unites States can be corrected by providing more food to those in need and by improving food selections or eating habits for those who take in sufficient calories.

WHO NEEDS VITAMIN SUPPLEMENTS?

"Do I need vitamin supplements?" you may ask. No firm answer is possible without a thorough analysis of your individual lifestyle and eating habits.

You need to treat true vitamin deficiencies with vitamin supplements, whether the deficiency results from a faulty diet or a disease condition. In either case, a qualified physician should diagnosis the deficiency. If precipitated by disease, the doctor also will treat the disease to correct the underlying problem. If the problem is poor eating habits, you can discontinue the supplements once they restore you to a healthy nutritional state and your dietary habits improve. If you are taking supplements to treat a disease, continue them until your physician advises otherwise.

Whether using vitamin supplements can successfully prevent conditions other than deficiency diseases is difficult to prove or disprove. Much of what we know about the effects of vitamins on disease is from studies of food, not supplements. A person who takes vitamins and does not develop a certain disease may attribute the good fortune to the supplement, but the mere absence of disease is not sufficient evidence to prove anything. It could have been coincidence.

Many people end up taking vitamin supplements as "nutrition insurance." They don't know what their actual vitamin status is, and they don't know the amount of vitamins in the foods they eat, so they take vitamin supplements "just to be sure."

Most nutritionists agree that people can get all the vitamins they need from foods—if they make the right food choices. However, nutritionists often do not argue with the use of supplements for extra insurance, as long as the supplements do not exceed 100 percent of the RDAs. Some nutrition experts, such as those representing The American Dietetic Association, do not support the use of supplements, especially if they contain megadoses of vitamins.

If you want to know if you really *need* to take vitamin supplements, CONSUMER GUIDE®

recommends that you consult a registered dietitian or your doctor. With help from qualified professionals, you can determine your nutrient needs based on your health, diet, activity, and lifestyle.

FOODS VERSUS SUPPLEMENTS

Wouldn't it be nice to be able to get all your nutrition needs met by swallowing a single pill? If you answered yes, you probably care about your health but do not want to worry about what you eat. Unfortunately, it doesn't work that way. Food is essential for a healthy life. No matter how much we think we know about what it is in foods that's vital to good health, we will never know it all. For example, scientists have already identified more than 10,000 nonnutrient compounds in plant foods. These compounds may not be essential, but each has a positive effect on health.

Another reason for preferring food to supplements as a primary source of vitamins is that it's much more difficult to get too much of a vitamin from food, making overdosing unlikely. At the very high doses typical of megadose supplements, the druglike effects of vitamins can be harmful. Although vitamin toxicity rarely causes death, it can cause discomfort and interfere with the healthy functioning of the body.

Some people think that as long as they take vitamin supplements, they don't need to worry about how or what they eat. This is unfortunate. To ensure good nutrition and good health, all essential nutrients, not just vitamins, must be supplied in adequate amounts.

Nutrients are all part of a team, and vitamins are just some of the players. *Vitamin supplements are not substitutes for good food.* Do not use them as an excuse for making poor food choices or developing bad eating habits.

VITAMINS AND DIETERS

Diets that include a variety of foods usually supply an adequate amount of vitamins. In attempting to lose weight, however, many people follow weight-reduction diets that do not include the variety of foods outlined in the Pyramid eating plan. (If you need a quick review of the Pyramid plan, see Chapter 1.) Even without restricting the types of foods you eat, when you cut down on calories, you inevitably find yourself eating less food. And less food means missed chances to meet nutrient needs.

For this reason, vitamin intakes may be less than desirable among calorie-conscious people. Vitamin supplements *may* provide a bit of insurance against possible deficiency in this situation. However, your doctor should evaluate your general health before you begin any:

• weight-reduction diet
• exercise program accompanying the diet plan
• vitamin supplementation

VITAMINS AND THE ELDERLY

Concern is growing among nutrition experts about the threat of inadequate or inappropriate diets and their effects on the vitamin status of elderly people. Data from several surveys suggest that many older people's diets contain less than two thirds of the RDAs for many vitamins and minerals. And in a continuing study of more than 700 senior citizens in the Boston area, researchers are finding that the seniors' diets provide less than two thirds of the RDAs for vitamins B_6, B_{12}, and D, as well as folate and the minerals zinc, calcium, and magnesium.

Elderly people often do not eat well for a variety of reasons: economic problems, loneliness, physical handicaps, and reduced mobility. Even among elderly people who do eat well, changes that occur with age can make it difficult for their bodies to absorb or use vitamins properly. Moreover, some medications, including those commonly prescribed for blood pressure, can interfere with vitamin use.

For the elderly, daily multivitamin/mineral supplements that supply 100 percent of the RDAs may be the answer. A doctor's supervision in both the choice and the dosage of these supplements is necessary to ensure their proper use and effectiveness. Even so, supplements can never substitute for food. Supplements obviously lack carbohydrate, fat, protein, fiber, and many other substances that the elderly may also have trouble obtaining. Older individuals should make every attempt to eat a balanced diet whether they take supplements or not.

VITAMINS FOR PREGNANT WOMEN, INFANTS, AND CHILDREN

Vitamin supplements are almost routinely prescribed for pregnant women, since pregnancy increases the need for vitamins. The use of supplements provides a certain degree of assurance that vitamin requirements will be met.

Vitamin supplements are often prescribed for infants as well. At birth, newborns receive a vitamin K injection to hold them over until they develop the intestinal bacteria that will make their own. An infant who is breast-fed may not get enough vitamin D, especially if his exposure to sunlight is limited. Consequently, pediatricians frequently prescribe a supplement that contains vitamin D. Often, it also includes vitamin C—a holdover from when vitamin C–poor evaporated formula was popular. The supplement may contain vitamin A as well.

Chewable vitamin supplements are popular for young children. They're available in a variety of flavors, sizes, and shapes to entice children into taking them. However, this very appeal—their candylike appearance and taste—has caused concern about possible accidental ingestion. Even though sold with childproof caps, chewable children's vitamins can cause accidental poisoning from overconsumption. They have also been known to cause a number of choking deaths. Small children—younger than three years old—should be given only liquid supplements or chewable tablets that have been crushed. *These, as well as any other vitamin/mineral supplements or drugs—particularly iron-containing supplements, which can be deadly—must be kept capped and out of the reach of children.*

Like adults, children can ordinarily acquire most of the vitamins they need from food. Nutritionists emphasize the importance of introducing children to the Food Guide Pyramid to foster good eating habits early in life. Still, children can and do go on eating jags, when variety is hardly the name of the game, providing reason for a daily supplement. Indeed, pediatricians frequently recommend the use of vitamin and mineral supplements during a child's formative years. Still, *don't use supplements as an excuse to allow a child to develop bad eating habits.*

SUPPLEMENTS AND ATHLETIC PERFORMANCE

With fitness and training programs at a peak, it is no wonder that many athletic hopefuls are searching for additional ways to get an edge over their rivals. Dietary supplements have always held an allure for athletes, beginning with the myth that salt tablets are necessary.

Many athletes believe that vitamin supplements can boost their energy. The truth is, only carbohydrates, fat, and protein can provide energy. The only way energy can be derived from supplements is if the supplement corrects a deficiency of a vitamin involved in the metabolism of carbohydrates, fat, or protein.

Athletes do have greater needs for some nutrients than their less-active friends. For one, their needs for energy can be considerable, ranging up to 6,000 calories a day for marathon runners. As a result, thiamin, riboflavin, niacin, iron, and copper requirements are higher to support the increase in energy metabolism. But these athletes also consume greater quantities of foods than nonathletes, which should be enough to provide them with the additional amounts of the vitamins and minerals they need.

Athletes who do not require such large amounts of calories do need to watch their intake of the vitamins and minerals that support energy metabolism. Concentrating on nutrient-rich, low-calorie foods—such as skim milk, broccoli, tomatoes, strawberries, whole-grain breads and cereals, kidney beans, turkey, chicken, and fish—is a good idea.

Female athletes may have special needs for iron and calcium. The requirement for iron is greater for women athletes than for men athletes. Athletes perspire a lot, losing iron in the process. Yet athletes need more iron to make the greater number of red blood cells needed to transport the larger amount of oxygen they need during exercise. Furthermore, in the blood vessels of the feet, the force of activity can destroy red blood cells, which then need replacing. These things happen to male athletes, too, but men do not lose blood through menstrual flow and, therefore, rarely have to concern themselves with iron loss.

Athletes may also benefit from higher intakes of antioxidant nutrients because they are exposed to large volumes of oxygen during exercise. (For more about antioxidants, see Chapter 5.)

SYNTHETIC VERSUS NATURAL

If you're going to take supplements, here's something to think about. Vitamins derived from foods are obviously natural. Those created in a laboratory are synthetic. Both are sold in supplement form. Which is better?

Synthetic vitamins are copies of the natural vitamin isolated from food. They're usually cheaper in price than natural vitamin supplements, and their potency can be controlled. Yet a vitamin is a vitamin regardless of its source. A vitamin made by a plant is essentially identical to one made by a drug company. As far as we know, our bodies cannot tell the difference once absorbed into the blood. Foods do, however, have additional ingredients that can either enhance or depress the amount of vitamin absorbed. For example, to absorb beta-carotene efficiently, some fat must be present.

Synthetic supplements sometimes have the advantage of being able to offer a vitamin in a more chemically stable form or in a form more readily usable by the body, but these advantages may be balanced by other considerations. For example, alpha-tocopherol acetate, a form of vitamin E found in supplements, is more stable than forms of vitamin E found in foods. However, the body retains the natural form of vitamin E longer than the synthetic form.

Folate in its supplement form, pteroyl monoglutamic acid, does not require modification first by an intestinal enzyme before being absorbed into the body, but the forms more commonly found in foods do. Orange juice, however, is rich in this easily absorbed form of folate.

CHECKING THE LABEL

Just as the labels on food have been changed to a uniform style, labels on supplements will soon have to conform as well. The latest proposals were published December 28, 1995. Though the details are still being worked out, the new supplement labels are expected to look much like food labels, bearing the title: Supplement Facts (see sample label, page 66).

The Supplement Facts label will likely convey information like a conventional food label does. The serving size will be clearly listed in common units, such as one tablet, one teaspoonful, or one capsule.

As proposed, the "Amount Per Serving" section will contain the actual nutrient information. In this section, the ingredient, the amount per serving, and the percent of the Daily Value will be listed. The amounts of the nutrients in a supplement are expected to be listed in a separate column, making them easier to read. They are usually given in milligrams (mg), micrograms (µg or mcg), or international units (IU). It's been proposed that biotin and folate (folic acid) be listed in micrograms (instead of a fraction of a milligram), with calcium and phosphorus listed in milligrams (instead of a fraction of a gram).

Another column will provide the percentage of the Daily Value (%DV) for each nutrient. The %DV reveals how the amount of a nutrient in one serving of the supplement relates to the amount you should get in an entire day. For most nutrients, the Daily Values are the highest RDA for all age and sex categories, excluding pregnant and lactating women. Unfortunately, this won't be as useful as it could be, because even when the new labeling guidelines are finalized and the regulations go into effect—perhaps as early as 1997—supplement labels will still express vitamin and mineral doses in terms of the outdated 1968 RDAs, as do food labels (except for the six nutrients for which

Supplement Facts

Serving Size   1 tablet

	Amount Per Serving	% Daily Value
Vitamin A (as retinyl acetate and 50% as beta-carotene)	5000 IU	100%
Vitamin C (as ascorbic acid)	60mg	100%
Vitamin D	400 IU	100%
Vitamin E (as di-alpha tocopheryl acetate)	30 IU	100%
Thiamin (as thiamin mononitrate)	1.5 mg	100%
Riboflavin	1.7 mg	100%
Niacin (as niacinamide)	20 mg	100%
Vitamin B_6 (as pyridoxine hydrochloride)	2.0 mg	100%
Folate (as folic acid)	400 µg	100%
Vitamin B_{12} (as cyanocobalamin)	6 µg	100%
Biotin	30 µg	10%
Pantothenic Acid (as calcium pantothenate)	10 mg	100%

Other ingredients: Gelatin, lactose, magnesium stearate, microcrystalline cellulose, FD&C Yellow No. 6, propylene glycol, propylparaben, and sodium benozate.

standards were added). This will not change until the Daily Values for nutrients are updated to reflect the most recent RDAs.

Until then—which is probably not in the near future—iron, for example, will be labeled 100%DV only when a serving of food or supplement contains 18 milligrams, even though the current 1989 RDAs lowered the maximum RDA for iron to 15 milligrams. Such confusion will continue for all nutrients that have had their RDAs changed drastically. The new proposals do establish standards for six nutrients that were included in the 1989 RDAs, but were not included in the 1968 RDAs at all: vitamin K, selenium, manganese, chromium, molybdenum, and chloride (but not fluoride, which is technically not an essential nutrient).

As before, when the supplement is for a specific group—such as infants, children under four years old, or pregnant or lactating women—the %DV column will have to state specifically the intended group and provide percentages based on that group's needs.

The new labels may also provide certain extra information. The vitamin A listing, for example, will be allowed to reveal what percentage of the vitamin A is provided as beta-carotene.

Other things to look for on both current and future labels include:

- The ingredients that supply each vitamin or mineral (listed in descending order by weight of the nutrient).
- Ingredients used to form the tablet or capsule—for example, cornstarch may be used as a filler, binder, or disintegrating agent; propylparaben may be used as a coating; and vanillin may be used as a flavoring agent.
- A warning—for example, "Keep out of the reach of children."
- An expiration date. (Taking a vitamin past this date is not dangerous, but the supplement's potency may be reduced. If you notice any

change in the color, smell, or taste of a vitamin supplement, discard it. Minerals, on the other hand, are very stable and may be used for an indefinite period.)

- Storage instructions. (Store vitamins in their original container in a cool, dry place. The kitchen and bathroom are not the best places because heat and humidity hasten deterioration.)

Read all supplement labels carefully. It is best to choose a supplement that provides about 100 percent of the U.S. RDA (100%DV on new labels) for vitamins, avoiding those supplements that supply excessive or unbalanced quantities of vitamins.

CHAPTER 4

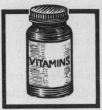

Megavitamin Therapy

We've all heard claims for megavitamin therapy: "You should take extra B vitamins when your body is under stress," they say, or "Schizophrenia can be controlled with large amounts of niacin," or even "You can eliminate the symptoms of menopause by taking lots of vitamin E."

Today, claims for miracle cures bombard us from all directions. Some megavitamin therapy promoters say that vitamin supplements—sometimes containing as much as several thousand percent of the recommended amount—are effective in treating many physical and mental disorders. Although some of these claims may have merit, many are not supported by controlled clinical research. The result is confusion about what might work and what might not.

Just what is megavitamin therapy? A megavitamin is a vitamin in a dose ten or more times its Recommended Dietary Allowance (RDA). For example, the RDA for vitamin C for adults is 60 mg, so 600 mg or more of vitamin C is a megavitamin dose. And by definition, therapy refers to a remedy. So megavitamin therapy does not usually apply to the use of vitamins for protection from disease.

The popular but misguided idea that "if a little is good, a lot must be better" needs a particular caveat when applied to vitamins. As discussed in Chapter 2, when you take in much larger amounts of a vitamin than you need, the excess acts more like a drug in the body and less like a nutrient. This is why you run the risk of experiencing side effects, just as you would if you overdosed on a drug. And some of these side effects can be dangerously toxic.

Not being labeled as drugs complicates the regulation of vitamin and mineral supplements. They are considered "food supplements"—subject to no more scrutiny than any other health food store cure-all. There are a few exceptions. The Food and Drug Administration (FDA) does have the authority to limit the potency or composition of folate, as well as vitamin and mineral supplements used by children and pregnant or nursing women. But all other vitamins in supplements are essentially unregulated. Vitamin and mineral supplements that are considered to be drugs, such as prenatal vitamins, *are* controlled by other divisions of the FDA.

The FDA and the Federal Trade Commission jointly police the advertising of vitamin and mineral supplements. However, only minimal regulation polices supplement advertising. Development of needed regulations was dealt a setback by the Food Supplement Act of 1994 that categorized most supplements as food supplements, and not as drugs.

Some people may be able to take megadoses of some vitamins without serious side effects. But there are definite potential hazards associated with the intake of large doses of some vitamins. We'll refer to these hazards in the individual vitamin profiles later in this book (see Chapter 7).

When promoters of megavitamin therapy raise false hopes, they are little better than hawkers at a frontier medicine show. The book, *Life Extension*, by Durk Pearson and Sandy Shaw, suggests that taking megadoses of about 25 different supplements daily can prevent or significantly delay heart disease and cancer. Jack Z. Yetiv, M.D., Ph.D., in his book *Popular Nutritional Practices: A Scientific Appraisal*, evaluates the Pearson-Shaw book and finds it "... extremely inaccurate; some of the recommendations in the book are potentially life threatening."

The references given in the Pearson-Shaw book *do not support the claims* they make and at times even contradict them. The book is typical of many that promote megavitamin therapy. They tempt the public with false claims and false hopes, while in reality, they offer little more than unproved, expensive regimens that might even harm the user.

Perhaps the most serious danger in using unsubstantiated megavitamin therapies to treat disease is the possible delay of necessary medical treatment that they can precipitate. Do not use vitamin and mineral supplements in place of legitimate medical treatment.

Large amounts of vitamins are not cure-alls. And, large amounts of vitamins can be very dangerous. Indeed, most anything can be poisonous if you take enough, even water. And vitamins are not different.

Because vitamins in large doses might have drug-like effects, they could compromise the effectiveness of standard medical treatment in the same way that taking two different drugs might. It is safest to seek medical care first if you have a disease or other condition, and always let your doctor know your interest in taking vitamins to augment your treatment. Often, forms of vitamins that are effective in treating diseases, such as the vitamin A–like retinoids, are not available without a prescription from your doctor.

The bottom line is that a vitamin supplement can cure a deficiency of a vitamin and it may even offer some protection against certain diseases. However, excessive amounts of vitamins—especially the thousand-percent megadoses some supplements have—can:

- interfere with medications
- interfere with the absorption of other vitamins
- disrupt body functions
- be toxic to your body

So, the simple rule to remember about the use of vitamins is—*DON'T OVERDOSE*.

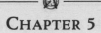

CHAPTER 5

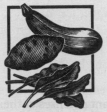

Antioxidants

Oxygen is essential for sustaining life. Without it, we could not support the basic functions of our body. But every breath of oxygen-laden air we take in exposes us to one of the most toxic of all biological compounds. It is a true irony that the substance we depend on for life may actually be responsible for shortening it.

How can something as vital as oxygen be so lethal? Oxygen itself is not the problem, but once oxygen transforms into a *free radical*, it assumes destructive powers. Free radicals are highly unstable forms of oxygen—they have lost an electron from their molecular structures. Normally these electrons exist in pairs. To replace the lost electron, free radicals actively seek out electrons from other substances in the body. When these materials give up an electron to the free radical, their structures, in turn, become damaged. Sometimes these damaged materials themselves steal electrons from other nearby substances, creating a domino-like path of destruction.

Fortunately, our bodies are armed with the means to protect us from the oxygen damage. A key part of our armament is a class of molecular compounds called *antioxidants*. These substances can neutralize free radicals. Our cells have a number of different antioxidant defenses at their disposal, some of which happen to be vitamins and minerals. Vitamin C, vitamin E, and the carotenoid beta-carotene (provitamin A) are antioxidants, as are three minerals: selenium, manganese, and zinc. (For specific information about these nutrients, see Chapter 7 and Chapter 11.)

Among the favorite targets of free radicals are cell proteins, enzymes, the fatty acids in cell membranes, and the genetic material DNA. Damage to these structures can trigger the development of conditions as diverse as cataracts, arthritis, diabetes, heart disease, and cancer. Much of the illness and loss of vitality we experience with age may result from the unchecked accumulation of free-radical damage to cells.

The forces that act on oxygen to create free radicals are called *oxidative stresses*. Some of these stresses arise as a normal part of cell reactions. Everyday reactions that help fight infection are also capable of causing oxidative stress.

Although we can't eliminate all oxidative stresses, the good news is we can take steps to avoid some of them. Cigarette smoking, drinking excessive amounts of alcohol, and eating excessive amounts of unsaturated fat impose unnecessary free-radical burdens on us. Air pollution and ultraviolet radiation from sunlight add more. We can't avoid them entirely. However, we can minimize our exposure to them by not exercising on heavily polluted days and by using sunscreens. Lead coverings also protect us from oxidative stress produced by X rays.

Luckily for us, antioxidants can protect us from unavoidable oxidative stresses. Our exposure to these stresses is probably much higher today than even a few years ago because of the pollution produced by our crowded, high-technology world. Thinning of the ozone layer has also left us more vulnerable to ultraviolet radiation than before. So our need for antioxidant nutrients is greater than ever. Yet our intake of these nutrients is at an all-time low.

How Do Antioxidants Work?

Antioxidants tackle free radicals by using a variety of tactics. One strategy is to run interference between the free radical and the cell material it has targeted to attack for an electron. By giving the free radical one of its own electrons, the antioxidant spares the cell material from damage. Antioxidants that work this way are called *free-radical scavengers*. Vitamin C, beta-carotene, and vitamin E all work as scavengers.

Mineral antioxidants use another tactic. They work attached to enzymes; the enzymes take out the free radicals through chemical reactions. Selenium works with an enzyme called *glutathione peroxidase*, while zinc works with *superoxide dismutase*, or SOD. A protein in the blood called *ceruloplasmin*, which contains copper, may also act as an antioxidant. Each of these enzymes has a particular free radical it keeps under surveillance.

The various antioxidants cooperate with one another to protect against free-radical damage. They require this team effort because antioxidants exist in different places in the cell and attack different free radicals. Vitamin E usually protects the fat in the cell membranes, while vitamin C protects mostly proteins. Beta-carotene is the most powerful defense we have against free radicals formed by ultraviolet light. Selenium enzymes protect the cell machinery that generates energy. Zinc enzymes take up stations at other points to halt free radicals that might slip by other antioxidants.

Vitamin C also helps put vitamin E back in action by giving it another electron once vitamin E loses its electron to a free radical. Likewise, vitamin E steps in to help out if selenium supplies are insufficient. So taking in adequate selenium frees vitamin E to be more effective in its other duties.

FREE-RADICAL DISEASES

The vast array of diseases and conditions believed to have a free-radical connection is daunting—

from heart disease and cancer to arthritis and cataracts. You can trace the aging process itself to lifelong free-radical damage. By squelching free radicals, antioxidants come as close as anything ever has to the fountain of youth.

Heart Disease

Several clinical trials have recently reported evidence that vitamin E can protect against heart disease. We already know about the link between blood levels of cholesterol—in particular low-density lipoprotein (LDL) cholesterol—and coronary heart disease. But now scientists know that only oxidized LDL cholesterol damages the walls of arteries. And it's thought that vitamin E may be able to prevent that oxidation.

Other clinical studies are now testing whether beta-carotene and vitamin C can also reduce heart disease. We know fruits and vegetables provide such protection, but until a few years ago we thought the reason was because these foods were low in fat. Low-fat diets work by keeping LDL cholesterol levels low. Now it appears these foods may be just as important for the antioxidant protection they provide from vitamins and maybe phytochemicals too.

Cancer

All cancers begin with an injury to a cell's genetic material, DNA. As these injured cells reproduce with the wrong genetic blueprint, a tumor takes form. Our immune systems fight cancer by destroying tumor cells while tumors are still very small, but free radicals deal a double blow in promoting the growth of cancer. Not only can they cause the initial damage to the DNA, but they can also sabotage the immune system, making it a less effective defense against tumors. It is not surprising that every one of the chemicals we know to cause cancer is either a free radical itself or triggers the formation of one.

Cataracts

The eye is particularly vulnerable to free radicals that form as a result of exposure to sunlight. Unless we wear eye protection that screens out ultraviolet radiation, we are constantly exposing our eyes to these penetrating rays from the sun. The free radicals formed from ultraviolet radiation most likely damage the protein-rich lens of the eye. Ordinarily, protective enzymes remove these damaged proteins from the eye. But as we age, these enzymes become less efficient. If the amount of damaged protein is large, it begins to build up in the lens. As it accumulates, it forms an opaque, solid mass—a cataract—that does not allow light to pass through. The diminished vision can eventually lead to blindness. About 45 percent of adults over age 75 develop cataracts.

Arthritis

Not as much is known about free-radical links to other diseases, but researchers suspect a link between free radicals and arthritis. Free-radical damage to important organs and tissues may contribute to a loss of function, with subtle consequences like a loss of energy or difficulty in getting around.

Antioxidants and Athletes

An athlete's level of activity creates a greater need for energy and, thus, a much greater demand for oxygen, than that of less-active people. Heavy exercise generates an additional free-radical burden because of the extra energy produced. Indeed, free-radical damage may trigger some of the muscle soreness that develops after a strenuous bout of exercise.

But do athletes have special needs for antioxidants to give them protection? This question is unanswered as yet, though many researchers think they do. One study from Tufts University Human Nutrition Research Center on Aging found that taking an antioxidant supplement appeared to benefit active people over the age of 50 after they exercised more than it benefited younger active people.

The question remains, however, whether younger, more athletic persons would also benefit. Until further research resolves the question, athletes certainly have as much to gain from adequate intakes of antioxidant vitamins and minerals as nonathletes. Megadoses of vitamins, however, may not be the answer.

MEASURING UP TO THE DIETARY REQUIREMENTS

The richest dietary sources of vitamin C and beta-carotene are fruits and vegetables. A recent study on the dietary habits of Americans revealed that most of us aren't eating enough fruits and vegetables to get the levels of antioxidants needed to protect us against free-radical–related diseases. According to the Second National Health and Nutrition Examination Survey, on a given day, only 21 percent of Americans ate any fruits or vegetables rich in carotenoids and only 28 percent consumed a good source of vitamin C.

Breads and cereals made from whole grains also provide antioxidants, but most people eat bread made from refined or white flours. Some nutritionists conclude that most Americans do not take in adequate amounts of these key nutrients for them to serve as antioxidants.

ARE WE GETTING ENOUGH?

Even if you eat food sources of antioxidants, it does not always guarantee that your body will get sufficient amounts. Citrus fruits, strawberries, potatoes, green peppers, and tomatoes contain substantial amounts of vitamin C, but high temperatures destroy the vitamin when these foods are heated.

Yellow-orange fruits and vegetables, such as carrots, squash, apricots, and mangoes, are concentrated sources of beta-carotene. Dark-green, leafy vegetables such as spinach, broccoli, asparagus, and mustard or beet greens are also rich in beta-carotene. Cooking does not affect this compound much, but extended storage in sunlight or air can destroy it.

Whole grains provide vitamin E, selenium, and zinc. The body does not absorb zinc well from whole grains because it is tightly bound to a substance in the grains. Vegetable oils made from corn, safflower, sunflower, and soybean are rich sources of vitamin E, but they also deliver a potential oxidative stress because they are polyunsaturated fats.

At a time when so many Americans are not choosing the right foods to provide the antioxidants they need, scientists are beginning to believe our requirements for these compounds may be higher than previously thought.

SUPPLEMENT PITFALLS

Although taking an antioxidant supplement can help meet your needs for these nutrients, take care not to rely on supplements alone. That's because most studies that have uncovered health benefits for antioxidants actually measured intake of foods, not antioxidants. Many researchers have just assumed that because these foods—mostly fruits and vegetables—are rich in antioxidants, then antioxidants must be the protective factor. But then again, maybe not.

Fruits and vegetables are also rich in fiber and low in fat. They also sport phytochemicals. It could be any one of these things, or all of them together that help prevent disease.

If you take an antioxidant supplement on the assumption that it holds the key, you eliminate the possible benefits these other substances might contribute. Besides, antioxidants work as a team to protect the body from free-radical damage. Taking extra amounts of one will not substitute for lack of another. Take care to ensure that you consumed sufficient quantities of all antioxidants—vitamins and minerals—to receive their full benefits.

A word of caution: If you take extra antioxidants, don't get a false sense of security. For optimal health, you need a total commitment to eliminating unhealthy behaviors like smoking, eating a high-fat diet, and getting no exercise. Taking an antioxidant without tackling these other problems will not get you far.

Indeed, some research has cast doubt on the benefits of antioxidant supplements. A 1994 Finnish study showed that supplementation with beta-carotene had no protective effect against lung cancer. This study was far from conclusive, however. Other researchers severely criticized it, because the volunteers were all heavy smokers, and the supplementation may have been a case of too little, too late. Those who did the best were those who had the highest level from dietary sources before the study began. Score another one for real food.

Because all these questions are still up in the air, for now, it seems best to stick with food sources of antioxidants. Just be sure to eat lots of fruits and vegetables—you can't overdose on them. And one thing you'll be sure of getting is plenty of phytochemicals.

PHYTOCHEMICALS TO THE RESCUE

Phytochemicals are the antioxidants of the future. That is, researchers are beginning to study how phytochemicals may prevent disease, just as they have done with antioxidants. The possibilities are infinitely larger in scope, though, because phytochemicals are more pervasive.

Just what *are* phytochemicals? *Phyto* means plant. So phytochemicals are natural substances—chemicals—found in plants. Researchers believe that many of them have disease-fighting properties. If that sounds preposterous, just think of all the medicines we have isolated from plants.

Sure enough, foods long rumored to protect from disease—like garlic—have turned up chemicals that appear to fight disease in lab conditions. In garlic's case, there are *allylic sulfides*, plus dozens more. In tea, that miracle beverage your grandma foisted on you to make you well, there are *polyphenols*. While soy has *genistein* and apples and strawberries contain *ellagic acid*, broccoli includes *sulforaphane* and celery contains *psoralens*. And there are hundreds, probably even thousands more, that are undiscovered. An orange, alone, contains about 150 different phytochemicals, estimate scientists.

Take beta-carotene, for instance. It's actually a phytochemical, as are all the carotenoids, also known as carotenes. Study after study has linked foods high in beta-carotene to a lower risk of cancer, particularly lung cancer, while suggesting protection against heart disease as well. You may even have started taking beta-carotene supplements based on all the news.

Now, researchers admit the foods high in beta-carotene that are associated with better health may be high in other carotenoids too. Unfortunately, even though other carotenoids might be more powerful than beta-carotene, we know little about their content in foods. This illustrates the potential pitfall of relying on beta-carotene supplements, because by doing so, you're missing out on almost 500 other members of the carotenoid family. Such tunnel vision may come back to haunt you, in the names of other carotenoids like *alpha-carotene*, *beta-cryptoxanthin*, *canthaxanthin*, and *lutein*.

Lycopene is another example. This carotenoid, found particularly in tomatoes, has twice the antioxidant power of beta-carotene. A study of 47,000 men recently found tomatoes and tomato products to be protective against prostate cancer. Men who ate ten or more servings a week of tomato products—tomatoes, tomato sauce, pizza—were 45 percent less likely to develop prostate cancer than those who rarely ate them. Cooked tomatoes were particularly protective. This is common to the other carotenoids as well, as heat can release carotenoids.

Previously, raw tomatoes were cited as lowering the risk of cancers of the mouth, esophagus, stomach, colon, and rectum. In a study of 3,000 people, those who ate seven or more servings a week had only half the cancer risk of those eating two servings or less. Researchers assume the protective substance in this case is lycopene, though they cannot be sure.

How can phytochemicals quell cancer? Scientists have suggested that these natural substances exert double-barreled action by blocking pro-cancer enzymes in the body and stimulating anti-cancer enzymes at the same time.

Some researchers hope that by isolating phytochemicals, they can then create phyto-fortified foods, or so-called "designer" foods, "functional" foods, or "nutraceuticals." But this poses the same potential trap that taking supplements of vitamins and minerals does. How do we know we've isolated the important ones? And what if certain phytochemicals need to work together to be effective? Or maybe they work best with vitamins and minerals? Isolating them may be the worst thing we could do. Better to take them in their natural form—as fruits and vegetables.

Indeed, there is no lack of studies linking fruit and vegetable consumption to lower risk of cancer. And phytochemicals may even help prevent heart disease, high blood pressure, cataracts, and infection. One class of phytochemicals called *flavonoids*—present in high amounts in tea, wine, apples, and some vegetables—may protect against heart disease. In a study of over 800 men, those who consumed the most flavonoids suffered half the heart attacks of those who consumed the least. Researchers speculate that flavonoids, which are antioxidants, prevent LDL cholesterol from becoming oxidized LDL cholesterol—the form that clogs arteries.

In light of all the evidence pointing more to fruits and vegetables than to single nutrients or phytochemicals, the National Institutes of Health has instituted a program called Five A Day. It encourages the public to eat five to nine servings of fruits and vegetables each day for better health. Surprisingly, most people eat only a total of two or three servings a day, even though juice counts toward that total as well as potatoes. A banana even counts as two servings. For other fruits, one piece or a half cup is a serving. Why not see how close you can come to the five to nine optimal range? It's almost guaranteed to improve your health.

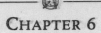

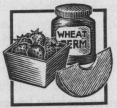

CHAPTER 6

Vitamins and Disease

After years in the background, diet has finally entered the ring as a serious contender in the fight against disease. First, the focus was on the leading roles of fat, cholesterol, sodium, and calories, while the supporting roles of vitamins and minerals went largely unnoticed. That's finally changing, because now we can detect and observe minute quantities of substances in the body, and we can explore activities of vitamins and minerals we never knew existed.

These explorations have led to a startling revelation: Vitamins (and minerals, too) may be more important than we ever dreamed in protecting us against some of our most common and deadly diseases. We have known for a while that the healthiest populations in the world eat diets low in fat and refined sugars and high in fiber. We've also known that fruits, vegetables, and whole grains are the cornerstone of a diet high in fiber and low in fat and refined sugars. Now we realize it is no coincidence that these diets are also richest in vitamins and minerals. So perhaps it's time to shift our attention from what we need to take out of the diet to what we need to boost in it.

This chapter reviews the latest findings on vitamins and their roles in protecting against disease. Chapter 10 reviews the findings for minerals. As you read through these fascinating discoveries, keep in mind that research is ongoing. New discoveries may change current thinking.

Before you run out to stock up on supplements, remember that *foods should always be your primary source of nutrition*. Supplements cannot provide you with the spectrum of benefits possible from foods, because they contain only a fraction of the natural compounds foods possess—the ones we know about. We are still learning about the promising potential of these other natural substances in foods called phytochemicals.

HEART DISEASE

As the leading cause of death in the United States, heart disease is the perfect target for prevention efforts. The dietary approach has traditionally centered around lowering dietary fat, saturated fat, and cholesterol; increasing fiber intake; and maintaining a lean body weight.

Now it appears that increasing your intake of vitamins—particularly antioxidants and certain B vitamins—may be just as important. Antioxidant vitamins play a key role in protecting the heart and blood vessels because low-density lipoprotein (LDL) cholesterol must be oxidized before it can do damage. And antioxidants prevent that oxidation.

For example, the blood normally carries vitamin E, an antioxidant, along with LDL cholesterol, perhaps as nature's intended arrangement for our protection. But when LDL cholesterol levels get too high or when vitamin E levels are too low, the protection may not be sufficient. Two recent studies, one in men and one in women, found that those who consumed the most vitamin E had the lowest risk of heart disease. In the studies, vitamin E came from both food and supplements, though protection didn't require megadoses. The average intake among those with the lowest risk of heart disease was 60 to 100 IU, or six to ten times the Recommended Dietary Allowance (RDA) for an adult man.

Vitamin C is another antioxidant vitamin that appears to protect against heart disease. People at higher risk for heart disease have lower vitamin C levels. For instance, men have lower levels than women, smokers lower than nonsmokers, and older adults lower than younger adults. It also so happens that heart disease peaks during the winter and spring months, just when availability of vitamin C–rich fruits and vegetables is lowest—a co-incidence? Maybe. Maybe not.

One way vitamin C apparently works is by diminishing the tendency for blood clots to form. These clots can block blood flow in the heart or brain, causing a heart attack or stroke. Reactions that rid the body of cholesterol may also involve vitamin C. Even in animals with satisfactory but marginal intakes of vitamin C, the body did not remove LDL cholesterol as quickly as in well-nourished animals. In people with low blood levels of vitamin C, high-density lipoprotein (HDL) cholesterol (sometimes called the "good" cholesterol) is frequently below protective levels. A few studies have also found higher blood pressure in people with low levels of vitamin C in their blood. Because vitamin C also assists vitamin E, it may also prevent heart disease by boosting vitamin E's effectiveness.

Beta-carotene may also benefit the heart, but the evidence is less convincing than that for the other antioxidant vitamins. One study in men found that beta-carotene supplements decreased the risk of a repeat heart attack. And that's important, because the risk of a second heart attack is much higher than the risk of a first, and the chances of surviving it are even poorer. However, two large clinical trials just concluded that beta-carotene offers no benefit to healthy people, while suggesting that high-dose supplements may even be harmful to smokers.

While antioxidants have claimed the limelight for some time, attention is now turning to several B vitamins for possible protection against heart disease. Vitamin B_6, vitamin B_{12}, and folate all help return blood levels of the amino acid homocysteine to normal. Experts believe homocysteine damages blood vessels. They now consider a high blood level of homocysteine to be an important risk factor for heart disease—as important as elevated blood cholesterol levels.

How convenient that a diet rich in these heart-healthy vitamins is also rich in fiber and low in fat, saturated fat, and cholesterol. To reap the benefits of such a diet, focus on whole grains, yellow-orange and dark-green leafy vegetables, and citrus fruits. You can also include chicken, lean meats, fish, and skim milk.

CANCER

As with heart disease, antioxidant vitamins may also reduce the risk of cancer in several different ways. One way is by interfering with the growth of tumors. Antioxidants may keep the immune system operating at its peak so it can seek out and destroy tumor cells.

Another way antioxidants may protect against cancer is by preventing chemicals from being transformed into cancer-causing substances, or carcinogens, in the first place. For example, vitamin C can stop the transformation of nitrates—chemicals added to processed meats and found in cigarette smoke—into powerful carcinogens called *nitrosamines*. But nitrates discourage the growth of microorganisms in meats—and, therefore, perform an important function. So instead of eliminating nitrates, manufacturers now add vitamin C to these foods to prevent their transformation into carcinogenic nitrosamines.

More than 40 studies have documented an association between eating foods rich in vitamin C and a decreased risk of cancer. Indeed, gastric cancer rarely occurs in people with high intakes of this nutrient. However, because vitamin C–rich diets are also rich in other nutrients, it's difficult to attribute benefits specifically to vitamin C. Unlike beta-carotene and vitamin E, which are found in relatively few foods, vitamin C is widely distributed among foods, from oranges and strawberries to tomatoes, green peppers, and potatoes. Its widespread presence in the diet makes it difficult to pinpoint the specific benefit of vitamin C. Other than gastric cancer, cervical cancer is the only type of cancer consistently associated with a low vitamin C intake. Vitamin C may work indirectly; it may be that vitamin C's most significant contribution to preventing cancer is by boosting immune system function.

It's been difficult to find a specific role for vitamin E as well. One study found that people with poor vitamin E nutrition had two to four times the risk of getting cancer or dying from it than people with good vitamin E nutrition. Most studies yield mixed results, though. Some evidence hints at possible benefits from vitamin E for breast and lung cancers.

High beta-carotene intakes, on the other hand, appear to benefit cancers of the cervix, esophagus, stomach, intestines, bladder, and head and neck. Beta-carotene has been thought to be especially protective against lung cancer, particularly among smokers. Recent studies, however, have cast some doubt on whether it is really beta-carotene or something else that is protective. Much of the support for beta-carotene's connection to lung and bladder cancers is from studies measuring consumption of foods rich in beta-carotene. More reliable research measures actual blood levels of the nutrients, which reflect nutrient intake from food as well as from supplements. Most important, a recent study of heavy smokers suggested an *increase* in lung cancer among those given beta-carotene supplements. Researchers are now urging caution for smokers taking beta-carotene.

The track record for vitamin A in protecting against cancer may be the most impressive of all. Unlike beta-carotene, vitamin A is not an antioxidant, so its benefits relate to its possible roles in reversing tumor development and boosting immune function. In fact, in the early stages of vitamin A deficiency, changes occur in cells of the skin, mouth, lungs, and intestines that resemble the early stages of cancer. Vitamin A directs cells to produce new cells that are identical reproductions of the originals. Tumors form when new cells that are different from the original cells begin to reproduce. Drug companies have harnessed this role of vitamin A to produce powerful synthetic forms of the vitamin called *retinoids*. They have used them in the treatment of cancer, with some success for cancers of the lung, mouth, and cervix.

Vitamin D may also protect against cancer. In one study, people with the lowest intakes of vitamin D and calcium were those who developed colon and rectal cancers during a year-long period. It is not clear whether low vitamin D has a specific effect on the development of these cancers or whether its effect stems from aggravating a calcium deficiency. Vitamin D is necessary to absorb calcium, and a low calcium intake increases the risk of colon and rectal cancers.

A study in the United States that measured differences in rates of breast cancer between the Northeast and the South raised a possible link between vitamin D and breast cancer. The rates of breast cancer in the Northeast were almost twice the rates of the sunnier South. Dietary intakes of the vitamin did not differ between regions, but women in the South are exposed to more sunlight and thus make more vitamin D in their skin.

Folate, too, shows some potential in fending off cancer. Folate supplements reversed an ominous change in cervical cells called *cervical dysplasia—*

believed to be a forerunner of cervical cancer. Folate may influence cell development through DNA, the genetic material of cells.

DIABETES

Keeping blood sugar, or glucose, from getting too high is the goal of diabetes treatment. The damage high blood sugar wreaks on tissues causes the majority of the complications from this disease, including heart disease and cataracts. Low intakes of antioxidants may worsen the risk of developing these complications, because free radicals may contribute to this damage in ways not yet understood. Antioxidants also might protect the cells of the pancreas that produce insulin from free-radical damage. This damage might be responsible for type I diabetes—the kind that develops in childhood and depends on insulin injections to control blood sugar levels.

Vitamin C and vitamin E may offer some benefits for people with diabetes. The structure of vitamin C is similar to that of glucose. Because of this similarity, the vitamin may bind to proteins before glucose can. This may change the structure of some tissues and alter their functions. Vitamin C levels in the blood of a person with diabetes are as much as 80 to 85 percent lower than in people without the disease.

By protecting cell membranes from oxidation, vitamin E may improve the effectiveness of insulin, which is responsible for removing glucose from the blood. Indeed, in one study, blood sugar control improved after vitamin E supplements were administered at druglike doses of 90 times the RDA for adult men. These were people with type II diabetes—who do not require insulin injections. People with type I diabetes are due for study next.

AGING

Rumors have long been rampant that vitamin E holds the secret to everlasting youth and virility. Though claims of increased virility haven't panned out, vitamin E's antioxidant properties have renewed interest in its anti-aging potential.

As we age, our organs and tissues begin to break down slowly with the wear and tear of continued use. This deterioration—caused, at least in part, by free-radical damage to cells—contributes to an erosion of vitality and health. As an antioxidant, vitamin E may be able to slow down or even prevent this destructive process by protecting cells from free-radical damage.

While nothing can really stop the aging process, vitamin E may be able to prevent or at least delay a number of conditions common among older people, such as Parkinson disease. The heart, brain, eyes, lungs, kidneys, and liver all might benefit from adequate vitamin E intake. It may not be the fountain of youth, but vitamin E, along with other antioxidants, may play a role in keeping you young at heart—literally.

IMMUNE FUNCTION

A healthy immune system fights off tumors as well as infection. It stands to reason, then, that a declining immune system leaves you vulnerable not only to colds, but to cancer as well. It can also sap your energy. Because immunity declines with age, older adults (over age 50) usually suffer from more infections, tumors, and lack of energy than younger adults, and thus are more likely to benefit from immune-boosting vitamins.

The immune system requires the production of large numbers of immune cells, or white blood cells, to mount attacks against bacteria or other foreign substances. These immune cells produce free radicals in response to the ensuing inflammation. So while other vitamins—such as folate and vitamins A, B_6, and D—may have important roles in preserving immune function, antioxidant nutrients are the most important because they quash these free radicals.

Surprisingly, of the antioxidants, it is vitamin E and beta-carotene—and not vitamin C—that appear to have the most impact on immune functioning. Older people with high levels of vitamin E in their blood are less susceptible to diseases such as influenza and pneumonia than people of the same age with lower blood levels of vitamin E.

In a study of older adults, supplements of vitamin E and beta-carotene (at levels two to three times recommended amounts) strengthened the immunity they received from a flu vaccine. Whether a similar boost to the immune system might lower the risk of cancer is still under study.

A recent study raised the possibility that beta-carotene might improve immune function in people infected with the human immunodeficiency virus (HIV). At doses of 180 milligrams (mg) of beta-carotene, or 30 times the recommended amount, the immune cells targeted by HIV—helper T cells—increased in number. It is still too early to predict if the body can sustain this benefit over a long period of time.

Vitamin C and the common cold has been a hot topic of controversy for a long time. Ever since Linus Pauling first suggested the vitamin could prevent colds over 30 years ago, rigorous scientific studies have failed to confirm his belief. But these studies did find that the symptoms of a cold may be less severe and may not last as long after taking vitamin C. How? As an antioxidant, vitamin C protects specific immune cells called *macrophages* from the free radicals released when these cells battle bacteria or viruses. This protection lets the macrophages be more effective in combating infection.

When the presence of bacteria, viruses, tumor cells, or other foreign substances in the system calls immune cells into action, they must increase their numbers to challenge these foreign substances successfully. Vitamins that are important to cell reproduction, such as vitamin B_6 and folate, play a vital role in this aspect of immune function. Vitamin B_6 also helps produce antibodies—proteins that recognize and attack specific foreign substances. Research shows maximum benefit from vitamin B_6 supplements at doses of 3 mg— only slightly higher than the 2-mg requirement for adult men. Other evidence points to the possible involvement of vitamin D.

Vitamin A's role in immune function is especially critical to children, whose need for this vitamin during growth is especially high. In developing countries where vitamin A deficiency is common, children commonly die from infections. A single vitamin A supplement given to children in Nepal resulted in a substantial reduction in deaths among those under five years of age.

The effect of vitamin A on immune function is far-reaching. Every aspect of immunity is dependent in some way on this vitamin, even though it is not functioning as an antioxidant in this case. So powerful are its effects that high doses of vitamin A are now being tested to stimulate normal immune responses into more aggressive activity. These tests use druglike synthetic forms of the vitamin, which are toxic at high doses. Do not attempt such supplementation without the supervision of a physician.

CATARACTS

The lens of the eye is exceedingly vulnerable to free-radical damage caused by sunlight. With age, the damage accumulates, and the lens becomes cloudy from the continuous bombardment of ultraviolet rays. Between the ages of 52 and 64, about 5 percent of adults have some form of cloudiness, or cataracts. Between ages 75 and 85, that increases to 46 percent. As cataracts worsen, they reduce vision. Indeed, cataract formation is now one of the major causes of blindness in the elderly.

The antioxidant vitamins C and E protect against cataracts. Animals who come out only at night—and thus aren't exposed to light rays—have much lower concentrations of vitamin C in their lenses than animals who are active during the day. One study found that middle-aged adults who had high blood levels of two of three antioxidants—vitamin C, vitamin E, or beta-carotene—had a reduced risk of cataracts. In another study, adults aged 55 or older who took supplements of vitamins E and C reduced their risk of cataracts by 50 percent or more. A very large study examining 1,380 eye patients in Massachusetts found that the use of multivitamin supplements also reduced the risk of all types of cataracts by more than 67 percent.

NEURAL TUBE DEFECTS

A neural tube defect is a birth defect of the developing nervous system of a fetus, causing the spine not to close properly. Spina bifida and anencephaly are examples of such birth defects. About 0.1 percent of American women of childbearing age are at risk of giving birth to a child with a neural tube defect.

Researchers from the United Kingdom first believed genetic predisposition was responsible for that country's unusually high rate of neural tube defects. But then multivitamin supplements showed promise in lowering the rate. Finally, researchers zeroed in on folate in particular. Subsequent studies reinforced the link between increased folate consumption and prevention of neural tube defects. The protection afforded by folate against neural tube defects was so striking in one study that researchers stopped the trial early so that the control group could reap the rewards of folate supplementation too.

Because folate acts in the very early stages of pregnancy—usually before a woman realizes she is pregnant—it is important for any woman who might get pregnant to get adequate folate. The U.S. Public Health Service now recommends that all women in their childbearing years consume at least 400 micrograms (µg) of folate daily. However, this level can be hard to attain from food sources alone, so supplementation may be necessary. The Food and Drug Administration has moved to require that folate be added to the B vitamins and iron now added to enriched flour.

Although too much folate does not appear to have any major toxic effects, there is a danger associated with exceeding the 400-µg level without a physician's supervision. Excess folate can mask a vitamin B_{12} deficiency, and an undetected deficiency of vitamin B_{12} can permanently damage the nervous system.

OSTEOPOROSIS

Osteoporosis usually brings to mind the need for the mineral calcium, but vitamins are just as important in a behind-the-scenes way. This disease, which involves a loss of considerable amounts of bone, primarily affects postmenopausal white and Asian women of slight build. There are many factors contributing to this disease, but experts recognize dietary intake of certain nutrients earlier in life as one of the most important. Dietary calcium is, indeed, the primary nutrient involved because it is so important to bone composition, but so are other nutrients, whose supporting roles cannot make up for inadequate calcium intake.

Among the vitamins that support healthy bone are vitamins A, C, D, and K. Vitamin D has a crucial role because it influences the amount of calcium absorbed from the diet and how well the body uses calcium. Reactions that occur in the liver and kidney activate vitamin D. A decline in kidney function with age can decrease the amount of active vitamin D. For people who have trouble activating the vitamin, calcium supplements will not prevent bone loss. Taking a vitamin D supplement or getting more sunlight to increase the vitamin in the skin will not be particularly helpful either. In this case, only taking the active form of the vitamin will help.

Some of the structures that support bone require vitamin A. This vitamin also helps regulate the rate at which bone breaks down and is replaced by new bone. Upsetting this balance could contribute to bone loss. Indeed, bones develop abnormally in children with severe vitamin A deficiency. Paradoxically, excessive vitamin A also promotes the breakdown of bone.

Connective tissue called *collagen* surrounds and supports bone, as long as it is healthy. Vitamin C contributes to bone development by ensuring that collagen is strong.

The role of vitamin K is not clear but may involve the depositing of calcium into bone. In research studies, vitamin K supplements reduced the amount of calcium lost from the body in the urine of women around or past menopausal age. Less calcium lost means more calcium retained by bone, and that means stronger bone.

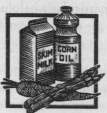

CHAPTER 7

Vitamin Profiles

Vitamin A: Retinol

As far as vitamin A is concerned, the eyes have it. The essential nutrient vitamin A, or retinol, plays a vital role in vision.

HISTORY

As indicated by its position at the head of the vitamin alphabet, vitamin A was the first vitamin discovered. In the early 1900s, researchers recognized that a certain substance in animal fats and fish oils was necessary for the growth of young animals. Scientists originally called the substance *fat-soluble A* to signify its presence in animal fats. Later, they renamed it *vitamin A*.

FUNCTIONS

The most clearly defined role of vitamin A is the part it plays in vision, especially the ability to see in the dark. Metabolites of the vitamin combine with certain proteins to make visual pigments that help the eye adjust from bright to dim light. This process, however, uses up a lot of vitamin A. If it's not replaced, night blindness can result.

Moreover, a deficiency of vitamin A dries out the transparent coating of the eye (the cornea) and the "whites" of the eye (the conjunctiva). If not treated, this condition, called *xerophthalmia*, causes irreversible damage and blindness. Vitamin A deficiency is a major cause of blindness in the world.

Vitamin A is also important for normal growth and reproduction—especially proper development of bones and teeth. Animal studies show that vitamin A is essential for normal sperm formation, for growth of a healthy fetus, and perhaps for the synthesis of steroid hormones.

Another important, but misunderstood, role of vitamin A involves preserving healthy skin—inside and out. Taking extra vitamin A won't make your sagging skin suddenly beautiful, but a deficiency of it will cause major skin problems. Furthermore, an adequate vitamin A intake ensures healthy mucous membranes of the gastrointestinal and respiratory tracts. In this way, vitamin A helps the body resist infection.

SOURCES OF VITAMIN A

Both animal and plant foods have vitamin A activity. Retinol, also called *preformed* vitamin A, is the natural form found in animals. Carotenoids, found in plants, are a group of pigmented compounds, including provitamins, that the body can convert to vitamin A. Bright-orange beta-carotene is the most important carotenoid, because it yields more vitamin A than alpha- or gamma-carotenes.

Some carotenoids, such as lycopene, do not convert to vitamin A at all. Lycopene, the orange-red pigment found in tomatoes and watermelon, is still of value, however, because it's an antioxidant even more potent than beta-carotene. (See Chapter 5 for more on antioxidants.)

Liver is the single best food source of vitamin A. However, many experts recommend not eating liver more than once or twice a month because of the toxic substances it can contain. Environmental pollutants tend to congregate in an animal's liver. Egg yolk, cheese, whole milk, butter, fortified skim milk, and margarine are also good sources of vitamin A. All these foods except fortified skim milk are also high in total fat and saturated fat. And all except margarine are high in cholesterol. Red palm oil, used for cooking in many tropical countries, and fish liver oils taken as supplements are also rich in vitamin A. One tablespoon of cod liver oil contains over 12,000 international units (IU), more than twice the daily recommended intake for adults.

Because of the high fat and cholesterol content of these foods, as well as the potential for overdosing,

Sources of Vitamin A

Food	Quantity	International Units (IU)
Sweet potatoes, baked (peeled after baking)	1 medium	28,805
Pumpkin, canned	½ cup	27,018
Sweet potatoes, candied	1 medium	25,188
Beef liver, cooked	2 ounces	20,230
Spinach, canned, drained	1 cup	18,781
Sweet potatoes, canned	1 cup	15,966
Spinach, cooked, fresh or frozen	1 cup	14,790
Carrot, raw	1 medium	12,767
Cantaloupe	½ medium	12,688
Peas and carrots, frozen (boiled, drained)	1 cup	12,418
Liverwurst, fresh	2 slices (¼-inch thick)	9,960
Apricot halves, dried	1 cup	9,412
Beef and vegetable stew	1 cup	8,984
Turnip greens, cooked	1 cup	7,917
Apricots, dried, cooked, unsweetened	1 cup	5,908
Vegetarian soups, ready to serve	1 cup	5,878
Cabbage, spoon or bok choy, cooked	1 cup	4,366
Collards, cooked	1 cup	3,491
Broccoli, cooked, drained	1 cup	3,481
Apricots, canned in heavy syrup	1 cup	3,173
Vegetable beef soup, ready to serve	1 cup	2,611

Food	Quantity	International Units (IU)
Red pepper, cooked	½ cup	2,577
Watermelon, raw	1 wedge (4×8 inches)	1,764
Chili con carne with beans	1 cup	1,511
Asparagus	1 cup	1,472
Tomatoes, canned (solids and liquid)	1 cup	1,450
Apricots, raw	3 medium	1,110
Macaroni and cheese (made with whole milk)	1 cup	1,071
Clams	1 dozen	855
Tomatoes, raw	1 medium	841
Lettuce, cos or romaine	1 cup	780
Tomato juice, canned	½ cup	674
Plums, canned with syrup	1 cup	668
Prunes, dried, medium	1 cup	649
Margarine	1 tablespoon	621
Peach halves, dried, cooked, unsweetened	1 cup	508
Milk, skim (fortified with vitamin A)	1 cup	500
Peaches, raw	1 medium	465
Butter	1 tablespoon	435
Milk, whole	1 cup	307
Endive, curly	½ cup	297
Corn, fresh or frozen	½ cup	203
Orange juice, unsweetened, fresh or frozen	½ cup	194
Tuna salad	1 cup	175
Corn	1 ear	167

it is recommended that you do not look to these sources to fulfill your need for vitamin A. (Recent studies suggest that vitamin A, as retinol, can be toxic at much lower doses than previously thought.) Instead, rely on the provitamin plant forms of carotenoids, which do not accumulate in your liver. Currently, Americans get about half their vitamin A as retinol from animal sources and half as carotenoids from plant sources.

Orange and yellow fruits and vegetables have high vitamin A activity because of the carotenoids they contain. Generally, the deeper the color of the fruit or vegetable, the higher the concentration of carotenoids it has. Carrots, for example, are especially good sources of beta-carotene, and therefore, are high in vitamin A value. Green, leafy vegetables such as spinach, asparagus, and broccoli also contain large amounts of carotenoids, but their intense green pigment, courtesy of chlorophyll, masks the tell-tale orange-yellow color. (See the table on pages 108–109 for a list of good food sources of vitamin A.)

DIETARY REQUIREMENTS FOR VITAMIN A

The Recommended Dietary Allowance (RDA) for vitamin A is 1,000 retinol equivalents (RE) for men and 800 RE for women. (The RDAs for vitamin A for children are listed in RDA Table 1, page 19.) Retinol equivalents are the preferred measure for vitamin A, because this method takes into account both forms of the vitamin—retinol and carotenoids. One RE is equal to 3.33 international units (IU) of retinol or 10 IU of beta-carotene. Assuming you get the vitamin from both sources, the RDAs are equivalent to about 5,000 IU for men and 4,000 IU for women.

It's not necessary to obtain the RDA amount for vitamin A each day. Since vitamin A is not soluble in water, you do not excrete excess amounts of the vitamin. The liver stores vitamin A, and the body can tap into the reserves whenever dietary intake is too low. For most adults it takes months to deplete stored amounts. As long as you have a well-balanced diet that includes milk and large amounts of yellow and green vegetables, your overall intake should be sufficient to provide the vitamin A your body needs.

The tables on pages 112–113 identify the vitamin A content of two typical daily diets—one is not unusual for a woman and the other is that of a teenage boy.

DEFICIENCY OF VITAMIN A

Vitamin A deficiency is common in the United States among low-income groups. Children are especially vulnerable because they are still growing rapidly. People who eat very-low-fat diets and those who experience fat malabsorption from conditions like celiac disease or infectious hepatitis can also become deficient in vitamin A. A zinc deficiency

Vitamin A Content in Two Daily Diets

Typical Day's Diet for Woman (1,700 Calories)*		International Units (IU) of Vitamin A
Breakfast	4 ounces orange juice	270
	1 ounce enriched cornflakes	1,250
	1 slice whole-wheat toast	none
	1 pat fortified margarine	170
	1 cup low-fat milk	500
	Black coffee	none
Lunch	Sandwich: 2 slices whole-wheat bread, 1 slice Swiss cheese,	
	2 ounces turkey breast	490
	1 cup skim milk (fortified)	500
	½ cup coleslaw	60
Dinner	½ chicken breast, fried	70
	1 medium baked potato	none
	1 cup tossed green salad	180
	½ cup peas, cooked	480
	1 enriched dinner roll	none
	2 pats fortified margarine	340
	1 cup frozen yogurt	150
	Black coffee	none
Total		**4,460**
RDA		**4,000**

*This diet represents what is typical for a woman between the ages of 18 and 35, not what is recommended.

112

Vitamin A Content in Two Daily Diets

Typical Day's Diet for Teenage Boy (3,000 Calories)*		International Units (IU) of Vitamin A
Breakfast	½ medium pink grapefruit	540
	2 scrambled eggs	620
	2 slices whole-wheat toast	none
	1 pat fortified margarine	170
	1 cup whole milk	310
Lunch	1 cheeseburger	360
	2 cups whole milk	620
	10 large french fries	none
	1 medium banana	230
Dinner	4 ounces round steak	25
	1 cup green beans	780
	1 cup mashed potatoes	40
	Lettuce and tomato salad	400
	2 slices whole-wheat bread	none
	1 pat fortified margarine	170
	1 cup whole milk	310
	4 chocolate chip cookies	50
Snacks	Cola drink	none
	½ cup ice cream	270
	¼ of 14-inch cheese pizza	200
Total		**5,095**
RDA		**5,000**

*This diet represents what is typical for a teenage boy, not what is recommended.

can also trigger a vitamin A deficiency by making it difficult to use the body's own stores of the vitamin.

An early warning sign of vitamin A deficiency is the inability to see well in the dark, a condition called *night blindness*. If the deficiency is not corrected, the outer layers of the eyes become dry, thickened, and cloudy, leading to blindness if left untreated.

Vitamin A deficiency also causes dry and rough skin, causing it to take on a kind of "goose flesh" appearance. In addition, one can become more susceptible to infectious diseases. That's because a lack of vitamin A damages the linings of the gastrointestinal and respiratory tracts, so they can't act as effective barriers against bacteria. Infections of the vagina and the urinary tract are also more likely.

USE AND MISUSE
OF VITAMIN A

Treatment for children with xerophthalmia starts with large doses of vitamin A, decreasing to smaller amounts after a few days.

Diseases such as obstructive jaundice or cystic fibrosis cause poor absorption of dietary fat and the fat-soluble vitamins that fat carries. So even if people with these diseases take in adequate vitamin A, they may still develop a deficiency because of poor absorption. To overcome this obstacle, doctors may prescribe large amounts of a water-soluble form of vitamin A.

A disease accompanied by prolonged fever, such as infectious hepatitis or rheumatic fever, can rapidly deplete the liver's reserves of vitamin A. As part of the treatment, a doctor may prescribe vitamin A in amounts greater than the RDA to prevent deficiency.

Vitamin A derivatives are used to treat skin disorders. Isotretinoin acne medicine (brand name: Accutane) is an oral medication used for severe cystic acne. Because of the possibility of such serious side effects as liver damage and elevated blood triglycerides, a doctor must closely monitor treatment with this medication. Any woman capable of becoming pregnant needs to use reliable birth control when taking this medicine because it can cause spontaneous abortion or serious birth defects. Pregnant women must avoid it.

Tretinoin (brand name: Retin-A) is a topical medication primarily used for acne, with less potential for serious side effects than oral isotretinoin. It treats baldness when prescribed along with minoxidil. It also may reduce the appearance of wrinkles and reverse the effects of sun damage on the skin. Another vitamin A derivative, etretinate, may treat psoriasis.

Research shows that people with a high intake of foods rich in beta-carotene—the carotenoid with the greatest vitamin A value—are less likely to develop lung cancer. Even among smokers, lung cancer is less likely to occur in those people who eat a diet that includes lots of vegetables containing beta-carotene.

Taking a beta-carotene supplement in pill form does not appear to have the same effect, however, perhaps because of other poorly understood substances in these foods, which offer protection as well. A recent study was halted nearly two years early because the data suggested that lung cancer was *increased* in smokers taking high doses of beta-carotene.

Vitamin A is not an antioxidant, so the protective effects of beta-carotene that are due to its antioxidant properties (see Chapter 5) do not apply to retinol. But vitamin A may have other protective roles. Among them are a possible reversal of damaged DNA and a boost in immunity, both of which may help prevent cancer.

Large amounts of vitamin A are clearly toxic. One massive dose or large doses taken over an extended period of time can cause hair loss, joint pain, nausea, bone and muscle soreness, headaches, dry and flaky skin, diarrhea, rashes, enlarged liver and spleen, cessation of menstruation, and stunted growth. Doses of only five to ten times the RDA for vitamin A can cause toxicity when taken over a long period.

Two recent studies indicate that toxicity can occur at levels far lower than previously thought. Researchers report that daily doses of 25,000 IU over a period of time have caused lasting liver damage. And a recent study of pregnant women found a fivefold increase in the risk of giving birth to a baby with a birth defect for women taking more than 10,000 IU than for those getting less than 5,000 IU.

The industry practice of "overage" compounds the danger of toxicity. This refers to the manufacturers' practice of including in supplements more than the labeled amount of some vitamins to ensure their stated potency throughout their shelf life. For example, the overage may be as high as 40 percent for vitamin A. This means that a supplement with a labeled dose of 25,000 IU may actually provide as much as 35,000 IU when first purchased.

In a few reported instances, vitamin A toxicity has occurred after eating large amounts of liver. (Polar bear liver is especially high in vitamin A; it contains as much as 560,000 IU per ounce!) Because liver stores vitamin A, eating it daily is not wise.

While the liver stores retinol, excess carotenoids accumulate in the fat just beneath the skin. If you eat a lot of carotene-rich foods, you may notice a yellowing of your skin, especially on the palms of your hands and soles of your feet. This is generally considered to be harmless, though carotene-containing tanning pills used in Europe reportedly cause infertility in women.

Vitamin B₁: Thiamin

The 1930s heralded the discovery of many of the B vitamins. Thiamin was discovered in 1934, a year after riboflavin. In 1937, researchers discovered niacin, and then vitamin B_6 in 1939.

The discovery of thiamin was the key that unlocked the mystery of a disease—a disease born of technology, but called by the simple name *beriberi*. The word itself means weakness in an East Indian dialect.

HISTORY

Beriberi, a debilitating, often fatal ailment, wasn't a serious health problem among the rice-eating peoples of Asia until the end of the 19th century. But then mills began to polish rice—a process that removes the outer brown layers of the grain, leaving behind smooth, white kernels. Rice stripped of this outer layer of bran has lost much of its thiamin.

Not surprisingly, soon after this refining practice began, the incidence of beriberi rose to epidemic levels in Asia. A similar situation occurred in countries where wheat was a dietary staple when refined white flour began to replace whole-wheat flour. The increased prevalence of beriberi spurred efforts to find its cause and cure. Still, the search took almost 50 years and did not end until thiamin was discovered.

A medical officer in the Japanese navy, named K. Takaki, was the first to suspect the relationship between diet and beriberi. In the 1880s, Takaki sought the root of this disease, which afflicted large numbers of Japanese sailors on long voyages—a situation reminiscent of scurvy. To test his belief that diet was at fault, Takaki added meat and milk to the rice diet of the sailors. Only a few men came down with the malady—those who refused to eat the milk and meat.

Further evidence came from Java, where the Dutch physician Cristiaan Eijkman found that chickens fed polished rice exhibited symptoms similar to those of beriberi. When he fed the chickens unpolished rice, the symptoms disappeared. Eijkman then tried the same thing on people and confirmed that unpolished rice could prevent and cure beriberi.

Still, it wasn't until 1910 that a search for the mystery substance in unpolished rice began in earnest. Chemist Robert Williams analyzed liquid extracted from rice polishings, painstakingly testing each substance from it for its effect on polyneuritis, the chicken disease similar to beriberi. In 1934, Williams isolated the substance that would solve the beriberi riddle—the vitamin thiamin.

FUNCTIONS OF THIAMIN

Like other B-complex vitamins, thiamin acts as a biological catalyst, or coenzyme. As a coenzyme, thiamin participates in the long chain of reactions that provides energy for the body and heat. Thiamin helps the body manufacture fats and metabolize protein. It's also needed for normal functioning of the nervous system.

SOURCES OF THIAMIN

The term *enriched* on food labels means that three B vitamins (thiamin, niacin, and riboflavin) plus one mineral (iron) have been added back to that food to make up for the nutrients lost in processing. Enriched breads and cereals are, therefore, very good sources of thiamin. Pork, oysters, green peas, and lima beans are also good sources. Most other foods contain only very small amounts of thiamin.

High cooking temperatures easily destroy thiamin. As a water-soluble vitamin, thiamin also leaches out of food into cooking water. In order to preserve the thiamin in foods, cook food over low temperatures in as small an amount of water for the shortest time possible. Steaming and microwaving keep losses to a minimum and often preserve the natural flavor best, too.

To help preserve their bright green color, some people add baking soda to vegetables when they cook them. This is not a good idea. Not only does the baking soda make the vegetables lose their shape and consistency, but it destroys the thiamin content. Sulfites, used as preservatives, also destroy thiamin.

Sources of Thiamin

Food	Quantity	Milligrams (mg)
Pistachio nuts	½ cup	0.54
Watermelon	1 slice	0.39
Filberts or hazelnuts	½ cup	0.34
Oatmeal, ready-to-serve	1 cup	0.28
Macaroni, cooked, enriched	1 cup	0.28
Cashews, roasted	½ cup	0.28
Peas, green, cooked	1 cup	0.28
Fish	3 ounces	0.27–0.57
Rice, enriched, cooked	1 cup	0.25
Sunflower seeds	1 tablespoon	0.21
Cantaloupe	½ medium	0.18
Pecan halves	½ cup	0.17
Sausage	3 links	0.15
Macadamia nuts	½ cup	0.14
Orange	1 medium	0.14
Potato, baked, with skin	1 medium	0.13
Bacon	3 slices	0.12
Bread, enriched white	1 slice	0.10
Liverwurst	2 slices	0.10
Lamb chop	3 ounces	0.09
Okra	½ cup	0.09
Yogurt, low-fat frozen	1 cup	0.08
Bread, whole-wheat	1 slice	0.07
Chicken, dark meat, no skin	3 ounces	0.06
Peanut butter	1 tablespoon	0.03
Orange juice, unsweetened	4 ounces	0.02

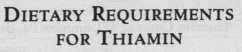

Dietary Requirements for Thiamin

The amount of thiamin your body requires depends on the number of calories you eat, particularly the calories you get from carbohydrates. You need 0.5 milligrams (mg) of thiamin for every 1,000 calories (assuming an average intake of carbohydrates). Thiamin intake should be at least 1.0 mg per day even if the total calorie intake is less than 2,000. By increasing your intake of carbohydrates, you also increase your need for thiamin, but your intake of thiamin usually increases.

The RDA for thiamin is 1.5 mg for men and 1.1 mg for women until age 50. Unless older adults are very active, their calorie needs usually decrease. So after age 50, the requirement decreases to 1.2 mg for men and 1.0 mg for women. A pregnant or nursing woman, who needs more calories, requires more thiamin than other women. A varied, well-balanced diet easily supplies the thiamin needed.

Deficiency of Thiamin

Numbness, muscle weakness, loss of appetite, and disorders of the nervous system characterize the form of beriberi known as "dry beriberi." In contrast, "wet beriberi" features fluid accumulation, especially in the lower legs. This severe form of the disease interferes with the heart and the circulatory system, and can eventually cause heart failure.

Thiamin Content of Common Foods

Food	Quantity	Milligrams (mg)
Meat-Protein Group		
Ham	3 ounces	0.60
Pork chop	3 ounces	0.54
Pork roast	3 ounces	0.48
Bologna	2 slices	0.24
Dried beans or peas, cooked	1 cup	0.21
Beef liver	3 ounces	0.18
Peanuts	½ cup	0.18
Frankfurter	1	0.09
Chicken, white meat, no skin	3 ounces	0.06
Roast beef	3 ounces	0.06
Ground beef	3 ounces	0.03
Tuna, canned in water	3 ounces	0.03
Milk-Dairy Group		
Milk, whole or skim	1 cup	0.10
Yogurt, low-fat	1 cup	0.10
Cottage cheese, low-fat	1 cup	0.05
Ice cream	1 cup	0.05
Bread-Cereal/Grain Group		
Breakfast cereals (enriched)		
Total cereal	1 ounce	1.75
Raisin Bran cereal	1 ounce	0.49
Wheaties cereal	1 ounce	0.37
Macaroni, noodles, or spaghetti, cooked, enriched	1 cup	0.28
Pancakes	3 medium	0.24
Bran muffin	1 medium	0.20
Dinner roll	1 medium	0.14

Thiamin Content of Common Foods (cont.)

Food	Quantity	Milligrams (mg)
Fruits-Vegetables Group		
Peas, cooked	½ cup	0.28
Orange	1 medium	0.12
Orange juice, unsweetened	4 ounces	0.10
Asparagus	½ cup	0.06
Carrot, raw	1 medium	0.06
Banana	1 medium	0.05
Green or snap beans	½ cup	0.04
Cabbage, raw	1 cup	0.03
Iceberg lettuce	1 cup	0.03
Apple	1 medium	0.03
Potatoes		
Baked	1 medium	0.15
French fries	10 pieces	0.10
Chips	15 pieces	0.06

Severe thiamin deficiency seldom occurs today in the Western world, except among alcoholics, who eat little or no food for extended periods of time. They can develop a pattern of neurologic symptoms known as Wernicke-Korsakoff syndrome, involving the nervous system and causing a form of psychosis.

Deficiency may also occur in people who make poor food choices through ignorance, neglect, or poverty. Diets deficient in thiamin are often deficient in other B vitamins as well, because the B vitamins exist in many of the same foods compounding the problem.

USE AND MISUSE OF THIAMIN

You need doses of thiamin two to five times the RDA to treat a deficiency. Fortunately, large amounts of thiamin are not toxic.

Because thiamin plays a part in the reactions that supply the body with energy, "stress formula" supplements often tout it as a cure for stress and fatigue, but thiamin does not provide instant energy. It has no known effect on fatigue unless a true thiamin deficiency is causing the fatigue. Some doctors use thiamin to treat mild depression, with some success. However, it is effective only when the depression itself results from inadequate thiamin intake.

Vitamin B₂: Riboflavin

In the 1920s and 1930s, nutritionists were searching for a growth-promoting factor in food. Their search kept turning up yellow substances. Meanwhile, biochemists who were busy trying to solve the mysteries of metabolism, kept encountering a yellow enzyme. The yellow substances in food and the enzyme that the researchers kept encountering were all *riboflavin*.

HISTORY

Most nutritionists in the 1920s believed that there were only two unidentified essential nutrients—a fat-soluble A and a water-soluble B. Soon, however, they found there was a second water-soluble B compound waiting to be identified.

As nutritionists gradually isolated growth-producing substances from liver, eggs, milk, and grass, all of the substances were yellow. In 1933, L. E. Booher obtained a yellow growth-promoting substance from milk whey, observing that the darker the yellow color, the greater its potency. Booher's observation led nutritionists to discover that all the yellow growth-producing substances in foods were one and the same—riboflavin.

While nutritionists zeroed in on the yellow substance in food, biochemists studied a yellow enzyme found to be essential for the body's energy needs. Biochemists were eventually able to separate the enzyme into two parts: a colorless protein and a yellow organic compound that turned out to be the riboflavin itself. This was the first clue scientists had that there is more than one B vitamin. They also learned that these B vitamins function as coenzymes.

FUNCTIONS OF RIBOFLAVIN

Riboflavin acts as a coenzyme—the nonprotein, active portion of an enzyme—helping to metabolize carbohydrates, fats, and proteins to provide the body with energy. Riboflavin doesn't act alone, however; it works in concert with its B-complex relatives. Riboflavin also has a role in the metabolism of other vitamins.

SOURCES OF RIBOFLAVIN

Milk is the best source of riboflavin in the American diet. A glass of milk provides one quarter of the RDA of riboflavin for men and one third of the RDA for women. Other dairy products such as cheese, yogurt, and ice cream are also good sources of the vitamin. Meats, especially liver and kidney, and some green leafy vegetables are other rich sources. Enriched breads and cereals have riboflavin added to them. (See the table on page 128 for riboflavin sources.)

Heat and oxygen do not easily destroy riboflavin, but light does. Milk can lose one half or more of its riboflavin content when exposed to light for four to six hours. To prevent this from occurring, it's important not to store milk in clear glass or translucent plastic containers. Milk in cardboard containers or colored plastic jugs are better choices.

DIETARY REQUIREMENTS FOR RIBOFLAVIN

The RDA for riboflavin is 0.6 mg for every 1,000 calories. This works out to be 1.7 mg each day for the average adult man and 1.3 mg for the average adult woman. A pregnant woman needs an additional 0.3 mg. During a baby's first six months, a nursing mother needs an additional 0.5 mg daily; during the second six months, she needs only 0.4 mg more. Recommended levels decrease slightly to

Sources of Riboflavin

Food	Quantity	Milligrams (mg)
Milk shake, thick	1 cup	0.50
Cottage cheese, low-fat	1 cup	0.41
Milk, whole	1 cup	0.39
Buttermilk, from whole milk	1 cup	0.38
Buttermilk, from skim milk	1 cup	0.37
Yogurt, low-fat frozen	1 cup	0.37
Pancakes	3 medium	0.36
Sweet potatoes	1 cup	0.33
Pretzels	1 cup	0.25
English muffin	1 medium	0.24
Cornbread	1 piece	0.24
Mushrooms	½ cup	0.24
Chicken, dark meat, no skin	3 ounces	0.21
Avocado	1 small	0.21
Almonds	½ cup	0.20
Almonds, whole, shelled	½ cup	0.20
Brussels sprouts	1 cup	0.17
Wild rice	1 cup	0.15
Corn chips	1 cup	0.13
Honeydew melon	½ medium	0.13
Sherbet	1 cup	0.13
Lima beans	1 cup	0.10
Dried peas, beans	1 cup	0.09
Tomatoes, canned	½ cup	0.07
Corn	½ cup	0.06
Turnip greens, cooked	½ cup	0.05

1.4 mg for men and 1.2 mg for women over age 50 as energy needs decrease.

DEFICIENCY OF RIBOFLAVIN

In riboflavin deficiency, the skin becomes greasy, scaly, and dry. There may be cracks, or fissures, at the corners of the mouth, inflammation and soreness of the lips, and a smooth, reddish-purple tongue.

Because prolonged deficiency of riboflavin causes severe eye damage in animals, some say eye problems in people, such as cataracts, might be due to a lack of this vitamin. However, there is little evidence to support this idea.

Hypersensitivity to light is a sign of riboflavin deficiency, but it is more likely due to a deficiency of several B vitamins. Since the B vitamins work together in a sequence of reactions, a deficiency of one vitamin affects the entire sequence.

USE AND MISUSE OF RIBOFLAVIN

Riboflavin deficiency requires treatment with doses as high as two to five times the RDA. Therapeutic doses of riboflavin are not used to treat any other condition.

Large doses of riboflavin are not toxic. However, large doses will cause the urine to appear bright yellow.

Riboflavin Content of Common Foods

Food	Quantity	Milligrams (mg)
Meat-Protein Group		
Beef liver	3 ounces	3.48
Tuna, canned in water	3 ounces	0.57
Pork chop, cooked	3 ounces	0.27
Egg	1 whole	0.25
Mixed vegetables	1 cup	0.22
Ground beef	3 ounces	0.18
Roast beef	3 ounces	0.15
Ham	3 ounces	0.15
Chicken, white meat, no skin	3 ounces	0.09
Bologna	2 slices	0.08
Peanuts	½ cup	0.08
Frankfurter, beef and pork	1	0.05
Milk-Dairy Group		
Milk shake, thick	1 cup	0.50
Yogurt, low-fat	1 cup	0.44
Milk, skim	1 cup	0.34
Ice cream	1 cup	0.25
Cheese, natural	1 ounce	0.10
Cheese, processed	1 ounce	0.07
Bread-Cereal/Grain Group		
Breakfast cereals (enriched)	1 ounce	0.4–1.7
Macaroni, enriched, cooked	1 cup	0.14
Bread, white, enriched	1 slice	0.06
Oatmeal, cooked	1 cup	0.05
Bread, whole-wheat	1 slice	0.03
Rice, cooked	1 cup	0.02

Riboflavin Content of Common Foods (cont.)

Food	Quantity	Milligrams (mg)
Fruits-Vegetables Group		
Spinach, cooked	½ cup	0.16
Banana	1 medium	0.11
Asparagus, cooked	½ cup	0.09
Broccoli, cooked	½ cup	0.08
Strawberries, raw	½ cup	0.05
Orange	1 medium	0.05
Carrot, raw	1 medium	0.04
Green or snap beans	½ cup	0.04
Potato, baked, with skin	1 medium	0.04
Squash, winter, baked	½ cup	0.03
Apple	1 medium	0.01

Niacin

Niacin, a member of the B complex family, has found many uses in the treatment of disease, and it may have more undiscovered roles.

Cardiologists prescribe megadoses of niacin to lower blood cholesterol and triglyceride levels in some people. Psychiatrists have thought that large doses of the vitamin might be useful in the treatment of schizophrenia, but scientific evidence supporting this use is lacking.

In moderate doses, niacin can benefit one other disease—the one that led investigators to discover this vitamin.

HISTORY

In the early part of the 18th century, a disease characterized by red, rough skin began to appear in Europe. Almost 200 years later, the disease was still a scourge—at least for people in the southern United States. The disease, called *pellagra*, was almost epidemic in the South by the early part of the 1900s.

It was so common that many believed it was an infectious disease spread from person to person. Others thought eating spoiled corn or flies could cause it, because outbreaks of the malady were more severe in the spring months, when flies hatched.

Few people believed that pellagra was a simple dietary deficiency, even though corn-based diets apparently made people susceptible to the disease. One person who did was Dr. Joseph Goldberger. He proved the link between diet and the disease by experimenting with the diets of children in a Mississippi orphanage who suffered from pellagra and 11 volunteers from a Mississippi prison farm. In both groups, when Goldberger added lean meat, milk, eggs, or yeast, their symptoms vanished.

This was in 1915, yet many physicians remained skeptical until 1937. When Conrad Elvehjem and his coworkers at the University of Wisconsin cured dogs with symptoms similar to pellagra by giving them nicotinic acid—a form of niacin. Soon doctors were using nicotinic acid to cure pellagra in humans.

FUNCTIONS OF NIACIN

Niacin occurs in two forms—nicotinic acid and nicotinamide (also called *niacinamide*)—both found in food. Nicotinic acid converts to nicotinamide in the body.

Like the other B vitamins, thiamin and riboflavin, niacin acts as a coenzyme, assisting other substances in the conversion of proteins, carbohydrates, and fats into energy.

SOURCES OF NIACIN

The niacin value of foods includes niacin itself—called *preformed* niacin—and the amino acid tryptophan, which converts to niacin in the body. Food composition tables, however, list only preformed niacin. *Niacin equivalent* is the term used to refer to either 1 mg of niacin or to 60 mg of tryptophan (it takes 60 mg of tryptophan to make 1 mg of niacin).

Most proteins contain tryptophan. In the average protein-rich American diet, tryptophan provides about 60 percent of the niacin you need. If a diet is adequate in protein, then it will surely supply enough niacin equivalents from both sources to meet daily needs. The best sources of niacin are foods with a high protein content, such as meat, eggs, and peanuts. Other good sources of niacin

Sources of Niacin

Food	Quantity	Milligrams (mg)
Peanut halves, roasted, salted	1 cup	20.6
Product 19 cereal	1 ounce	20.0
Tuna, canned in water, drained	3½ ounces	12.2
Chicken, white meat, no skin	3½ ounces	9.5
Beef liver	3 ounces	9.1
Turkey, light or dark meat, no skin	3½ ounces	7.3
Lamb chops, cooked	3½ ounces	6.1
Beef round, bottom, broiled	4 ounces	5.3
Cheerios cereal	1 ounce	5.0
Ground beef	3 ounces	5.0
Chicken, dark meat, no skin	3½ ounces	4.9
Pork chops, cooked	3½ ounces	4.4
Ham, baked	3 ounces	3.5
Salmon, broiled or baked	3 ounces	3.4
Roast beef	3 ounces	3.4
Peanut butter	1 tablespoon	2.1
Chicken liver, cooked	2 ounces	1.2
Frankfurter, all beef, cooked	1	1.1
Dried beans or peas, cooked	1 cup	1.0
Cheese, blue	1 ounce	0.29
Yogurt	1 cup	0.29
Cottage cheese, creamed	1 cup	0.27
Milk, whole or skim	1 cup	0.21
Ice cream	1 cup	0.16
Egg	1 whole	0.03
Cheese, cheddar	1 ounce	0.02

equivalents, such as milk, actually provide more tryptophan than niacin. Mushrooms and greens are good vegetable sources. Niacin is also added to enriched breads and cereals to replace that lost during processing.

DIETARY REQUIREMENTS FOR NIACIN

The RDA takes into account both preformed niacin and that available from tryptophan. Together they account for the recommendation of 6.6 mg of niacin for each 1,000 calories eaten. For women, this should total no less than 13 mg (niacin equivalents) and for men, no less than 18 mg (niacin equivalents). Pregnant and lactating women require slightly more. Human milk contains about 7 niacin equivalents per 1,000 calories, which is enough for infants.

DEFICIENCY OF NIACIN

The first symptoms of pellagra are weakness, loss of appetite, and some digestive disturbances. As the deficiency disease progresses, the skin becomes rough and red in areas exposed to sunlight, heat, or irritation. Later, open sores, diarrhea, dementia, and delirium may develop. And finally, death results if the condition is left untreated.

This disease, now rarely seen in the United States, is still common in parts of the world where corn is the major cereal grain. Corn is deficient in trypto-

Niacin Content in Two Daily Diets*

Typical Day's Diet for Woman (1,700 Calories)**		Milligrams (mg) of Niacin
Breakfast	4 ounces orange juice	0.25
	1 ounce enriched cornflakes	0.1
	1 slice enriched white toast	0.8
	1 pat margarine	none
	1 cup skim milk	0.2
	Black coffee	none
Lunch	Sandwich: 2 slices whole-wheat bread, 1 slice Swiss cheese, 2 ounces turkey breast	7.1
	1 cup skim milk	0.2
	½ cup cole slaw	0.3
Dinner	4-ounce pork chop	4.4
	1 medium baked potato	1.3
	1 cup tossed green salad	0.1
	½ cup peas, cooked	1.2
	1 enriched dinner roll	1.2
	2 pats margarine	none
	½ cup low-fat frozen yogurt	1.6
	Black coffee	none
Total		**18.8**
RDA		**15.0**

* Values for preformed niacin. Totals would be higher if tryptophan contribution were included.

** This diet represents what is typical for a woman between the ages of 18 and 35, not what is recommended.

Niacin Content in Two Daily Diets*

Typical Day's Diet for Teenage Boy (3,000 Calories)**		Milligrams (mg) of Niacin
Breakfast	½ medium pink grapefruit	0.4
	2 scrambled eggs	0.2
	2 slices enriched white toast	1.7
	1 pat margarine	none
	1 cup whole milk	0.2
Lunch	1 cheeseburger (¼ lb.)	7.0
	2 cups whole milk	0.4
	10 large french fries	0.9
	1 medium banana	0.6
Dinner	4 ounces round steak	5.3
	1 cup green beans	0.3
	1 cup mashed potatoes	2.3
	Lettuce and tomato salad	0.4
	2 slices enriched white bread	1.7
	1 pat margarine	none
	1 cup whole milk	0.2
	4 chocolate chip cookies	1.2
Snacks	Cola drink	none
	½ cup ice cream	0.08
	¼ of 14-inch cheese pizza	4.2
Total		**27.1**
RDA		**20.0**

* Values for preformed niacin. Totals would be higher if tryptophan contribution were included.

** This diet represents what is typical for a teenage boy, not what is recommended.

phan, and the niacin it contains is difficult to absorb. In Latin American countries, they combine cornmeal with the mineral lime when making tortillas, the alkalinity of the lime frees the niacin so that it can be absorbed.

USE AND MISUSE OF NIACIN

Treatment for niacin deficiency involves giving 25 to 50 mg of the vitamin.

Some practitioners still recommend megavitamin niacin therapy for mental illness and learning disorders in children, but no scientific studies support either use.

Large doses of nicotinic acid, in amounts from 500 mg to 3 or 4 grams (g) daily, are effective in lowering blood cholesterol and triglycerides levels. The use of nicotinic acid to treat this condition is becoming increasingly popular to reduce the risk of heart attack and stroke. It is actually safer and more effective than many other cholesterol-lowering drugs.

Used in such large doses, however, nicotinic acid is no longer working as a vitamin, but as a drug, and side effects can occur. Doses of 75 mg or more cause blood-vessel dilation, which can result in tingling, itching, and flushing of the face, neck, and chest—a condition called *nicotinic acid flush*. It is uncomfortable, but not dangerous. A slow-release form of nicotinic acid can reduce skin flushing but carries the risk of liver toxicity.

In addition, large doses of nicotinic acid can cause indigestion, peptic ulcers, injury to the liver, and an increased blood level of both uric acid and glucose. This can lead to misdiagnoses of diabetes or gout.

High doses of the other form of niacin, niacinamide, do not cause any adverse reactions. However, niacinamide also does not lower blood cholesterol and triglyceride levels.

Some headache specialists prescribe niacin in daily doses of 150 mg to help treat migraines, in the hopes that the dilating effects of niacin will help stabilize the overdilating-constricting cycle of cerebral blood vessels.

Pantothenic Acid

Pantothenic acid is everywhere. It occurs in all living cells and can be found, at least to some extent, in all foods. Appropriately, its name comes from the Greek word *pantos*, meaning "everywhere."

Although discovered more than 40 years ago, nutritionists have never gotten too excited over the vitamin because deficiency in humans is very rare. In fact, symptoms of pantothenic acid deficiency in people occur only after long periods of food restriction.

That hasn't stopped authors of some popular nutrition books from blaming pantothenic acid deficiency for arthritis, Addison disease, and allergies. Others tout the vitamin as improving mental processes, getting rid of gray hair, and ensuring normal births.

HISTORY

Unlike the discovery of other vitamins, when investigators discovered pantothenic acid in the 1930s, they weren't looking for the cause of a specific human disease. They were looking for a substance necessary for yeast to grow. Along the way, researchers noticed that diets lacking this substance caused certain disorders in animals, including a retarded growth rate, anemia, degenerated nerve tissue, decreased production of antibodies, ulcers, and malformed offspring.

Since many animal species proved to have a dietary requirement for pantothenic acid, scientists believed that people probably needed it, too. Experiments in the 1950s tested how a diet without pantothenic acid affected humans. After three or four weeks on a highly purified diet that lacked only pantothenic acid, volunteers complained of weakness and an overall "unwell" feeling. One person had burning cramps.

A few volunteers received a diet not only deficient in pantothenic acid, but also containing a compound that specifically interfered with the vitamin. These people developed symptoms faster than those in the other group and complained of in-

Pantothenic Acid Content of Common Foods

Food	Quantity	Milligrams (mg)
Meat-Protein Group		
Beef liver, raw	3 ounces	3.90
Beef kidney, raw	3 ounces	1.44
Liverwurst	1 ounce	0.82
Ham, cured	3 ounces	0.66
Egg, fresh, raw	1 whole	0.63
Pork chop, meat only, cooked	3 ounces	0.48
Salmon, canned	3 ounces	0.47
Ground beef	3 ounces	0.30
Round steak	3 ounces	0.30
Almonds, dried, shelled	3½ ounces	0.24
Milk-Dairy Group		
Yogurt, low-fat	1 cup	1.57
Milk, whole or skim	1 cup	0.81
Ice cream	1 cup	0.77
Cottage cheese, low-fat	1 cup	0.54
Blue cheese	1 ounce	0.49
Swiss cheese	1 ounce	0.12
Cheddar cheese	1 ounce	0.12
Bread-Cereal/Grain Group		
100% Bran cereal	½ cup	0.49
40% Bran Flakes cereal	¾ cup	0.21
Bread, whole-wheat	1 slice	0.17
Bread, rye	1 slice	0.13
Bread, white, enriched	1 slice	0.07

Pantothenic Acid Content of Common Foods (cont.)

Food	Quantity	Milligrams (mg)
Fruits-Vegetables Group		
Cauliflower, raw	1 cup	0.65
Grapefruit	½ medium	0.41
Orange	1 medium	0.33
Banana	1 medium	0.30
Tomato juice	4 ounces	0.30
Asparagus, fresh	1 cup	0.29
Corn, frozen	½ cup	0.18
Cabbage, shredded, raw	1 cup	0.10
Apple	1 medium	0.08
Green beans, fresh or frozen	1 cup	0.07
Carrot, raw	1 medium	0.06

somnia, depression, gastrointestinal problems, leg cramps, and a burning sensation in the hands and feet.

In both groups, volunteers showed signs of reduced antibody production. In everyone, symptoms disappeared after adding back pantothenic acid, proving that pantothenic acid was indeed an essential vitamin for humans.

FUNCTIONS OF PANTOTHENIC ACID

Pantothenic acid is part of coenzyme A, which helps release energy from carbohydrates, fats, and proteins. It also helps form some compounds, including fats.

SOURCES OF
PANTOTHENIC ACID

All foods contain this vitamin in some amount. The best sources include an eclectic mix: eggs, salmon, liver, kidney, peanuts, wheat bran, and yeast. Fresh vegetables are good sources—better than canned vegetables, because the canning process reduces the amount of pantothenic acid available. (See the table on pages 141–142.)

DIETARY REQUIREMENTS
FOR PANTOTHENIC ACID

The estimated safe and adequate daily intake for adults is 4 to 7 mg. The average American gets about 10 to 20 mg. Bacteria living in the intestinal tract make some pantothenic acid, but no one knows yet if this contributes to the body's supply.

DEFICIENCY OF
PANTOTHENIC ACID

Pantothenic acid deficiency is not likely to occur as long as people eat ordinary diets that consist of a variety of foods. Symptoms of deficiency, such as insomnia, leg cramps, or burning feet, have only occurred in experimental situations. Even then, severe symptoms occur only if people also take a drug that interferes with the vitamin.

USE AND MISUSE OF PANTOTHENIC ACID

Pantothenic acid isn't used to treat any health problem or condition other than its own deficiency, in the rare chance it might actually occur.

A deficiency of pantothenic acid in black laboratory rats results in gray hair. This finding led some people to surmise that pantothenic acid deficiency was the root cause of graying. If so, then supplements of the vitamin might prevent people's hair from turning gray. Unfortunately, this just isn't true. Pantothenic acid does not prevent or reverse graying.

Massive doses of pantothenic acid (as much as 10 to 20 g a day) have been reported to cause diarrhea in some people, but serious toxicity is not known to occur.

Vitamin B₆: Pyridoxine

Nutritionists aren't sure whether Americans get enough vitamin B_6 or not. Although there's no evidence of widespread deficiency, some nutritionists believe the usual intake of the vitamin is just barely enough, perhaps causing borderline deficiency.

HISTORY

It's called simply vitamin B_6, but researchers discovered early on that this vitamin is not one substance, but three: pyridoxine, pyridoxamine, and pyridoxal. All three have the same biological activity and all three occur naturally in food.

FUNCTIONS OF PYRIDOXINE

Pyridoxine functions mainly by helping to metabolize protein and amino acids. Though not directly involved in the release of energy, like some other B vitamins, pyridoxine helps remove the nitrogen from amino acids, making them available as sources of energy. Pyridoxine also helps manufacture other important compounds, such as antibodies, hemoglobin, and hormones.

Pyridoxine has a role in lowering dangerous homocysteine levels (see heart disease in Chapter 6). In fact, new research suggests that a deficiency of pyridoxine all by itself is a risk factor for heart disease.

SOURCES OF PYRIDOXINE

Vitamin B_6 is in all foods, in one form or another. Plant foods are generally high in pyridoxine; pyridoxamine and pyridoxal are more common in foods of animal origin. All three forms of vitamin B_6—pyridoxine, pyridoxamine, and pyridoxal—appear to have the same biological activity.

Whole wheat, salmon, nuts, wheat germ, brown rice, peas, and beans are good sources. Vegetables contain smaller amounts, but if eaten in large quantities, they can be an important source. Even though pyridoxine is lost during the milling of grains to make flour, manufacturers do not regularly add it back to enriched products, except some highly fortified cereals.

DIETARY REQUIREMENTS FOR PYRIDOXINE

The amount of protein you eat determines your dietary requirement for this vitamin, because it functions in protein metabolism. The RDA for pyridoxine is 2.0 mg for men and 1.6 mg for women. Pregnant and nursing women require more. Children under ten years all require slightly less. Even with the large amount of protein Americans eat, the RDAs for pyridoxine are sufficient for most people. The problem is that many people are not even meeting the RDA.

DEFICIENCY OF PYRIDOXINE

The 1980 Nationwide Food Consumption Survey showed that pyridoxine intake was below 70 percent of the RDA in half of the people surveyed. A 1990 survey showed that intake of the vitamin was still inadequate for most men and women. Other studies show reduced blood levels of pyridoxine in some pregnant women, elderly adults, alcohol abusers, and people with disorders such as kidney disease and Down syndrome.

Some prescription medications, including birth control pills, steroids, and the antibiotics isoni-

Sources of Vitamin B₆ (Pyridoxine)

Food	Quantity	Milligrams (mg)
Banana	1 medium	0.66
Corn Flakes cereal	1 cup	0.52
Instant breakfast drink	1 envelope	0.50
Brussels sprouts, cooked	1 cup	0.45
Halibut	3 ounces	0.43
Cheerios cereal	1 cup	0.41
Avocado	½ medium	0.36
Pork chop	3 ounces	0.33
Potato, baked, without skin	1 medium	0.28
Roast beef	3 ounces	0.27
Cantaloupe	¼ melon	0.26
Cottage cheese, low-fat	½ cup	0.18
Lamb chop	3 ounces	0.15
Tomato	1 medium	0.14
Brewer's yeast	1 tablespoon	0.14
Sunflower seeds	2 tablespoons	0.14
Yogurt, low-fat	8 ounces	0.10
Lima beans, fresh or frozen	½ cup	0.10
Wheat germ	2 tablespoons	0.10
Summer squash, fresh or frozen	½ cup	0.10
Ice cream	1 cup	0.07
Egg	1 whole	0.07
Spoon Size Shredded Wheat cereal	1 cup	0.07
Frankfurter	1	0.06
Peanut butter	1 tablespoon	0.06
Oatmeal	1 cup	0.05
Liverwurst	1 slice	0.03
Asparagus	½ cup	0.02
Peanuts	2 tablespoons	0.05

azid and penicillamine, can increase the need for pyridoxine. If you take one of these medicines, discuss with your doctor whether you should also take a pyridoxine supplement.

USE AND MISUSE OF PYRIDOXINE

People who need more pyridoxine because of a medical condition are often treated with supplemental pyridoxine, in doses of 10 to 50 mg per day. In addition, some people are born with metabolic errors that increase their need for the vitamin. Supplements of pyridoxine are also used for people with sickle-cell disease.

It is popular to recommend pyridoxine supplements for many disorders, including:

- nausea of pregnancy
- premenstrual symptoms
- sensitivity to the flavor enhancer monosodium glutamate
- carpal tunnel syndrome.

Controversy dogs pyridoxine's usefulness in these situations, however, because supporting data are lacking and the potential danger from large doses does exist.

Despite being water-soluble, pyridoxine is toxic in high doses, causing reversible nerve damage to the extremities. For example, women taking doses of 500 mg—250 times the RDA—or more of pyri-

Vitamin B$_6$ Content of Common Foods

Food	Quantity	Milligrams (mg)
Meat-Protein Group		
Beef liver	3 ounces	0.78
Chicken, white meat, no skin	3 ounces	0.48
Round steak	3 ounces	0.36
Tuna, canned in water	3 ounces	0.32
Chicken, dark meat, no skin	3 ounces	0.30
Salmon, canned	3 ounces	0.25
Ground beef	3 ounces	0.21
Ham	3 ounces	0.18
Egg, fresh	1 whole	0.07
Milk-Dairy Group		
Cottage cheese	1 cup	0.15
Milk, whole or skim	1 cup	0.10
Cheddar cheese	1 ounce	0.02
Bread-Cereal/Grain Group		
Ready-to-eat breakfast cereals (enriched)		
Total cereal	1 cup	2.34
Special K, Grape-Nuts Flakes, Raisin Bran, or Wheaties cereals	1 cup	0.60
Bread, whole-wheat	1 slice	0.04
Bread, white, enriched	1 slice	0.01
Fruits-Vegetables Group		
Banana	1 medium	0.66
Boiled potatoes	1 cup	0.42
Spinach, fresh or frozen	½ cup	0.14
Potato chips	10 chips	0.13

Vitamin B₆ Content of
Common Foods (cont.)

Food	Quantity	Milligrams (mg)
Fruits-Vegetables Group (cont.)		
Grapefruit	½ medium	0.12
Lima beans, fresh or frozen	½ cup	0.10
Tomato juice	4 ounces	0.10
Corn, frozen	½ cup	0.08
Orange	1 medium	0.08
Green or snap beans, fresh or frozen	1 cup	0.08
Cabbage, chopped, raw	1 cup	0.07
Apple, unpared	1 medium	0.07

doxine for an extended period of time developed such tingling and numbness in their hands and feet, they were unable to walk. When they discontinued the supplement, the symptoms began to disappear.

Excessive pyridoxine may also increase excretion of oxalate in the urine, increasing the risk of developing kidney stones.

Biotin

"Caution! Egg whites may be hazardous to your health." No, the Surgeon General has not gone so far as to print that phrase on egg cartons, and no one is in any real danger. Unless, of course, you plan to eat nothing but egg whites, like the man who reportedly lived on nothing but six dozen raw eggs a week. However, almost 50 years ago, raw egg whites caused a real problem for some experimental animals. And the cure for the animals' problem turned out to be a previously undiscovered essential nutrient for people.

HISTORY

In the 1930s, an investigator at the Lister Institute of Preventive Medicine in London, England, was experimenting with the diets of rats. After feeding the rodents raw egg whites for several weeks, he noticed they developed an eczemalike skin condition, lost their hair, became paralyzed, and began to hemorrhage under the skin.

Later, another team of investigators fed rats different foods to see which ones prevented or alleviated the "egg-white syndrome." Various foods (such as dried yeast, milk, and egg yolk) cured the rats' conditions. But what did all of these foods have in common?

It was 1940 before scientist Paul Gyorgy identified the common denominator as a vitamin. At first, thinking that it was an isolated substance, he named it *vitamin H*. Soon after, however, scientists realized it was actually another member of the B complex. They did away with *vitamin H* and renamed it *biotin*.

Biotin Content of Common Foods

Food	Quantity	Micrograms (µg)
Meat-Protein Group		
Beef liver, raw	3½ ounces	100
Oysters, raw	3½ ounces	10
Sardines, in oil	3½ ounces	5
Clams, raw	3½ ounces	2
Frankfurter	1	1
Milk-Dairy Group		
Whole milk	1 cup	8
Blue cheese	3½ ounces	7
Brie	3½ ounces	7
Skim milk	1 cup	5
Yogurt	1 cup	3
Cheddar	3½ ounces	3
Cottage cheese	3½ ounces	2
Bread-Cereal/Grain Group		
Raisin Bran cereal	¾ cup	3
Bran Flakes	¾ cup	3
Wheat Chex cereal	⅔ cup	2
Fruits-Vegetables Group		
Cauliflower	1 cup	17
Banana	1 medium	4
Grapefruit	½ medium	3

FUNCTIONS OF BIOTIN

Biotin acts as a coenzyme in several metabolic reactions. It plays a role in the manufacture of body fats, the metabolism of carbohydrates, the breakdown of proteins to urea, and the conversion of amino acids from protein into blood sugar for energy.

SOURCES OF BIOTIN

Milk, liver, egg yolk, yeast, and dried peas and beans are good sources of biotin. Nuts and mushrooms contain smaller amounts of the vitamin. (See page 152 for the biotin content of common foods.) Bacteria can also make biotin in the intestinal tract.

DIETARY REQUIREMENTS FOR BIOTIN

The safe and adequate intake of biotin is 30 to 100 micrograms (µg) per day. The typical varied diet of Americans provides about 100 to 300 µg. This is plenty for healthy people, especially when added to that produced by intestinal bacteria.

DEFICIENCY OF BIOTIN

A deficiency of biotin occurs only in unusual circumstances. People on bizarre diets that include large amounts of raw egg whites exhibited symptoms of a deficiency. The deficiency resulted, not because of a lack of biotin, per se, but because raw egg whites contain a substance called *avidin* that ties up biotin, preventing its absorption. Cooking egg whites deactivates the avidin.

A biotin deficiency can also result from prolonged use of antibiotic medications that destroy intestinal bacteria, but this only leads to true deficiency when combined with a diet that lacks sufficient biotin.

Some people are born with an inherited disorder that increases their need for biotin. In this situation, a supplement may be necessary to prevent a biotin deficiency.

USE AND MISUSE OF BIOTIN

Biotin supplements may be needed in the rare instances cited above. Large doses of biotin are not toxic.

Folate

Folacin, folic acid, and folate all refer to the same B vitamin, which occurs in foods in all three forms. The term *folate* covers all three, and the term *folate activity* describes the actual biological potency, or vitamin value, of a food.

Folic acid is the simplest form of the vitamin. It's found in only small amounts in foods, but it's the form used in most vitamin supplements.

HISTORY

The discovery of folate was closely tied to the discovery of vitamin B_{12}. These two vitamins work together in several important biological reactions. A deficiency of either vitamin results in a condition known as megaloblastic or macrocytic (large-cell) anemia.

In 1930, researcher Lucy Wills and her colleagues reported that yeast contained a substance that could cure macrocytic anemia in pregnant women. But it wasn't until the early 1940s that folate was finally isolated and identified.

FUNCTIONS OF FOLATE

Folate functions as a coenzyme during many reactions in the body. It has an important role in making new cells, because it helps form the genetic material DNA (deoxyribonucleic acid) and RNA (ribonucleic acid). DNA carries and RNA transmits the genetic information that acts as the blueprint for cell production.

We especially need folate when new cells are manufactured. This function of folate helps to explain why the vitamin is necessary for normal growth and development, and why anemia occurs when there's not enough. The body makes large numbers of red blood cells each day to replace those it destroys. DNA is essential for this process; therefore, folate is as well.

SOURCES OF FOLATE

Folate is rich in green leafy vegetables, such as broccoli, spinach, and asparagus (its name comes from the word *foliage*). Seeds, liver, and dried peas and beans are other good sources. Orange juice

Sources of Folate

Food	Quantity	Micrograms (µg)
Product 19 cereal	1 cup	400
Brewer's yeast	1 tablespoon	280
Asparagus	1 cup	242.5
Brussels sprouts	1 cup	156.9
Cocoa Krispies cereal	1 cup	133.1
Instant breakfast drink	1 envelope	99.9
Avocado	½ medium	80.3
Crispix cereal	¾ cup	75.0
Beets	½ cup	68.0
Orange juice, unsweetened	½ cup	54.5
Wheat germ	2 tablespoons	45.4
Romaine lettuce, chopped	1 cup	40.7
Orange	1 medium	39.7
Cantaloupe, diced	1 cup	39.2
Cabbage, cooked	½ cup	30.0
Sweet potato	1 medium	29.9
Strawberries	1 cup	26.4
Yogurt, low-fat	8 ounces	22.0
Red pepper	1 medium	21.8
Beer	12 ounces	21.4
Whole-wheat bread	1 slice	15.7
Grapefruit juice, unsweetened	½ cup	12.8
Milk, nonfat or whole	1 cup	12.7
Cucumber	1 small	10.1
Baked potato, without skin	1 medium	8.5

contains less, but is a good source because it contains the most readily absorbed form of the vitamin. It also contains vitamin C, and vitamin C helps preserve folate. Also, with orange juice, you avoid the problem of destroying folate by cooking it. With vegetables, you must take care not to overcook or use much water, as the folate can be lost.

DIETARY REQUIREMENTS FOR FOLATE

The RDA for folate is 200 µg for adult men and 180 µg for adult women. Pregnant women require 400 µg, because so many new cells are being made. The average American diet provides about 200 to 250 µg of the vitamin.

Foods contain folate both in free form and bound to amino acids. To absorb folate, however, it must be freed. Vitamin B_{12} helps to free the folate.

DEFICIENCY OF FOLATE

Folate deficiency can result from either inadequate intake or reduced absorption. It may also occur during periods of increased need, such as multiple pregnancies, cancer, or severe burns.

Some medications can interfere with the body's ability to use this vitamin. These medications include aspirin, oral contraceptives, and drugs used to treat convulsions, psoriasis, and cancer. In addition, abuse of alcohol can damage the intestine so that less folate is absorbed.

Symptoms of folate deficiency include diarrhea, weight loss, anemia, and a red, sore, and swollen tongue. The macrocytic anemia caused by folate deficiency is prevalent in underdeveloped countries, among low-income pregnant women. Macrocytic anemia caused by folate deficiency rarely occurs in the United States, because of the routine use of supplements during pregnancy.

Experts now emphasize the importance of folate supplementation in the very early stages of pregnancy, because the vitamin plays an important role in early fetal development. Inadequate amounts during the first few weeks of pregnancy can cause birth defects of the spinal cord, known as neural tube defects. Because folate is so important at a time when many women might not even know they are pregnant, women planning to conceive—and any women capable of becoming pregnant—should be sure they are getting enough folate.

USE AND MISUSE OF FOLATE

Over-the-counter vitamin supplements generally contain about 400 μg of folic acid, because they follow standards based on the previous RDAs. The most recent edition of the RDA halved the folate RDA. Why? Since deficiency was not common in the United States, the experts set the RDA within the range typical diets were providing—180 μg or 200 μg. With the new evidence of folate's importance to fetal development, and with even newer evidence of folate's protective role in heart disease, this may have been shortsighted. The next edition of the RDAs may well return folate requirements to their original levels. And fortification of flour with folate—along with three B vitamins and iron—has been mandated.

Doctors prescribe folate supplements if they diagnose a folate deficiency and have ruled out a vitamin B_{12} deficiency. Excessive intake of folate may actually mask a deficiency of vitamin B_{12} or an underlying case of pernicious anemia. Large doses of folate cause the blood to appear normal, which, in turn, may delay diagnosis and treatment of vitamin B_{12} deficiency, resulting in serious, irreversible damage to the nervous system. The longer the delay, the more serious the damage.

Under normal circumstances, large amounts of folate are not toxic. They can, however, interfere with the action of antiseizure and anticancer medications.

Vitamin B_{12}: Cyanocobalamin/ Cobalamin

Vitamin B_{12} is unique. It differs from other vitamins, even those of the B complex, in many ways. The vitamin has a chemical structure much more complex than that of any other vitamin. It's the only vitamin to contain an inorganic element (the mineral cobalt) as an integral part of its makeup. And only microorganisms and bacteria can make vitamin B_{12}—plants and animals can't.

A substance made in the stomach—called intrinsic factor—must be present to absorb vitamin B_{12} from the intestinal tract in significant amounts. This factor combines with the vitamin B_{12} that is released from food during digestion. It carries the vitamin to the lower part of the small intestine, where, assisted by calcium, it attaches itself to special receptor cells. This carrier then releases vitamin B_{12} so it can enter these cells and be absorbed into the body. Without intrinsic factor, vitamin B_{12} misses its connection with the receptor cells and passes out of the body.

Some people have a condition known as *pernicious anemia* and can't make intrinsic factor. As a result, they can't absorb vitamin B_{12} even when there's plenty of the vitamin in their diets. Eventually, they show symptoms of a vitamin B_{12} deficiency. Pernicious anemia is a macrocytic, or large-cell, anemia similar to the anemia caused by folate deficiency.

HISTORY

The pursuit of vitamin B_{12} began in 1926, when two investigators found that patients who ate almost a pound of raw liver a day were effectively relieved of pernicious anemia. Scientists correctly speculated that liver contained a substance that prevents the disorder, but they wondered why victims of pernicious anemia needed it in such large quantities.

William Castle suggested that liver contained an antipernicious anemia (APA) factor. He also believed that people who had the disease lacked a factor intrinsically necessary to use the APA factor. By eating about a pound of liver a day, these people could counteract the lack of the intrinsic factor and absorb the APA factor they needed.

For the next 20 years, scientists searched for the APA factor. Progress was slow until 1948, when testing began on an experimental "animal"—the microorganism *Lactobacillus lactis*. Instead of testing liver extracts on people, researchers tested them on the microorganisms. Since these microorganisms reproduce so quickly, many generations could be tested in a short period of time.

In less than a year, two research groups—one in England and one in the United States—both managed to isolate pure vitamin B_{12}. It turned out that vitamin B_{12} was the APA factor.

FUNCTIONS OF VITAMIN B_{12}

Vitamin B_{12} is essential to cells because it's needed to make DNA (deoxyribonucleic acid) and RNA (ribonucleic acid), which carry and transmit genetic information for every living cell. This information tells a cell how to function and must be passed along each time a cell divides. Rapidly dividing cells need a continuous supply of vitamin B_{12}. This vitamin works along with the vitamin folate in this important role.

Vitamin B_{12} also helps maintain normal bone marrow. And it functions in the production of a material called *myelin*, which covers and protects nerve fibers. Vitamin B_{12} also plays a central role in folate metabolism. It releases free folate from its bound form so it can be absorbed, and it helps in the transportation and storage of folate. A deficiency of vitamin B_{12} can create a folate deficiency even when dietary intake of folate is adequate. That is why a deficiency of either vitamin causes a similar type of anemia.

SOURCES OF VITAMIN B_{12}

Vitamin B_{12} is found mostly in animal foods, such as liver, meat, clams, oysters, sardines, and salmon. Fermented bean products, such as tempeh, contain some vitamin B_{12}. Manufacturers also add vitamin B_{12} to some cereals.

Bacteria in the intestines make some vitamin B_{12}, but far less than the amount needed daily.

DIETARY REQUIREMENTS FOR VITAMIN B_{12}

The RDA for vitamin B_{12} is 2 µg daily for adults and 2.2 µg daily for women who are pregnant or

Sources of Vitamin B₁₂

Food	Quantity	Micrograms (µg)
Liver, beef	3½ ounces	70.4
Clams, canned	½ cup	24.7
Liver, chicken	3½ ounces	19.2
Oysters, raw	3½ ounces	19.0
Sardines	3½ ounces	8.7
Product 19 cereal	1 cup	6.0
Liverwurst	2 slices	4.8
Salmon, canned	3½ ounces	4.3
Grape-Nuts cereal	½ cup	3.0
Hamburger	3 ounces	2.3
Tuna, canned in water	3½ ounces	2.2
Lamb	3½ ounces	2.1
Haddock	3½ ounces	1.7
Beef steak	3 ounces	1.6
Veal, lean	3½ ounces	1.4
Yogurt, low-fat	8 ounces	1.4
Flounder	3½ ounces	1.2
Ham	3½ ounces	0.9
Milk, nonfat	1 cup	0.9
Cottage cheese, low-fat	½ cup	0.8
Pork sausage	3 links	0.7
Instant breakfast drink or breakfast bar	1 envelope or bar	0.6
Egg	1 whole	0.5
Crabmeat, canned	3½ ounces	0.5
Swiss cheese*	1 ounce	0.5
Buttermilk	8 ounces	0.5
Camembert cheese*	1 ounce	0.4
Blue cheese*	1 ounce	0.4
Cheddar cheese*	1 ounce	0.2

*As cheese ripens, the amount of B vitamins increases.

breast-feeding. The average American diet provides 7 to 30 μg of the vitamin.

DEFICIENCY OF VITAMIN B$_{12}$

When the supply of vitamin B$_{12}$ in the body is low, it slows down the production of red blood cells (causing anemia) and the cells that line the intestine. This is similar to what happens as a result of insufficient folate. But unlike folate deficiency, a lack of vitamin B$_{12}$ can also cause serious damage to the nervous system. If the condition persists for long, the damage is irreversible.

A deficiency of vitamin B$_{12}$ caused by insufficient intake is not common. The average well-fed person has a supply of the vitamin stored in the liver that can last five years or longer. Dietary deficiency of vitamin B$_{12}$ is seen only in strict vegetarians who don't eat foods of animal origin—not even milk or eggs.

Such a restricted diet is a particular problem for pregnant or breast-feeding women, since the baby can develop a vitamin B$_{12}$ deficiency even if the mother remains healthy. For this reason, all vegetarian mothers should eat foods fortified with vitamin B$_{12}$. Vegetarians who regularly eat eggs or drink milk get all the vitamin B$_{12}$ they need.

Pernicious anemia is usually an inherited disease in which a deficiency of vitamin B$_{12}$ occurs despite adequate amounts in the diet. People with this disease cannot produce intrinsic factor, the substance needed to absorb vitamin B_{12}. They need to receive injections of vitamin B_{12} so the vitamin can bypass the stomach and intrinsic factor and enter the bloodstream directly.

Because intrinsic factor originates in the stomach, partial or total removal of the stomach reduces absorption of vitamin B_{12}. Moreover, removal of the end of the small intestine (ileum) also creates a deficiency, because that's where absorption of the vitamin takes place. In these cases, pernicious anemia results from the surgery, not an inherited gene.

Stomach acid frees vitamin B_{12} from the proteins it is bound to in foods, but for the one third of adults who experience a decline in stomach acid as they age, this can be a problem. They risk a vitamin B_{12} deficiency late in life. If undetected, the problem can cause nerve damage. An unexplained unsteady gait and loss of coordination often signal this type of vitamin B_{12} deficiency.

USE AND MISUSE
OF VITAMIN B_{12}

Physicians treat pernicious anemia with an injection of 50 to 100 μg of vitamin B_{12} three times a week until symptoms subside. These injections may be lifelong.

Other people believe injections of vitamin B_{12} are a tonic, providing energy. More likely, they act as a placebo. Its use for this purpose is controversial.

There are no reports of vitamin B_{12} causing toxicity or adverse effects even when taken in large amounts. Taking the vitamin orally, however, will not help those people with undiagnosed pernicious anemia because they cannot absorb the nutrient.

Vitamin C: Ascorbic Acid

When you hear the words *vitamin C*, you may instinctively think of the common cold. For that you can thank Linus Pauling and his 1970 book, *Vitamin C and the Common Cold*. In it, Pauling recommended megadoses of vitamin C to reduce the frequency and severity of colds. The book triggered a sales boom for vitamin C that is still going strong. It also prompted nutritionists to begin a series of carefully designed studies of the vitamin and its functions.

Today, some people still swear by vitamin C. Nutritionists have found little proof of its effectiveness against catching the common cold, but there is evidence to suggest it can reduce the severity of a cold somewhat.

HISTORY

The story of vitamin C began centuries ago, with accounts of a disease called *scurvy*. The ailment causes muscle weakness, lethargy, poor wound healing, and bleeding from the gums and under the skin. As recounted in this book's introduction, scurvy was rampant around the world for centuries. Documents dating back before the time of Christ describe the disease. Ships' logs tell of its widespread occurrence among sailors in the 16th century.

History books report that scurvy was a common problem among the troops during the American Civil War. And records of Antarctic explorers recount how Captain Robert Scott and his team succumbed to the malady in 1912.

Almost as old as reports of the disease are reports of successful ways to treat it: green salads, fruits, vegetables, pickled cabbage, small onions, and an ale made of such things as wormwood, horseradish, and mustard seed. In the 1530s, French explorer Jacques Cartier told how the natives of Newfoundland cured the mysterious disease by giving his men an extract prepared from the green shoots of an evergreen tree.

However, the disease was still the "scourge of the navy" 200 years later, when the British physician James Lind singled out a cure for scurvy. Believing that acidic materials relieved symptoms of the illness, Lind tried six different substances on six groups of scurvy-stricken men. He gave them all the standard shipboard diet, but to one pair of men in each of the six groups he gave a different test substance. One pair received a solution of sulfuric acid each day; another, cider; and a third, sea water. The fourth pair received vinegar, and the fifth took a daily combination of garlic, mustard seed, balsam of Peru, and gum myrrh. The sixth pair in the experiment received two oranges and a lemon each day—lucky them.

Lind found that the men who ate citrus fruit improved rapidly; one returned to duty after only six days. The sailors who drank the cider showed slight improvement after two weeks, but none of the others improved.

Although Lind published the results of his experiment, 50 years passed before the British navy finally added lime juice to its sailors' diets. And it wasn't until 1932 that researchers isolated the vitamin itself. At the time, it carried the name *hexuronic acid*. Later, scientists renamed it *ascorbic* (meaning "without scurvy") acid.

FUNCTIONS OF VITAMIN C

A major function of vitamin C is its role as a cofactor in the formation and repair of collagen—the connective tissue that holds the body's cells and tissues together. Collagen is a primary component of blood vessels, skin, tendons, and ligments. Vitamin C also promotes the normal development of bones and teeth. Furthermore, it's needed for amino acid metabolism and the synthesis of hormones, including the thyroid hormone that controls the rate of metabolism in the body. Vitamin C also aids the absorption of iron and calcium.

These days, vitamin C is heralded for its antioxidant status. It prevents other substances from combining with oxygen by tying up oxygen itself. In this role, vitamin C protects a number of enzymes involved in functions ranging from cholesterol metabolism to immune function.

It is a useful food additive in many processed foods. When added to cured meats, vitamin C inhibits in the stomach the formation of nitrosamines—compounds known to cause cancer in laboratory animals.

SOURCES OF VITAMIN C

Of course, the famed citrus fruits—oranges, lemons, grapefruits, and limes—are excellent sources of vitamin C. Other often overlooked excellent sources of vitamin C are strawberries, kiwifruit, cantaloupe, and peppers. Potatoes also supply vitamin C in significant amounts because of the large numbers of potatoes Americans eat on a regular basis. Though cooking destroys some of the vitamin, you can minimize the amount lost if the temperature is not too high and you don't cook them any longer than necessary. Even potato chips and french fries retain some of the vitamin C from the raw potato.

Rose hips from the rose plant—used to prepare rose hip tea—are rich in vitamin C. Fruit juices, fruit juice drinks, and drink mixes may be fortified with vitamin C at fairly high levels. (Refer to the table on pages 170–174 for sources of vitamin C.)

More than with any other vitamin except folate, vitamin C is easy to destroy. The amount in foods falls off rapidly during transport, processing, storage, and preparation. Bruising or cutting a fruit or vegetable destroys some of the vitamin, as does light, air, and heat. Still, if you cover and refrigerate orange juice, it will retain much of its vitamin C value, even after several days. For maximum vitamin value, it's best to use fresh, unprocessed fruits and vegetables whenever possible.

Sources of Vitamin C

Food	Quantity	Milligrams (mg)
Cantaloupe	½ medium	194.7
Currant juice, black	½ cup	194.4
Guava, fresh	1 medium	165.2
Honeydew melon	½ medium	160.0
Peppers, red, raw	1 pod	142.5
Kohlrabi, cooked	1 cup	86.8
Papayas, raw	1 cup (½-inch cubes)	86.5
Strawberries, frozen or fresh	1 cup	84.5
Strawberries, raw	1 cup	84.5
Green pepper, cooked (without stem or seeds)	1 medium	84.4
Cranapple juice	1 cup	78.4
Kiwifruit	1 medium	74.5
Brussels sprouts, cooked	1 cup	70.8
Tomato soup, canned, condensed (with equal amount milk)	1 cup	66.5

Food	Quantity	Milligrams (mg)
Grape juice, sweetened	1 cup	59.8
Mango	1 medium	57.3
Cauliflower, cooked (flowerbuds)	1 cup	56.3
Grapefruit sections, canned in syrup	1 cup	54.1
Gazpacho	1 cup	52.7
Mandarin orange sections	1 cup	50.3
Orange juice, fresh or canned	1 cup	48.4
Beef and vegetable stew	1 cup	48.1
Watermelon, raw	1 wedge (4×8 inches)	46.3
Cranberry juice, sweetened	½ cup	44.8
Fruit cup, fresh (citrus, apple, grape)	1 cup	44.6
Asparagus, green, canned (solids and liquid)	1 cup	44.5
Cabbage, bok choy, cooked	1 cup	44.2
Gooseberries, raw	1 cup	41.6
Raspberries, red, frozen	1 cup	41.2
Spanish rice (homemade), meatless	1 cup	40.6
Turnip greens, cooked	1 cup	39.5
Cowpeas, cooked	1 cup	38.3
Broccoli, cooked	½ cup	36.9
Tomatoes, canned (solids and liquid)	1 cup	36.2
Grapefruit juice, fresh or canned	½ cup	36.1

Food	Quantity	Milligrams (mg)
Cole slaw with mayonnaise	1 cup	35.0
Sauerkraut, canned (solids and liquid)	1 cup	34.7
Tomato, raw	1 medium	34.4
Rutabaga	1 cup	32.0
Chard, Swiss, cooked, fresh or frozen	1 cup	31.5
Sweet potatoes, cooked	½ cup	31.4
Raspberries, red, raw	1 cup	30.8
Lemon, fresh	1 medium	30.7
Cabbage, cooked (common varieties)	1 cup	30.2
Blackberries, raw	1 cup	30.2
Sweet potatoes, candied	1 medium	28.0
Tomato paste	¼ cup	27.7
Tangerine, raw	1 medium	26.9
Pineapple, raw, diced	2 slices	25.9
Winter squash, baked, mashed	1 cup	23.5
Spinach, cooked	1 cup	23.4
Cabbage, raw (common varieties)	1 cup	22.5
Loganberries	1 cup	22.5
Okra, cooked	½ cup	22.4
Tomato juice, canned	½ cup	22.2
Sweet potatoes, canned	1 cup	21.2
Cabbage, celery or Chinese, raw	1 cup	20.5
Fruit cobbler	1 cup	20.4

Food	Quantity	Milligrams (mg)
Parsnips, cooked	1 cup	20.2
Potatoes, hash brown	1 cup	20.0
Beef liver, cooked	3 ounces	19.6
Blueberries, raw	1 cup	18.8
Arugula	1 cup	18.2
Turnips, cooked, diced	1 cup	18.1
Grapes	1 cup	17.3
Potato sticks	1 cup	17.0
Artichokes, cooked	1 cup	16.8
Peas, green, fresh or frozen	1 cup	15.8
Potato, baked	1 medium	15.7
Collards, cooked	1 cup	15.5
Spinach, canned (drained solids)	½ cup	15.3
Lemon juice, fresh	¼ cup	15.1
Cress, garden, raw	1 cup	14.6
Avocado, raw (late summer, fall: Florida)	1 medium	13.7
Pineapple juice, canned	1 cup	13.4
Spaghetti with meatballs and tomato sauce	1 cup	13.2
Potato, mashed (milk and butter added)	1 cup	13.0
Guacamole dip	2 tablespoons	12.0
Potatoes, boiled	1 cup	11.5
Beans, lima, fresh or frozen	½ cup	10.9
Tomatoes, sun-dried	½ cup	10.6
Cherries, sweet, raw	1 cup	10.2

Sources of Vitamin C (cont.)

Food	Quantity	Milligrams (mg)
Summer squash, cooked, diced	1 cup	9.9
Limeade, sweetened	1 cup	9.7
Lemonade concentrate, diluted, sweetened	1 cup	9.7
Beans, snap, green	½ cup	9.4
Peas, green, canned (solids and liquid)	½ cup	8.2
Rhubarb, cooked (sugar added)	1 cup	7.9
Peaches, dried, uncooked	1 cup	7.7
Lettuce, cos or romaine	1 cup	7.2
Plum	1 medium	6.3
Parsley	1 tablespoon	5.0
Celery	½ cup	4.2
Papaya juice, canned	½ cup	3.8
Lobster salad	1 cup	3.4
Apricot halves, dried, uncooked	1 cup	3.1
Soybeans, boiled, drained	1 cup	2.9
Cucumber, raw, pared	½ cup	2.8
Lettuce, iceberg	1 cup	2.1

DIETARY REQUIREMENTS FOR VITAMIN C

The RDA for vitamin C is 60 mg daily for adults, with an additional 20 mg for pregnant women and an additional 40 mg for women who are breast-feeding. The RDAs now indicate that smokers need at least 100 mg of vitamin C a day.

These amounts are several times what's needed to treat deficiency symptoms. Even so, many people believe these levels are not high enough for optimal nutrition, which deals more with vitamin C's antioxidant properties than with prevention of a deficiency.

DEFICIENCY OF VITAMIN C

The classic vitamin C deficiency disease is scurvy. Early signs of the disease are bleeding gums and bleeding under the skin, causing tiny pinpoint bruises. The deficiency can progress to where it causes poor wound healing, anemia, and impaired bone growth.

The body normally stores about 1,500 mg of vitamin C at a time, and symptoms of a deficiency do not occur until the body pool is less than 300 mg. It would take several weeks on a diet containing no vitamin C for this drop to occur in an otherwise well-nourished person.

Since only 10 mg of vitamin C is needed daily to prevent scurvy, the disease is rarely seen today, except in infants who are not given supplemental vitamin C. But even without signs of scurvy, low intakes of vitamin C can compromise many body functions, including the ability to rid the body of cholesterol and the immune system's ability to fight off infection and disease.

People who smoke cigarettes and women who use oral contraceptives have lower than normal blood levels of vitamin C. In light of these findings in smokers the current RDAs raised the amount of vitamin C required for smokers. They may need as much as 100 percent more vitamin C in their diets than nonsmokers.

Vitamin C Content of Common Foods*

Food	Quantity	Milligrams (mg)
Fruits-Vegetables Group		
Orange, fresh	1 medium	69.7
Grapefruit, fresh	½ medium	50.1
Broccoli, raw	½ cup	41.0
Vegetable juice	½ cup	33.5
Cauliflower, chopped, raw	½ cup	23.2
Asparagus, cooked	½ cup	22.0
Scallions	¼ cup	18.0
Spinach, raw	1 cup	15.7
Onions, raw	½ cup	15.1
Corn flakes	1 cup	15.0
French fries	1 cup (about 25 pieces)	12.1
Banana	1 medium	10.4
Apple	1 medium	7.9
Corn, canned	½ cup	6.9
Potato chips	1 cup	6.2
Zucchini	½ cup	4.1

*Milk and milk products, cereal foods (unless fortified), and meats contain little or no ascorbic acid. Organ meats are exceptions. Beef liver contains 23 mg ascorbic acid in a three-ounce serving.

Vitamin C Use and Misuse

Vitamin C supplements easily cure scurvy. Doctors sometimes use vitamin C to acidify the urine when treating certain bladder or kidney disorders. Sometimes physicians prescribe vitamin C supplements before surgery, ensuring a sufficient supply of the vitamin to promote wound healing.

Vitamin C is the most popular single vitamin. Besides taking it to try to prevent colds, people pop vitamin C capsules in the hopes it will ease schizophrenia, senility, cancer, and other medical problems. For some disorders, it's hard to separate the true effects of the vitamin from the psychological effects—the placebo effect.

Scientifically controlled studies testing the value of vitamin C in preventing or treating colds show only a slight benefit in reducing a cold's severity, similar to antihistamine's effect. For the most part, however, studies have not proved that megadoses of the vitamin prevent colds.

What about cancer treatment? A study testing the value of 10 g (10,000 mg) a day of vitamin C in cancer patients showed no effect on relieving symptoms or on prolonging survival. However, vitamin C may have a role in preventing cancer (see Chapter 6).

Large single doses of vitamin C are not toxic; the excess is simply excreted in the urine. However, large habitual intakes may cause problems. Some people develop cramps and diarrhea when taking 1,000 mg (1 gram) or more a day.

Large doses of vitamin C may decrease the amount of copper that the body absorbs. It also increases the amount of iron that is absorbed—a problem for people who have hemochromatosis, or iron-overload disease, an inherited defect in their ability to control iron absorption.

It's suspected that some susceptible people might develop calcium oxalate kidney stones after taking large doses of vitamin C. This may promote stone formation.

Increased excretion of uric acid can also result from large doses of vitamin C. This is a problem for those who suffer from gout. It can lead to a misdiagnosis of the condition.

Large doses of vitamin C can break down red blood cells in people with an inherited disease. Those with sickle-cell disease have an abnormal hemoglobin protein that's distorted by vitamin C; those with this condition should not take large amounts of vitamin C.

Chewable vitamin C tablets can erode tooth enamel if used over a long period of time. Large doses of vitamin C may also interfere with the action of some anticlotting medications.

Some nutritionists warn that if you take more than 1,000 mg per day of vitamin C, you risk developing rebound scurvy when you stop the supplements. Apparently your body develops a mechanism for breaking down and excreting the vitamin quickly, so that a deficiency may develop when you resume normal intake. Others argue that there's little evidence this condition ever occurs. To be safe, people taking large amounts of vitamin C should wean themselves gradually from it rather than stopping abruptly. The body can then become accustomed to lower intakes.

There have been cases of babies who developed scurvy after their mothers took large amounts of vitamin C during pregnancy. Apparently, the babies developed an increased requirement for the vitamin due to their exposure to large amounts before birth.

Vitamin C is chemically similar to glucose. Physicians need to know if you are taking megadoses of vitamin C, so that they won't misinterpret laboratory tests for the presence of glucose in the urine. This can also create problems for people with diabetes who need to monitor blood glucose levels. Large amounts of vitamin C can also cover up the presence of blood in the stool, distorting the results of tests designed to detect colon cancer.

Vitamin D: Cholecalciferol

Vitamin D is known as the sunshine vitamin—and for good reason. If you get enough sunshine your body can make its own vitamin D.

HISTORY

Years ago, few children in tropical countries developed the malformed bones and teeth characteristic of rickets. Yet many children in temperate climates and large industrial cities did. Why the difference? The sun.

Skin contains the substance provitamin D, which starts to convert to vitamin D when exposed to sunlight. In tropical countries, sunlight shone on children year-round. Since these children had ample opportunity for exposure, their skin formed adequate amounts of vitamin D and thus didn't experienced the symptoms of rickets.

Children in temperate zones, however, got little exposure to the sun during the winter months, and their skin could not make enough vitamin D. Neither could the skin of children in large, industrial cities because the smoke-filled air filtered out much of the sun's ultraviolet light.

At one time, rickets afflicted large numbers of children in this country as well. Researchers looking for the cause discovered that diets that prevented calcium from depositing in bones produced the soft bones characteristic of rickets. From this research, investigators concluded that rickets was actually a vitamin-deficiency disease.

However, researchers were perplexed when they discovered that ultraviolet light could also prevent the deficiency. In the 1920s, nutritionists were able to prevent or cure rickets by feeding children cod liver oil or food exposed to ultraviolet light. They also prevented rickets by exposing children to direct sunlight or the light from a sunlamp. The explanation for these findings didn't crystallize for several more years. Cod liver oil was effective against rickets because it contains vitamin D. Foods exposed to ultraviolet light were effective because the light changed a substance in plant foods into a form of the vitamin that the body can use—vitamin D_2.

Today, doctors seldom see cases of rickets in the United States. The few cases that do occur can usually be traced to poverty, neglect, or ignorance. The dramatic drop in rickets cases is primarily due to the increased availability of milk fortified with vitamin D. Choosing to fortify milk made sense because children usually drink lots of it. It's also the single best source of calcium in the American diet, and since vitamin D helps the body use calcium to build strong teeth and bones, milk was an appropriate food to select.

FUNCTIONS OF VITAMIN D

Vitamin D is necessary to help the body absorb the minerals calcium and phosphorus, which are needed for the proper growth and development of bones and teeth.

Whether it comes from food or is made in the skin, vitamin D must be activated before it's of use to the body. It first travels to the liver, where it undergoes a chemical change. Then it moves through the bloodstream to the kidneys, where it undergoes another change to become the active form of the vitamin. This active form—dihydroxy vitamin D—is the one that helps the body absorb calcium and phosphorus.

SOURCES OF VITAMIN D

Few foods contain significant amounts of vitamin D naturally. And the ones that do are not foods you want to overdo: butter, cream, egg yolk, and liver. But there are some good sources. All milk—including skim milk—is fortified with vitamin D at a level of 100 IU per cup. Some manufacturers also fortify cereals with vitamin D. Cod liver oil, as a supplement, contains over 1,200 IU of vitamin D per tablespoon.

A fair-skinned person can make a sufficient quantity of vitamin D with only 20 to 30 minutes of sun exposure a day. It would take three hours for a dark-skinned person to make an equal amount of the vitamin because skin pigment filters out ultraviolet rays.

You cannot overdose on vitamin D from sun exposure because it limits itself. Of course, you can get too much sun, increasing your risk of skin cancer. Unfortunately, because sunscreens filter out the ultraviolet rays that burn your skin, they block the manufacture of vitamin D as well. Exposing unprotected skin to the sun in the early morning or late afternoon hours solves both problems.

Clouds, smog, clothing, and even window glass also filter out ultraviolet rays. Housebound people, those with dark skin, and those who live in cloudy, northern climates—like London—are most likely to be deficient in vitamin D. These people must get vitamin D from foods.

Sources of Vitamin D

Food	Quantity	Micrograms (µg)
Tuna salad	1 cup	7.5
Skim milk, fortified	1 cup	2.5
Milk, fortified	1 cup	2.5
Egg Beaters egg substitutes	½ cup	2.1
Eggnog	½ cup	1.5
Raisin Bran cereal	1 cup	1.4
Total cereal	1 cup	1.2
Product 19 cereal	1 cup	1.2
Yogurt, low-fat, flavored	1 cup	1.2
Special K cereal	1 cup	1.2
Kix cereal	1½ cups	1.2
Liver, pork, cooked	2½ ounces	0.8
Malted milkshake	10 ounces	0.8
Liver, beef, cooked	2½ ounces	0.8
Egg	1 large	0.6
Ice cream bar	1 bar	0.5
Swiss cheese	1 ounce	0.3
Liver, calves', cooked	2½ ounces	0.2
Liver, chicken, cooked	2½ ounces	0.2
Butter	1 tablespoon	0.1

Dietary Requirements
for Vitamin D

Since 1980, we measure vitamin D in micrograms (µg) instead of International Units (IU). The RDA for children and for women who are pregnant or breast-feeding is 10 µg (400 IU). For other adults over the age of 24, the RDA is 5 µg (200 IU). One quart of fortified milk supplies 10 µg; one cup contains 2.5 µg.

Deficiency of Vitamin D

Vitamin D deficiency causes rickets in children. Because vitamin D is crucial to proper calcium absorption, the hallmark of rickets is the undermineralization of bones. One of its common signs is bowlegs. Another sign is beadlike swellings on the ribs—a condition called *rachitic rosary*. Teething is usually late in children with rickets, and what teeth do develop are susceptible to decay.

Though rickets is rare in the United States today, some cases do appear in low-income children, vegetarian children, and infants who were breast-fed for an extended period of time with no supplementation.

Vitamin D deficiency in adults is called *osteomalacia*. It involves the loss of calcium and protein from bones, due to insufficient vitamin D. Osteomalacia differs from osteoporosis in that bone loses only mineral. In osteoporosis, bone itself is lost. In developing countries, osteomalacia is prevalent in women who have low intakes of calcium and vitamin D and several closely spaced pregnancies, followed by long periods of breast-feeding.

USE AND MISUSE OF VITAMIN D

Breast-fed babies routinely receive vitamin D supplements. Formula-fed infants, on the other hand, receive the recommended amount of vitamin D in commercial infant formula and do not require additional supplementation. Strict vegetarians who do not get enough sunlight should consider taking vitamin D supplements.

The standard treatment for rickets is a fairly high dose of vitamin D given under a doctor's supervision. Doctors give the active form of the vitamin in cases where the conversion of vitamin D to the active dihydroxy form is inadequate.

Vitamin D is the most toxic of all the vitamins. As little as 2,000 IU a day—only five times required amounts—can be toxic to children. Symptoms of overdose include diarrhea, nausea, and headache. The most serious complication is the elevated blood calcium levels that too much vitamin D can cause. This condition can lead to calcium deposits in the kidneys, heart, and other tissues, causing irreversible damage.

Some people claim that natural sources of vitamin D, such as cod liver oil, are not toxic. This is not true. Toxicity symptoms have developed in children given large doses of cod liver oil. Avoid supplements—natural or synthetic—in amounts over the RDA, unless prescribed by a doctor.

Vitamin E: Tocopherol

Perhaps no other vitamin has received more attention lately than vitamin E. Retail sales of vitamin E supplements are soaring. Yet we lack scientific evidence for many of the claims for this vitamin, including those that it:

- promotes physical endurance
- enhances sexual potency
- smooths scars
- lowers blood fat levels
- relieves hot flashes and other menopausal symptoms.

What exactly is vitamin E? It's not a single compound, but several different compounds, all with vitamin E activity. One, alpha-tocopherol, has the greatest activity. Other compounds with vitamin E activity are beta-tocopherol, gamma-tocopherol, and delta-tocopherol.

HISTORY

Vitamin E's existence was first hinted at in 1922. Laboratory rats fed purified diets lost their reproductive ability; male rats became sterile, and female rats reabsorbed their fetuses or delivered deformed or stillborn offspring. Adding such foods as lettuce, wheat, meat, or butter to the animals' diets, though, supplied an unknown factor that prevented these reproductive problems. Isolated in 1936, the discoverers named it tocopherol, from the Greek meaning "to bring forth offspring." Later the substance became known as vitamin E.

Curiously, researchers noticed that deficiency symptoms varied from one species to another. In rabbits, for example, vitamin E deficiency resulted in a degenerative muscle disease. Because these symptoms were similar to those seen in humans with muscular dystrophy, researchers hoped vitamin E could cure or prevent this crippling disease. Hopes were also high that the vitamin might help human cases of infertility and sterility. Since 1938, however, studies in humans have failed to confirm any of these benefits.

FUNCTIONS OF VITAMIN E

Vitamin E functions as an antioxidant in the cells and tissues of the body. That means it combines with oxygen to prevent other body substances from doing so. It protects polyunsaturated fats and other oxygen-sensitive compounds such as vitamin A from being destroyed by damaging oxidation reactions.

Vitamin E's antioxidant properties are also important to cell membranes. For example, vitamin E protects lung cells that are in constant contact

187

with oxygen and white blood cells that help the body fight disease. A deficiency of vitamin E weakens the immune system, increasing susceptibility to infection.

But the benefits of vitamin E's antioxidant role may go much further. Evidence is starting to build that vitamin E can protect against heart disease and may slow the deterioration associated with aging. Critics scoffed at such claims in the past, but an understanding of the importance of vitamin E's antioxidant role may be beginning to pay off. (See Chapters 5 and 6 for more about the role of vitamin E in disease prevention.)

Vitamin E also acts as an antioxidant in foods. The vitamin E in vegetable oils helps keep them from being oxidized and turning rancid. Likewise, it protects vitamin A in foods from being oxidized. This makes vitamin E a useful food preservative.

SOURCES OF VITAMIN E

Oils and margarines from corn, cottonseed, soybean, safflower, and wheat germ are all good sources of vitamin E. Generally, the more polyunsaturated an oil is, the more vitamin E it contains, serving as its own built-in protection. Fruits, vegetables, and whole grains contain less. Refining grains reduces their vitamin E content, as does commercial processing and storage of food. Cooking foods at high temperatures also destroys vitamin E. So a polyunsaturated oil is useless as a vitamin E source if it's used for frying. Your best sources are fresh and lightly processed foods, as well as those that aren't overcooked.

These days, it's difficult to get much vitamin E in the diet, because of cooking and processing losses and because of the generally reduced intake of fat. Moreover, the current emphasis on monounsaturated fats, such as olive oil or canola oil, rather than vitamin E–containing polyunsaturated fats, further decreases our intake of vitamin E. Monounsaturated fats have other benefits for the heart, though, so you shouldn't stop using olive and canola oils. It is important to find other sources of vitamin E. Besides, the less polyunsaturated fats you eat, the less vitamin E you need, so your requirements may be lower if you switch to olive or canola oils.

DIETARY REQUIREMENTS FOR VITAMIN E

The RDA for vitamin E is 10 mg of D-alpha-tocopherol for adult men and 8 mg for women. One milligram of D-alpha-tocopherol is equal to 1.5 IU, so the RDA is equal to 15 IU and 12 IU for men and women, respectively. Food and supplement labels usually list amounts of vitamin E in milligrams rather than international units.

DEFICIENCY OF VITAMIN E

No obvious symptoms accompany a vitamin E deficiency, making it hard to detect. A brownish

Sources of Vitamin E

Food	Quantity	Milligrams (mg)
Just Right with Fiber cereal	1 cup	30.2
Wheat germ oil	1 tablespoon	24.6
Total cereal	1 cup	23.4
Hazelnuts	½ cup	16.1
Sunflower seeds	2 tablespoons	9.0
Sunflower oil	1 tablespoon	8.2
Peanuts	½ cup	6.6
Brazil nuts	½ cup	5.3
Cottonseed oil	1 tablespoon	5.2
Corn	1 ear	4.8
Safflower oil	1 tablespoon	4.7
Almonds	½ cup	4.0
Corn oil	1 tablespoon	2.8
Canola oil	1 tablespoon	2.8
Asparagus, fresh or frozen	1 cup	2.6
Soybean oil	1 tablespoon	2.0
Olive oil	1 tablespoon	1.6
Walnuts	½ cup	1.3
Brussels sprouts, fresh or frozen	1 cup	1.3
Wheat germ	2 tablespoons	1.1
Sweet potato	1 medium	1.1
Broccoli, fresh or frozen	1 cup	1.0
Pear	1 medium	0.9
Tomato	1 medium	0.8
Brown rice	1 cup	0.8
Plum	1 large	0.7
Oatmeal	1 cup	0.6
Apple	1 medium	0.5
Whole-wheat flour	⅓ cup	0.4

Food	Quantity	Milligrams (mg)
Walnut oil	1 tablespoon	0.4
Grapefruit	½ medium	0.4
Egg	1 large	0.4
Raspberries	½ cup	0.3
Banana	1 medium	0.3
Butter	1 tablespoon	0.2
Carrot	1 medium	0.2
Orange	1 medium	0.2
Cornmeal, uncooked	¼ cup	0.1
Beans, dried	½ cup	0.1

pigmentation of the skin, often called *age spots* or *lipofuscin*, may signal the problem, but only a blood test can confirm if vitamin E levels are actually too low.

When diseases of the liver, gall bladder, or pancreas reduce intestinal absorption, a mild deficiency of vitamin E can result. A diet of processed foods that's very low in fat might also cause a deficiency.

Vitamin E deficiency may occur in newborn babies, especially those born prematurely, because the mother doesn't transfer much vitamin E to the developing fetus until the last few weeks of pregnancy.

The deficiency can cause hemolytic anemia, a condition in which the red blood cells are so fragile they rupture.

USE AND MISUSE OF VITAMIN E

Premature babies receive vitamin E to reduce or prevent oxygen damage to the retina of the eye. Vitamin E therapy treats claudication—pains in the calf muscles that occur at night or during exercise. A controversial use of vitamin E supplements is to treat painful, benign breast lumps (fibrocystic breast disease).

Ongoing animal studies suggest that vitamin E may limit lung damage caused by air pollution. It appears that vitamin E can reduce the activity of such common air pollutants as ozone and nitrogen dioxide. There is no evidence, however, that vitamin E can treat fertility problems and muscle degeneration in humans like it does in animals.

Vitamin E applied to cuts may very well increase the healing rate because it minimizes oxidation reactions in the wound. The value of vitamin E in preventing the stretch marks of pregnancy is legendary, but this benefit has not been proved scientifically.

Many women report that vitamin E helps reduce hot flashes and other symptoms of menopause. These are considered anecdotal reports.

Though vitamin E can slow down the oxidation of fats that occurs in aging, experimental studies have not shown it to increase the life span of animals. Neither has it been shown to control such signs of aging as wrinkled skin or gray hair. However, the vitamin may indeed delay or prevent some diseases or a loss of function related to aging (see Chapter 6). While vitamin E may not make you live longer, it may help you live a little better as you get older.

Vitamin E seems to be fairly safe when taken in amounts of 400 IU daily for a long time. Amounts larger than this might delay blood clotting, possibly causing an increased risk of the bleeding type of stroke. People on anticoagulant therapy (blood thinners) should not take megadoses of vitamin E for this reason.

Vitamin K: Phylloquinone and Menaquinone

The *K* in vitamin K seems strange, but it came from the Danish word *koagulation*, meaning "blood clotting," which precisely reflects its function in the human body.

HISTORY

The importance of a dietary factor in blood clotting was first recognized by a Danish scientist. In 1929, he reported that chicks fed diets lacking a particular dietary factor hemorrhaged. Their blood was slow to form the clots needed to control bleeding. The missing factor was vitamin K.

FUNCTION OF VITAMIN K

The proteins used in blood clotting require vitamin K. When there isn't enough of the vitamin, blood takes longer to clot, which can increase the amount of blood lost. Vitamin K also helps make a protein that may help regulate blood calcium levels. Calcium, usually associated with keeping bones strong, is also necessary for blood clotting. Thus vitamin K may be doubly important for blood clotting.

SOURCES OF VITAMIN K

The best food sources of vitamin K are green leafy vegetables such as cabbage, turnip greens, broccoli, lettuce, and spinach. Beef liver is another good source; chicken liver, pork liver, milk, and eggs contain smaller amounts of the vitamin. Liver, however, may also contain environmental toxins. Other sources are better choices.

We get only about half of our vitamin K from the foods we eat. The other half comes from the bacteria living in our digestive tracts, which produce vitamin K. The extent to which we are able to use bacterially produced vitamin K, however, is still somewhat uncertain.

DIETARY REQUIREMENTS FOR VITAMIN K

For a long time, we didn't know enough about vitamin K to establish requirements. The first recommendation for the vitamin wasn't established until the 1989 edition of the RDAs. The requirement varies by age; for men, it ranges from 45 to 80 µg as age increases from 11 to over 50 years. For women, the range is from 45 to 65 µg. A typical well-balanced diet in the United States sup-

Sources of Vitamin K

Food	Quantity	Micrograms (µg)
Turnip greens, cooked	⅔ cup	650
Lettuce	¼ head	129
Cabbage, cooked	⅔ cup	125
Liver, beef	3 ounces	110
Broccoli, cooked	½ cup	100
Spinach, cooked	½ cup	80
Asparagus, cooked	⅔ cup	57
Liver, pork	3 ounces	30
Peas, cooked	⅔ cup	19
Ham	3 ounces	18
Green beans, cooked	¾ cup	14
Cheese	1 ounce	14
Egg	1 large	11
Ground beef, raw	4 ounces	10.5
Milk	1 cup	10
Liver, chicken	3 ounces	8
Peach	1 medium	8
Butter	1 tablespoon	6
Tomato	1 small	5
Banana	1 medium	3
Applesauce	⅓ cup	2
Corn oil	1 tablespoon	2
Bread	1 slice	1

plies 300 to 500 µg of vitamin K—more than enough to meet average dietary needs.

DEFICIENCY OF VITAMIN K

Liver or gall bladder disease, or any disease of the intestinal tract that interferes with absorption of fats, can cause a deficiency of vitamin K.

Long-term use of oral antibiotics kills off the bacteria in the intestines that manufacture the vitamin. This can lead to a deficiency, especially if coupled with a diet that doesn't provide enough vitamin K.

Use of mineral oil or medications such as cholestyramine to lower blood cholesterol can interfere with vitamin K absorption. With extended use, this can lead to a deficiency.

Newborn babies, especially those born prematurely, are born with little vitamin K. For the first couple of days after birth, the baby's intestinal tract has no bacteria to make the vitamin either. Moreover, the primary source of a baby's nutrition—milk—is not a good source of vitamin K. Because the lack of vitamin K could lead to bleeding problems, babies get a vitamin K supplement soon after birth.

VITAMIN K USE AND MISUSE

People who cannot absorb vitamin K and sometimes those on long-term antibiotic therapy take vitamin K supplements. When there's a known deficiency, vitamin K is given before surgery.

Anticoagulants (blood thinners, such as dicumarol) are used in the treatment of heart disease and other diseases that cause the blood to clot too easily. Blood thinners interfere with the action of vitamin K and slow down the clotting process. People taking anticoagulants may inadvertently reduce the action of the drug by eating vitamin K–rich foods.

Large doses of vitamin K have been reported to cause bleeding. Water-soluble forms of vitamin K have occasionally caused toxicity (red-cell breakdown, jaundice, and brain damage) when given to infants or pregnant women.

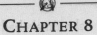

CHAPTER 8

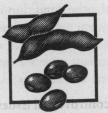

Vitaminlike Substances

There are many other substances in food that function much like vitamins. They do not, however, really fit the definition of vitamins, either because our bodies can make them or because we require them in larger amounts than vitamins. Most occur so widely in foods that a deficiency is unlikely.

CHOLINE

Choline is a substance in most animal tissues. It can exist by itself or as part of another substance. For example, it can be found in lecithin—a waxy material found in the protective myelin sheath that surrounds nerve fibers. It can also exist as part of the neurotransmitter acetylcholine—a substance essential for the transmission of impulses through the nervous system.

When experimental animals had their pancreases removed, researchers discovered the resulting lack of choline caused the condition hepatic cirrhosis, or fatty liver. When present, choline prevents the degenerative fatty changes that would otherwise occur. Could choline supplements do the same in humans? No one knows.

Other equally controversial issues involve the use of choline to lower cholesterol levels and improve memory.

Researchers have had limited success treating certain conditions with large doses of choline and lecithin. One of these conditions is Alzheimer disease. Another is tardive dyskinesia, a syndrome marked by involuntary movements of the face and jaw resulting from long-term use of psychiatric medications.

Egg yolks, liver, beef, and soybeans are good sources of choline. Under normal circumstances, choline and lecithin supplements are not necessary because the body manufactures choline. Infants, however, may need a dietary supply of choline. The American Academy of Pediatrics recommends that infant formula supply at least 7 mg of choline per 100 calories—the same amount present in human breast milk.

BIOFLAVONOIDS

Citrus fruits and their skins are the secret hiding places of bioflavonoids. In the 1930s, nutritionists thought bioflavonoids were essential to human nutrition and able to reverse the effects of vitamin C deficiency. This idea was later proved wrong; there is no evidence that bioflavonoids are essential to normal functioning.

They may, however, prove to have some disease-preventing powers. New research into how phytochemicals prevent disease may yet turn up evidence of what bioflavonoids might do for us in the preventive realm. (For more on phytochemicals, see Chapter 5.)

INOSITOL

Liver, wheat germ, citrus fruits, and meats are rich sources of inositol. The body can make inositol, concentrating it in hair and muscles. Perhaps because of this concentration in hair, inositol was rumored to be effective against baldness, but there's no scientific evidence for such a claim.

Of nine compounds related to inositol, the only one considered important to plants and animals is myoinositol. Researchers don't yet completely understand its function, but it's believed to aid the metabolism of fats. It's also useful in restoring nerve function to people with diabetes who experience nerve damage.

LIPOIC ACID

Lipoic acid functions as a coenzyme along with the vitamin thiamin. Yeast and liver are good sources of this substance, which the body can also make.

CARNITINE (VITAMIN B-T)

Carnitine plays a role in fat and energy metabolism in the body. Recently, carnitine received publicity for its potential usefulness in fighting heart disease. However, scientists need to study it further to establish what value, if any, it has for heart patients.

Carnitine is found mostly in foods of animal origin and in lesser amounts in foods of plant origin; therefore, a vegetarian diet is apt to be low in carnitine.

Under normal circumstances, though, the body makes this substance, so dietary sources are of little concern. Some people, however, may have an inherited inability to make sufficient amounts of carnitine and, therefore, would need dietary sources.

Symptoms of carnitine deficiency include muscle weakness, low blood sugar levels, and high blood ammonia levels. The treatment is not obvious, as carnitine supplements reduce the symptoms only in some people.

COENZYME Q

Coenzyme Q, also called *ubiquinone*, is a chemical relative of vitamin E. Coenzyme Q is made by the body and plays a role in energy metabolism. Current research is examining the benefit of coenzyme Q supplements in the treatment of certain types of heart disease, but answers are still not definitive.

Para-Aminobenzoic Acid (PABA)

Para-aminobenzoic acid (PABA) is part of the B vitamin folate and, therefore, isn't considered a separate vitamin. PABA is best known for its use in sunscreens; when applied to skin, it can help protect against sunburn. Taken orally, however, PABA does not have the same effect. Large doses taken over extended periods of time can cause nausea and vomiting. We do not recommend oral use.

CHAPTER 9

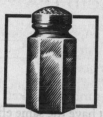

The Story of Minerals

Minerals, sometimes referred to as inorganic elements, make up about four percent, or about five pounds, of the body's weight. Even ancient peoples recognized the value and usefulness of minerals:

• Chinese writings from as early as 3000 B.C. recommended seaweed and burnt sponge to treat goiter, a deficiency of the mineral iodine. Both seaweed and sponges are rich in iodine.

• In ancient Greece, people soaked hot iron swords in water and then used the iron-enriched water to treat anemia.

• As many as 30 references to salt—sodium chloride—can be found in the Bible, including its use in purifying ceremonies and as an offering to God.

203

- A Greek slave said to be "worth his weight in salt" actually commanded this price—payment in salt.
- At banquets, important people sat at the table closest to the salt cellar. This was considered a position of honor.
- The word *salary* comes from the Latin word for salt, *saleria*.

Despite all these early references to minerals, many centuries passed before researchers clarified the role that minerals play in the body. In 1799, the French chemist Antoine Lavoisier—often called "the father of nutrition"—correctly predicted that scientists would isolate "elements" (known today as minerals) from the earth.

In 1804, another Frenchman, Theodore de Saussure, proved that the mineral makeup of soil influenced the mineral content of plants grown on that soil.

Research during the second half of the 19th century concentrated mostly on trace minerals—those needed only in tiny amounts. In the early 20th century, as scientists isolated and identified vitamins, they also demonstrated that many minerals were essential to human nutrition too.

Today, we are aware of 50 minerals in the body. Of these, 17 are definitely essential. The others are accidental contaminants or are waiting for us to discover their true importance. Recently, for example, researchers linked boron to mineral metabolism and bone development. It's possible that even small amounts of arsenic may prove to be useful to the body, perhaps in the metabolism of the amino acid methionine.

WHAT ARE MINERALS?

Minerals are different from vitamins; they are not organic substances made by plants or animals. They're actually inorganic elements found in soil. Plants absorb minerals directly from the soil, and animals get their supply indirectly, either by eating the plants or by eating other animals that have eaten the plants.

Minerals are grouped into two categories depending on the amount normally found in the body. *Macrominerals* are those found in significant amounts—about five grams or more—in the body. They include calcium, phosphorus, magnesium, chlorine, sodium, potassium, and sulfur. Calcium and phosphorus are present in the largest amounts—about one pound.

Microminerals consist of the trace elements found in smaller amounts in the body. The daily requirements for these minerals are only a few milligrams or less. They include the essential minerals: iron, iodine, zinc, fluoride, copper, chromium, manganese, selenium, molybdenum, and cobalt.

Research suggests that other trace minerals, such as nickel, tin, silicon, and vanadium, are essential for animals. It's possible they may prove to be necessary for humans as well. *Trace contaminants* is a better term for cadmium, aluminum, and lead. Although they exist in the body, experts do not consider them to be essential. In the future, that status may change, but at present, exposure to contaminants such as lead, cadmium, mercury, and arsenic is cause for concern as they are very toxic.

The National Research Council has established Recommended Dietary Allowances (RDAs) for seven minerals: calcium, iron, phosphorus, magnesium, zinc, iodine, and selenium.

Much less information is available about other minerals, making precise recommendations impossible. So, instead, the experts established ranges of "safe and adequate daily intakes" for sodium, potassium, chlorine, copper, fluoride, chromium, manganese, and molybdenum. (See page 21 for Table 2, "Estimated Safe and Adequate Daily Dietary Intakes of Additional Selected Vitamins and Minerals.")

WHAT MINERALS DO

Every cell in the body contains minerals. And almost everything the body does involves minerals in some way or another. Their main jobs are to help maintain the structure of living tissue and to regulate important body processes.

In their structural role, minerals contribute strength and firmness to bones and teeth. They're also part of essential body compounds. For example, iron is a part of hemoglobin (the oxygen-carrying substance in red blood cells) and is also a part of a number of different enzymes; iodine is a part of the thyroid hormone; and cobalt is a part of vitamin B_{12}.

In their role as regulators, minerals act as cofactors in enzyme-controlled body reactions. In other words, they keep enzyme reactions running up to speed. Iron, zinc, and copper are parts of enzymes. If the diet doesn't supply enough of these minerals, the body can't make enough enzymes.

Free mineral ions—particles with either a positive or negative electrical charge—have many important functions. These ions are important for:

• maintenance of normal acid–base balance
• transmission of nerve impulses
• regulation of normal cell membrane function
• regulation of muscle response to nerve stimuli

Some minerals have druglike effects. For example, fluoride prevents tooth decay and chromium helps control blood sugar in people with diabetes.

MINERAL DEFICIENCIES

Nutrition surveys often find that intakes of certain minerals, such as calcium, iron, and zinc, are lower than recommended. Part of the reason could be that refined and processed foods have fewer minerals. One way to remedy the loss is to replace those minerals lost in processing—a process called *enrichment*. In the 1920s, health authorities successfully prevented iodine-deficiency goiter by adding iodine to salt. And manufacturers currently add iron to cereals and breads that have the mineral stripped during processing. Many companies add calcium to fruit juices, breakfast cereals, and breads, too.

MINERAL TOXICITY

Excessive mineral supplements can be harmful. Large doses can:

- cause abnormal fluid accumulations in vital organs
- interfere with the functions of other minerals
- irritate the intestines, causing nausea and bleeding

A real danger is the replacement of one mineral with a similar one in an enzyme. The impostor enzyme doesn't function as the real one does or it doesn't function at all.

A WORD ABOUT WATER

In the body, metabolic reactions involving vitamins and minerals take place in water. Thus, water is essential for the maintenance of normal body function. Water makes up about 60 percent of an adult's body and an even greater percentage of a child's body. Men have slightly more water in their bodies than women do, and younger people have more than older people. About 70 percent of lean body tissue, or muscle, is actually water.

Water carries nutrients into cells and transports wastes out of them. It acts as a solvent for compounds such as vitamins, minerals, glucose, and amino acids (the building blocks of protein). It lubricates joints, acts as a shock absorber inside the eye and spinal cord, and helps the body maintain its temperature.

Most people drink about 2½ quarts of water daily. Normally, this comes from many sources: liquids (milk, tap water, noncaffeinated soft drinks, soups), animal foods (meat, fish, eggs), and fruits and vegetables. For example, cucumbers contain about 96 percent water; lettuce, 94 percent; watermelon, 93 percent; broccoli, 91 percent; and oranges, 84 percent.

Beverages such as coffee, tea, caffeine-containing soft drinks, and alcoholic drinks do not add to our total water intake. The caffeine and alcohol they contain are diuretics, causing the body to lose more water than is being added.

We also *lose* water in urine, stool, sweat, and the air we exhale. You can see the water when you exhale in the mist that forms on a mirror or pair of glasses when you blow on them, or the water vapor coming out of your mouth on a cold day.

People who are healthy generally excrete at least one quart of urine a day to rid the body of wastes.

During waking hours, this means urinating about every four hours. Less frequent urination is a sign that you're not consuming enough fluids. More frequent urination is good. The more water you consume, the easier it is on your kidneys.

Thirst partially controls the water content of the body, but often thirst lags behind the body's needs. That makes it even more important to pay attention to it. When you thirst for water, you're usually already behind in fluid intake. So indulge yourself (unless your doctor has advised you to do otherwise). Drinking too much water poses no danger to healthy people; they just excrete the excess, producing a more dilute urine.

ELECTROLYTES

When found in body tissues, minerals occur mainly as mineral salts. When these mineral salts dissolve in water, they may separate into ions—electrically charged particles called *electrolytes*. Sodium and potassium are the body's major electrolytes. They are extremely important. Electrolytes control the movement of nutrients into cells and wastes out of cells.

CHAPTER 10

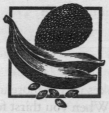

Minerals and Disease

Minerals are not getting the same attention vitamins have been getting lately—not because they don't deserve it, though. Minerals can protect you from some of the same diseases that vitamins can. And some minerals work cooperatively with vitamins: Selenium and vitamin E, calcium and vitamin D, and zinc and vitamin A are just a few examples of vitamin and mineral teamwork.

Part of the problem with minerals' reputations might be that minerals have the potential to be more toxic than vitamins. For many trace minerals, there is a fine line between not enough and too much. Most of the benefits attributed to minerals come from consuming the normal amounts found in foods. Unlike most vitamins, taking more than twice the recommended amount of a mineral may do more harm than good, unless you are correcting a deficiency under a doctor's supervision.

HEART DISEASE

Several essential minerals may have an effect on heart disease risk—not all of it good. Some protect the heart by acting as antioxidants, some benefit the circulatory system by other means, and some may do harm when overdone.

Selenium

In the tradition of vitamin antioxidants, the mineral selenium is also an antioxidant thought to protect against heart disease. Unlike vitamin antioxidants, which act directly on free radicals, mineral antioxidants work with enzyme proteins to ensure that these enzymes live up to their potential.

But the benefits of selenium are not unlimited. For example, providing more selenium than enzymes working at maximum capacity can use will not provide any further advantage. This limited benefit is probably a good thing, considering the toxicity of high doses.

The idea that selenium can protect the heart comes from a particular type of heart disease in China called *Keshan disease*. Keshan disease involves deterioration of heart muscle in children and pregnant women. The disease is much more common in areas of China with selenium-poor soil than in selenium-rich areas. Plants grown in selenium-rich soil have more selenium than plants grown in selenium-poor soil. The same is true of animals that feed on plants grown in these areas.

Could there be a connection between Keshan disease and the selenium content of the foods in the regions? In the United States, Keshan disease does not exist. Comparisons of soil selenium levels and rates of heart disease have not turned up consistent results. That may be because we eat foods from many regions, not just locally grown produce. Or perhaps another factor combines with low selenium intake to trigger the disease to appear.

Selenium does have other mechanisms that may protect the heart. The mineral controls the levels of hormonelike substances called *prostaglandins*. One of these substances promotes the tendency for blood vessels to constrict and clots to form. Working as part of an antioxidant enzyme, selenium controls how much of this prostaglandin is formed. Selenium also favors production of another prostaglandin, which has the opposite effect. When there is insufficient selenium, too much of the first type of prostaglandin forms. This could eventually lead to clogged arteries.

Chromium

Other minerals may also affect heart disease risk, even though they do not function as antioxidants. Investigators are looking at the potential for chromium supplements to lower blood cholesterol levels. Autopsies show that the blood chromium levels in people who died from heart disease are much lower than in people who died from accidents. People who live in countries where heart disease is common also have less chromium in their arteries than people from countries where heart disease is rare.

A recent study looked at people with high blood cholesterol levels who took 200 micrograms (µg) of chromium picolinate for six weeks. It lowered their total cholesterol about 19 percent and low-density lipoprotein (LDL) cholesterol by 21 percent, on average. Moreover, chromium lowered the blood level of bad LDL cholesterol, without lowering the blood level of good high-density lipoprotein (HDL) cholesterol.

Iron

Recently, scientists renewed fears that too much iron might increase the risk of heart attack. A single study from Finland found that heart attacks occurred more often in men with high blood levels of the storage form of iron, ferritin. This study unleashed a rash of publicity about too much iron in our diets and in supplements. It suggested that women might be at lower risk for heart attacks because they consume less iron than men. However, researchers have yet to test the effects of iron on heart attacks in women.

There is worry about iron and an inherited disease called *hemochromatosis*, or iron overload. One of the consequences of this insidious condition is heart disease. Most people do not absorb more iron than they need regardless of how much is in their diets because they have controls to prevent excessive absorption. But people who have this inherited defect, mostly men, do not have the normal controls and need to be careful about consuming too much iron.

Even people who haven't inherited the defect and should not have to worry can override their controls by consuming large amounts of alcohol. Indeed, in the Finnish study, alcohol intake was high in the men with high ferritin levels.

Until other investigators duplicate these results, a conservative approach toward iron is prudent. Yet it is unwise to avoid dietary iron because a deficiency of this mineral has serious implications. Lowered resistance to infection could be life threatening, especially for children. It might also interfere with their ability to learn.

HYPERTENSION AND STROKE

High blood pressure, or hypertension, increases the risk of heart disease and stroke. Mineral protection comes from calcium, magnesium, and potassium, all of which favor low blood pressure. Hypertension is less frequent in regions of the country with hard water, which is higher in calcium and magnesium. Soft water usually contains more sodium.

People who eat diets rich in fruits, dark-green leafy vegetables, and whole grains rarely suffer from high blood pressure. These foods contribute substantial amounts of potassium and magnesium to the diet. Consumption of calcium-rich milk is also directly related to a reduced risk of hypertension.

In addition to promoting lower blood pressure, dietary potassium may also protect against stroke. A study in southern California looked at the consumption of potassium and other minerals in adults between 50 and 79 years of age. The study found that the risk of dying from stroke over a 12-year period was 2½ times greater for the men who consumed the lowest amount of potassium and 5 times greater for the women who consumed the lowest amounts. The effect of potassium intake on stroke deaths was stronger than that of either calcium or magnesium.

CANCER

For a long time, the only mineral thought to offer protection against cancer was selenium. Now, calcium is a candidate as well.

Early studies of selenium were confusing. Some found reduced rates of cancers in people living in areas with selenium-rich soil, whereas others showed higher rates of cancers. In one study in Finland, cancer risk was six times greater for people with the lowest levels of selenium in their blood, with an even higher risk for those whose vitamin E level was also low.

Whether selenium promotes cancer may depend on which carcinogens are present. As part of an antioxidant enzyme, selenium stimulates the system in the liver responsible for detoxifying chemicals. This system takes some carcinogens out of action, but it also triggers others into action. Because of this dual effect, it's important not to consume too much or too little of this mineral.

The possibility that calcium may offer protection against colon and rectal cancers has generated excitement among researchers. They're finding low rates of colon cancer where calcium intakes are high. In the Northeast, for example, where calcium intakes are the lowest in the United States, many more people die from these cancers than in other regions. Fewer people die from colon cancer in the western United States, where calcium intakes are the highest.

Recently, researchers confirmed that people getting more calcium (1,500 milligrams [mg] in this case) produced less bile acid than people getting little calcium. Bile acids are believed to stimulate tumor growth in the colon; therefore, excessive bile acid production could mean an increased risk of colon cancer. Calcium is also thought to attach to bile acids, rendering them harmless.

Eating a diet rich in calcium might not be enough, however. A high fat intake might offset benefits from increased calcium intake. For this reason, turn to low-fat sources of calcium such as skim milk, yogurt, dried beans, dark-green leafy vegetables, and tofu (coagulated with calcium).

DIABETES

With age, some people find it more and more difficult to control blood sugar levels. It is not a lack of insulin that causes the difficulty, but a loss of insulin's potency or the body's ability to react to the hormone. Deficiencies of several minerals may contribute to the problem.

Chromium assists insulin in removing sugar from the blood, but blood chromium levels decline with age, particularly in people who consume a diet of mostly processed foods. (Processing removes chromium from foods such as whole grains, which are a particularly rich source of chromium before being refined.) At the same time, foods rich in refined sugars such as sweets, presweetened breakfast cereals, and baked goods increase the need for this nutrient.

In one study of older people with non–insulin-dependent diabetes, blood sugar returned to normal when they took chromium supplements. Generally, older people with mildly elevated blood sugar levels are the most likely to respond to these supplements.

Magnesium supplements may also benefit blood sugar levels in older adults. Magnesium levels are lower in the blood of people with diabetes compared with healthy people, and like chromium, blood magnesium levels decline with age. In a study of older people with non–insulin-dependent diabetes, insulin's action on blood sugar improved with magnesium supplements.

The best sources of magnesium are spinach, other greens, and nuts. Since these aren't necessarily everyday foods, you might have to make an effort to get enough magnesium in your diet.

IMMUNE FUNCTION

If you've suffered a cold or the flu lately, you are one of millions who can appreciate how important a properly functioning immune system is. But it does more than you may think. Your immune system not only fights off viruses and bacterial infections but also destroys cancer cells in the early stages of the disease. To ensure optimal immune function, several minerals, including iron, zinc, copper, and selenium, are also needed.

Iron-deficiency anemia is the most common nutritional deficiency disease in the world. Women during their child-bearing years and children are the most susceptible. Many people with iron-deficiency anemia die from infection because of weakened immune systems. Iron's role in maintaining immunity covers every aspect of how the system works. Iron is a vital component of a number of substances lethal to bacteria and is found in saliva, tears, and human breast milk. Iron also helps produce antibodies and maintain your white blood cell count. Iron promotes the activity of "natural killer" immune cells, which are responsible for destroying cancer cells.

Although you need to make sure you are getting sufficient iron to keep your immune system active, too much iron can have the opposite effect. Bacteria and other organisms gobble up any iron in excess of what you need and use it to help them thrive. The proper balance is important.

A robust immune system also calls for adequate zinc, though researchers aren't quite sure of its role. Zinc may help the functioning of two immune system organs: the thymic gland and the spleen. Blood zinc levels decline with age in some people, and when they do, a loss of immune function seems to follow. People with low blood levels of zinc suffer more from infection-related diseases than people with normal levels.

A few studies show improved immune function in elderly adults after taking zinc supplements, but other studies show no benefit. One study found that zinc supplements brought immune function in older adults back to levels seen in younger adults. As with iron, however, you must be careful not to take too much zinc. Levels twice the RDA boost immune function in men, but levels ten times the RDA actually depress it. Moreover, high doses of zinc can cause a copper deficiency to develop.

Though copper may be another key mineral for the immune system, we know even less about its role than we do about the role of iron and zinc. We do know that groups of people who experience clinical copper deficiency—preterm infants, children with genetic copper defects, and hospital patients experiencing inadequate tube feedings—all suffer from depressed immune function and all show improved immune response after taking copper supplements. Copper deficiency is rare, but intakes that are only marginally adequate are all too common.

OSTEOPOROSIS

Osteoporosis is a disease in which bone loss is so extensive that a bone can spontaneously fracture without any stress. These fractures are dangerous because they occur without warning and can cause falls or other accidents.

A calcium supplement will almost certainly be needed after menopause to help offset the bone loss caused by declining estrogen levels. Experts recommend getting 1,500 mg of calcium during the most susceptible time period—five to ten years after menopause.

An adequate magnesium intake is necessary to be sure the body is using calcium efficiently. Studies show that calcium supplements are not as effective in increasing bone density in people who are deficient in magnesium. In other words, calcium cannot correct bone loss if there is a magnesium deficiency. (The same is also true for vitamin D.)

Copper's contribution to bone strength receives little attention. The mineral network that supports bone depends on reactions involving copper. A weakness in this network weakens the entire structure. For example, preterm infants, who frequently develop copper deficiencies, suffer bone loss similar to that of adults with osteoporosis, despite their young ages. Though copper deficiency is rare in adults, many people may be getting suboptimal amounts, with unknown consequences.

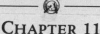

CHAPTER 11

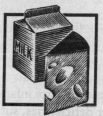

Mineral Profiles

Calcium

FUNCTIONS OF CALCIUM

Building strong bones and teeth is the most familiar function of calcium. Indeed, those bones and teeth contain 99 percent of all the calcium in your body. The remaining 1 percent circulates in blood or resides in the body's soft tissues. This 1 percent, however, plays many extremely important roles, including:

- blood clotting
- contraction and relaxation of muscles—including the heart muscle
- transmission of nerve impulses
- activation of enzymes
- hormone secretion

Because maintaining a normal blood calcium level is so important to vital functions such as heart rhythm, the body has a way to ensure a constant level of calcium in the blood, no matter how much your diet provides. The secret reservoir of calcium happens to be your bones, which release calcium into the blood as needed. But if this happens too often, your bones suffer the consequences.

SOURCES OF CALCIUM

Milk, yogurt, cheese, and other dairy products are rich sources of calcium. Dried beans and peas, and green vegetables such as broccoli, kale, bok choy, and chard are also good sources. Spinach, however, is not a good source; the calcium in spinach is not well absorbed because spinach contains a substance called *oxalic acid*, which attaches to calcium, preventing its absorption.

Phytic acid, a substance found in whole grains and dried beans and peas, also combines with calcium and other minerals, preventing their absorption. This presents a problem only for people who consume extremely large amounts of these foods and do not drink milk. For those people, a calcium supplement might be necessary to prevent a deficiency.

Recently, fruit juices, cereals, even bread are sporting added calcium. Fruit juices contain acids, such as citric acid, that boost the amount of calcium absorbed. For someone who does not, or cannot, drink milk, orange juice fortified with calcium can be a nutritious alternative. Mineral water may also contribute some calcium to the diet, as does hard water.

DIETARY REQUIREMENTS FOR CALCIUM

The Recommended Dietary Allowance (RDA) for adults over age 25 is 800 milligrams (mg) of calcium. For women who are pregnant or breast-feeding, the RDA is now 1,200 mg. This is also the requirement for children over age 11, adolescents, and adults up to age 25.

But, the RDAs are outdated. In 1994, the National Institutes of Health set higher standards for optimal calcium intake to help prevent or postpone osteoporosis: 1,000 mg per day for women aged 25 to 50; 1,500 mg per day for postmenopausal women (1,000 mg per day if on hormone replacement therapy); 1,000 mg per day for men aged 25 to 65; 1,500 mg per day for men and women over age 65. These daily levels may be difficult to meet from foods.

One quart of milk contains approximately 1,000 mg of calcium. Two cups of milk or its equivalent (as described in the Food Guide Pyramid in Chapter 1) contributes half an adult's daily requirement for calcium. Foods such as dark-green vegetables, breads, cereals, and dried peas and beans must provide the rest. If you cannot meet these levels through foods, you'll need a calcium supplement.

Calcium Content of Common Foods

Food	Quantity	Milligrams (mg)
Meat-Protein Group		
Sardines, canned, drained	4 ounces	428
Salmon, pink, canned	4 ounces	239
Chicken, roasted, white meat, no skin	3 ounces	140
Navy beans	1 cup	127
Tofu (bean curd)	4 ounces	119
Almonds, roasted	¼ cup	69
Hamburger with bun	4 ounces	68
Peanuts, roasted	¼ cup	64
Milk-Dairy Group		
Yogurt, low-fat	1 cup	372
Milk, skim	1 cup	302
Milk, whole	1 cup	291
Swiss cheese	1 ounce	272
Ice cream	1 cup	169
American cheese	1 ounce	142
Cream cheese	1 tablespoon	8
Bread-Cereal/Grain Group		
Farina	1 cup	56
Bread, whole-wheat	1 slice	23
Bread, white, enriched	1 slice	21
Rice, white, cooked	1 cup	16
Fruits-Vegetables Group		
Spinach, cooked, fresh or frozen	1 cup	277
Turnip greens	1 cup	197
Figs, dried	½ cup	144
Broccoli	1 cup	94

Calcium Content of
Common Foods (cont.)

Food	Quantity	Milligrams (mg)
Fruits-Vegetables Group (cont.)		
Green beans	1 cup	61
Cabbage, raw	1 cup	33
Olives, green	10	24
Apple	1 medium	10
Other		
Soup, chicken noodle	1 cup	31

DEFICIENCY OF CALCIUM

A deficiency of calcium can cause the development of bones and teeth to be stunted. A lack of vitamin D, which is needed for calcium's absorption and use, can have a similar effect. Without it, there's a softening of bones, called *rickets* in children and *osteomalacia* in adults.

Bones suffer the brunt of insufficient calcium, because they defer their needs to other functions, that demand a higher priority. Blood clotting and muscle contraction are critical functions of calcium that must be sustained to preserve life. If muscle contractions go awry, your heart can stop. So when the blood contains too little calcium, bones give up their calcium for these functions. If this happens too often, your bones become porous and weak.

The result of such weakening is *osteoporosis*, or adult bone loss. If you lose one third or more of your bone mass, fractures can spontaneously occur. One in four postmenopausal women develops osteoporosis; in men, the condition is less common, because they have a larger bone mass to work with and generally take in more calcium. Low calcium intake during childhood, teen, and early adult years can set the stage for osteoporosis in later life.

CALCIUM USE AND MISUSE

Doctors correct a calcium deficiency with calcium supplements, which often have vitamin D added to ensure calcium absorption. Doctors also prescribe calcium supplements to postmenopausal women to prevent osteoporosis, since it is so difficult to get as much calcium as is now recommended. Some use calcium as an adjunct to estrogen replacement therapy.

Recent research indicates that calcium supplements may benefit some people who have high blood pressure. They may also be useful in preventing a condition that sometimes occurs in pregnancy, called *toxemia*. In addition, studies show that people with higher intakes of calcium may be less likely to develop colon cancer (see Chapter 10 for more information).

The belief that large doses of calcium supplements will increase the risk of kidney stones is unfounded. Recent research showed that men who consumed more than 1,000 mg of calcium daily were only half as likely to get kidney stones as those who consumed less than 600 mg. This indicates that a high-calcium diet could actually protect against kidney stones rather than increase risk.

Calcium carbonate is the most common form of calcium found in supplements. This is the type of calcium in crushed oyster shells and some antacids. However, it is only 40 percent calcium. The label indicates this with a statement, such as: "Each tablet provides 1,250 mg of calcium carbonate, which yields 500 mg of elemental calcium."

Some people tout bone meal and dolomite as "natural" sources of calcium, but because they can be contaminated with lead, arsenic, or other toxic metals, we don't recommend their use. (See the Supplement Product Profiles in Chapter 12 for an evaluation of specific calcium supplements.)

Phosphorus

Besides calcium, phosphorus is vital for strong bones and teeth. Phosphorus also plays an important role in energy storage and release. It's found in DNA (deoxyribonucleic acid) and RNA (ribonucleic acid), the genetic materials that serve as the blueprints for the formation of new cells. Phosphorus is necessary for normal milk secretion and many metabolic reactions as well.

The RDA for phosphorus is 800 mg per day for adults over age 25. For pregnant and nursing women, the RDA increases to 1,200 mg. For most age groups, the RDA for phosphorus is the same as for calcium. The ideal ratio of calcium to phosphorus is one to one. Milk contains phosphorus and calcium in approximately this ratio.

Good sources of phosphorus are also good sources of protein—for example, milk and other dairy products, eggs, meat, fish, poultry, nuts, and whole grains. Even sodas and food additives supply this mineral. As a result, getting enough phosphorus is not a problem for most Americans. Perhaps getting too much is.

Although phosphorus deficiency has been reported in some infants fed cow's milk and in some people taking large amounts of antacids, a deficiency is most unlikely. Americans consume as much as four times the RDA for phosphorus. American diets are heavy in high-protein foods (such as meat, fish, or poultry), carbonated beverages, and ready-to-eat convenience foods—all of which increase the body's supply of phosphorus.

Some nutrition experts believe that excessive phosphorus intakes, when coupled with low intakes of calcium, may be a key factor in whether people develop osteoporosis, because high levels of phosphorus can interfere with calcium absorption. To be safe, consume phosphorus-rich foods or drinks in moderation.

Phosphorus Content of Common Foods

Food	Quantity	Milligrams (mg)
Meat-Protein Group		
Sardines, Atlantic, canned	3 ounces	412
Peanuts, roasted, salted	½ cup	375
Pork and beans	1 cup	296
Kidney beans, canned	1 cup	254
Lima beans, cooked	1 cup	209
Almonds, roasted	¼ cup	205
Roast chicken, white meat, no skin	3 ounces	185
Pistachio nuts	¼ cup	161
Tuna, canned in water	3 ounces	156
Beef, rib roast	3 ounces	138
Luncheon meat	2 slices	92
Frankfurter	1	39
Milk-Dairy Group		
Milk, skim	1 cup	247
Milk, whole	1 cup	228
Bread-Cereal/Grain Group		
Pancake, whole-wheat	1 medium	96
Rice, white, enriched, cooked	1 cup	68
Bread, whole-wheat	1 slice	65
Bread, white, enriched	1 slice	24
Fruits-Vegetables Group		
Broccoli	1 cup	101
Potato, baked with skin	1	70
Figs, dried	½ cup	68
Bean sprouts, cooked	½ cup	58
Cauliflower, cooked	1 cup	43
Corn, sweet, yellow, fresh	½ cup	38

Phosphorus Content of Common Foods (cont.)

Food	Quantity	Milligrams (mg)
Fruits-Vegetables Group (cont.)		
Beans, green, cooked	½ cup	16
Grapefruit	½ medium	12
Apple	1 medium	10
Peppers, sweet, raw, green, chopped	½ cup	10
Others		
Shake, vanilla	10 ounces	307
Pretzels, thin	1 cup	45
Soft drink, cola	12 ounces	44

Magnesium

Magnesium is another vital part of the mineral structure of bones and teeth. As with calcium, bones act as a reservoir for magnesium so that it will be available when needed.

Magnesium plays a role in protein synthesis, muscle relaxation, and energy release. It also triggers important metabolic reactions, including calcium metabolism. The parathyroid hormone needs magnesium to function normally; this regulates blood calcium levels.

Magnesium is found in most foods, particularly green leafy vegetables. This is because magnesium is part of chlorophyll, the pigment in plants that makes them green and fosters photosynthesis. Other good sources are dairy products, breads and cereals, nuts, chocolate, and dried peas and beans. Hard water also contains significant magnesium—one of the minerals that makes it "hard."

Magnesium Content of Common Foods

Food	Quantity	Milligrams (mg)
Meat-Protein Group		
Navy beans, cooked	1 cup	108
Black-eyed peas, cooked	1 cup	91
Beans, lima, boiled	½ cup	41
Lobster, Northern, meat	1 medium	36
Tuna, canned in water	4 ounces	32
Beef, chuck roast	3 ounces	23
Chicken, breast, no skin	½	20
Pork chop	3 ounces	20
Egg, hard-boiled	1 large	5
Milk-Dairy Group		
Yogurt, nonfat	1 cup	47
Milk, whole	1 cup	33
Ice cream, vanilla, plain	½ cup	9
Cheddar cheese	1 ounce	8
Bread-Cereal/Grain Group		
Oatmeal	1 cup	57
Granola, ready-to-eat	½ cup	55
Noodles, egg	1 cup	30
Bread, whole-wheat	1 slice	27
Rice, white, cooked	⅔ cup	13

Magnesium Content of Common Foods (cont.)

Food	Quantity	Milligrams (mg)
Fruits-Vegetables Group		
Figs, dried	½ cup	59
Broccoli, cooked	1 cup	37
Avocado	½ medium	34
Asparagus, fresh	½ cup	12
Strawberries, whole, fresh	⅔ cup	10
Cherries, raw, sweet	½ cup	8
Cauliflower, cooked	½ cup	8
Apple	1 medium	7
Mushrooms, raw	½ cup	4

The RDA for magnesium is 350 mg a day for men and 280 mg a day for women. Pregnant women need 20 mg per day more. Breast-feeding women require an extra 75 mg per day for the first six months to replenish the magnesium lost in breast milk. An additional 60 mg per day is enough during the second six months.

Magnesium deficiency can occur after prolonged vomiting or diarrhea, alcohol abuse, or long-term use of diuretics. A high intake of calcium can increase magnesium excretion and, if unchecked, can lead to problems such as nervousness, irritability, and tremors. Magnesium deficiency also causes muscles to remain contracted, leading to a loss of muscle control. It may also be the cause of hallucinations in people undergoing alcohol withdrawal.

Although a true dietary deficiency of magnesium is unusual, some experts believe suboptimal intakes may be common, with long-term consequences for bone health. Moreover, research suggests that people who regularly drink hard water, which is high in magnesium, have a lower incidence of sudden death from heart failure than do people who regularly drink soft water.

Magnesium may also benefit blood pressure. Pregnant women and people taking diuretics may be able to lower their blood pressure with supplemental magnesium. Consult with your physician if you think you might benefit.

Magnesium toxicity, on the other hand, is also a potential problem because magnesium is present in so many over-the-counter preparations. Recently, the government revealed 14 deaths from magnesium toxicity over the past two and a half decades; they involved people who misused magnesium-containing antacids and laxatives, taking much more than label directions indicate. The risk is greatest for those who absorb more magnesium than usual and those who cannot effectively excrete an excess. This group includes:

- older people
- people with long-standing diabetes
- people with kidney disease
- people who have had intestinal surgery
- people taking medication to slow intestinal motility

Chlorine

Chlorine is an important regulator of body systems, such as water balance, acid–base balance, and fluid pressure. For example, this mineral is part of hydrochloric acid, needed in the stomach for digestion. The acidity it creates ensures proper absorption of food and reduces the growth of harmful bacteria.

There is no RDA for chlorine. The recommended minimum safe intake is 750 mg. Regular table salt is 60 percent chlorine, as chloride. This source, along with the salt that occurs naturally in foods, provides all the chlorine that's needed. Even a diet restricted in sodium can supply adequate amounts of chlorine.

A chlorine deficiency is not likely because it's so prevalent in foods, but it can happen under certain circumstances. For example, several years ago, by mistake, some infant formula lacked chlorine. Children fed this formula as their sole source of food developed chlorine deficiencies.

Sodium

FUNCTION OF SODIUM

Sodium plays a critical role in regulating water balance in the body. It's also important for regulating acid–base balance, transmitting nerve impulses, maintaining cell membrane function and muscle activity, and absorbing and transporting certain nutrients. Sodium is also a part of body fluids such as sweat and tears.

SOURCES OF SODIUM

There's sodium in almost all the foods you eat; it's there either naturally or added in processing. Celery, carrots, greens, beets, eggs, and milk, for example, are naturally high in sodium. But natural sodium levels can't compare to the sodium in processed foods.

Foods such as pickles, luncheon meats, canned vegetables, soups, and frozen dinners are extremely high in sodium because processing adds so much salt (sodium chloride).

Unfortunately, you can't always tell food is high in sodium by tasting it. For example, cheese, cold breakfast cereal, ice cream, and prepared puddings are often high in sodium, even though they don't taste salty.

Even substances such as toothpaste and mouthwash contain sodium. So does the drinking water in many areas. Artificially softened water adds about 150 mg per quart of water—not a lot unless you are following a severely sodium-restricted diet. If so, run a separate line to your kitchen sink cold water faucet that bypasses the water softener. Your cooking and drinking water will then contain only the sodium naturally present in the water in your

Sodium Content of Common Foods

Food	Quantity	Milligrams (mg)
Meat-Protein Group		
Beef, ground	4 ounces	95
Pork, roasted	3 ounces	79
Peanut butter	1 tablespoon	76
Turkey, no skin, light or dark meat	3 ounces	66
Egg, whole	1 large	63
Chicken, white meat, without skin	3 ounces	60
Kidney beans, dried	1 cup	4
Milk-Dairy Group		
Cheddar cheese	1 ounce	176
Milk, whole	1 cup	120
Ice cream, 10% fat	1 cup	105
Butter, salted	1 tablespoon	76
Bread-Cereal/Grain Group		
Bread, white	1 slice	127
Brewer's yeast, dried	1 tablespoon	10
Fruits-Vegetables Group		
Sauerkraut	1 cup	1,560
Pickle, dill	1	993
Olives, green	5	480
Tomato juice	½ cup	438
Raisins, seedless	½ cup	9
Asparagus, cooked	1 cup	7
Zucchini, cooked	1 cup	5
Potato, baked, without skin	1 medium	5
Apple	1 medium	0

Food	Quantity	Milligrams (mg)
Others		
Soy sauce	2 tablespoons	2,057
Baking powder, sodium aluminum sulfate	1 tablespoon	1,140
Potato chips	1 cup	195
Jam or preserves	1 tablespoon	8

area. You'll also preserve the calcium and magnesium in your water, since hard water is rich in these nutrients.

How to tell how much sodium is in the foods you buy? Check the label. Though sodium has been on the label since 1986, specific guidelines for declaring sodium content and making health claims were only established in 1994.

Manufacturers may now use the following terms:

- *sodium free*—less than 5 mg per serving
- *very low sodium*—less than 35 mg per serving (for dehydrated soup mixes—less than 35 mg per 50-gram (g) serving after reconstituting)
- *low sodium*—less than 140 mg per serving
- *reduced sodium*—at least 25 percent less sodium than a comparable food (For example, potato chips would have to be compared with a similar salty snack.)

- *unsalted*—no salt added during processing (The salted version of the food it resembles and substitutes for must normally be processed with salt. An unsalted product has to state it is not sodium free if it contains sodium in forms other than sodium chloride.)
- *salt free*—must be sodium free

These rules apply to single foods only. For packaged main dishes, such as frozen dinners or entrées, the amounts of sodium are expressed per 100 g. Because of this, these products might be labeled low sodium but still have more sodium than the amounts given above.

DIETARY REQUIREMENTS OF SODIUM

Most of the sodium you eat comes from sodium chloride—common table salt. About 40 percent of table salt is sodium. On average, Americans eat about 4 to 5 g (4,000 to 5,000 mg) of sodium per day (your intake may be higher if your diet includes a lot of processed foods). But you only need one tenth of that—about 500 mg of sodium—to meet your body's actual need for this mineral. Experts recommend that total daily sodium not exceed 2,400 mg.

DEFICIENCY OF SODIUM

Because the body has a large sodium reserve and, under normal circumstances, people eat plenty of sodium-containing foods, a deficiency is not likely. However, salt depletion can temporarily occur through profuse sweating if you exercise strenuously for a prolonged time in warm weather or hot climates. Even in this situation, salt that's lost is easily replaced by eating salty foods. Salt tablets are not necessary and can be dangerous.

SODIUM USE AND MISUSE

High blood pressure rarely appears in cultures with low salt intakes. Is that a coincidence? Most researchers think not. Yet for all the population studies that link high salt intake with high blood pressure, it's never been proved that salt *causes* blood pressure to rise.

A new study in chimps—as biologically close to humans as you can get—proved that salt could raise blood pressure and could lower it when removed. The Australian researchers used salt levels that mimicked human levels. They also eliminated calcium and potassium as factors, by supplementing their diets with these minerals. The chimp study also confirmed the popular theory that some people are "salt sensitive"—more susceptible than others to developing high blood pressure because of salt intake.

Because a tendency toward salt sensitivity might be inherited, you'd be wise to cut back on the salt in your diet and check your blood pressure regularly if you have a family history of hypertension. Because Americans as a group consume a lot of salt and high blood pressure is widespread, a low-salt diet might be a wise choice for everyone (unless otherwise directed by a doctor).

Doctors generally advise people diagnosed with high blood pressure to reduce their salt intake. But because not everybody is salt sensitive, not everyone will benefit from salt restriction. The only way to know for sure is to try it. Moreover, experts say a low-sodium diet improves the response to some medications, such as diuretics, by making them more effective in treating high blood pressure.

Potassium

The body's potassium resides mostly inside body cells. Potassium plays an important role in maintaining water balance and acid–base balance. Its presence is crucial in the transmission of nerve impulses from nerves to muscles. It also acts as a catalyst in carbohydrate and protein metabolism. Because potassium is a constant part of muscle, measurements of potassium content can estimate body composition.

Studies are increasingly suggesting that a high intake of potassium-rich foods reduces blood pressure and the risk of stroke. Theoretically, when potassium intake is high, the body excretes more sodium, lowering blood pressure. Vegetarians, for example, have lower blood pressure than nonvegetarians. Though it is difficult to rule out all other factors, vegetarians do eat diets rich in fruits and vegetables, and thus rich in potassium.

Potassium Content of Common Foods

Food	Quantity	Milligrams (mg)
Meat-Protein Group		
Lima beans, cooked	1 cup	955
Pinto beans, cooked	1 cup	800
Kidney beans, canned	1 cup	713
Peas, split, cooked	1 cup	710
Sirloin steak, lean	6 ounces	674
Peanuts, dried, unsalted	½ cup	491
Sole/flounder, baked	3 ounces	394
Chicken breast, roasted, no skin	½	196
Milk-Dairy Group		
Yogurt	1 cup	624
Milk, whole	1 cup	370
Cheddar cheese	1 ounce	28
Bread-Cereal/Grain Group		
Brewer's yeast	1 tablespoon	224
Wheat germ	2 tablespoons	134
Bread, whole-wheat	1 slice	78
Fruits-Vegetables Group		
Cantaloupe melon	½ medium	1,426
Bok choy, cooked	1 cup	631
Spinach, cooked	1 cup	566
Watermelon	1 slice	559
Beets, cooked	1 cup	518

Potassium Content of
Common Foods (cont.)

Food	Quantity	Milligrams (mg)
Fruits-Vegetables Group (cont.)		
Potato, baked, with skin	1 medium	510
Zucchini, cooked	1 cup	455
Banana	1 medium	451
Winter squash, baked	1 cup	407
Asparagus	1 cup	392
Broccoli	1 cup	331
Apricots	3 small	314
Cauliflower	1 cup	250
Orange	1 medium	237
Orange juice	½ cup	236
Celery	½ cup	172
Peach	1 medium	171
Apple	1 medium	159
Red radishes	½ cup	135
Romaine lettuce	1 cup	87

Some diuretics commonly prescribed to treat high blood pressure cause the body to lose potassium. If you take such a diuretic, you can compensate for the loss by eating foods rich in potassium. While almost all whole foods contain some potassium, particularly good sources include milk, meat, potatoes, tomatoes, prunes, bananas, oranges, and dried peas and beans. As a group, fruits and vegetables reign supreme in the potassium-supply category. Processed foods, on the other hand, lose much of their potassium.

Potassium combined with chloride is effective at restoring potassium losses from the body and can satisfy a taste for table salt. Many salt substitutes are compounds of potassium chloride. People with kidney disease, however, should avoid them.

Because potassium is found in so many foods, dietary deficiency is unlikely. However, uncontrolled diabetes or a prolonged excessive water loss (as from sweating) may result in potassium depletion. Rapid weight loss—from liquid diets or fasting—can also deplete the body of potassium. Muscle weakness is an early sign of potassium depletion. It indicates a very serious situation. Not only can it interfere with muscle action and fluid balance, but it can lead to abnormal heart rhythm, possibly triggering a heart attack.

The safe minimum level of intake for potassium is 2,000 mg per day for adults. Some nutritionists think 3,000 mg per day would benefit those with high blood pressure.

Under normal circumstances, potassium supplements are not recommended. Physicians may prescribe them to prevent potassium depletion in people taking certain types of diuretics, though.

Sulfur

Sulfur is found throughout the body, especially in the skin, hair, and nails. Sulfur aids the storage and release of energy. It's part of the genetic material of cells, and helps promote enzyme reactions and blood clotting. Sulfur is part of two B vitamins, biotin and thiamin. Sulfur also combines with certain toxic materials so they can then pass out safely in the urine.

Although there is no RDA for sulfur, it's not because it plays an unimportant role. When protein intake is adequate, sulfur intake is adequate as well. That's because sulfur-containing amino acids (the building blocks of protein) supply the body with the amount of sulfur it needs. However, taking in adequate amounts of sulfur from other sources preserves these amino acids for their other vital functions.

A wide variety of foods contain sulfur. Cheese, eggs, fish, poultry, grains, nuts, and dried peas and beans are all rich sources.

Iron

FUNCTION OF IRON

Most of the body's iron resides in the hemoglobin of red blood cells—the pigment that makes these blood cells appear red. Hemoglobin carries oxygen to cells and transports carbon dioxide from cells. Iron is also essential to enzymes involved in energy release, cholesterol metabolism, immune function, and connective-tissue production.

Iron Content of Common Foods

Food	Quantity	Milligrams (mg)
Meat-Protein Group		
Liver, beef	2½ ounces	4.8
Liver, chicken	½ cup	4.5
Soybeans, cooked	½ cup	4.4
Peas, dried, cooked	2½ cups	2.0
Beef, lamb	3 ounces	1.8–2.4
Chicken breast	1 whole	1.7
Pork, veal	3 ounces	0.9–3.3
Fish	3 ounces	0.6–1.5
Bread-Cereal/Grain Group		
Farina	1 cup	10.0
Bread, whole grain	2 slices	1.7
Spaghetti, noodles, or macaroni, cooked	1 cup	1.5–2.0
Bread, enriched	2 slices	1.4
Cereals, enriched, ready-to-eat	1 cup	1.0–18.0
Fruits-Vegetables Group		
Spinach, cooked	1 cup	2.9
Figs, dried	½ cup	2.2
Potato, baked with skin	1 medium	1.7
Turnip greens, cooked	1 cup	1.2
Cherries, fresh	1 cup	0.6
Honeydew melon	½ medium	0.4
Grapes	1 cup	0.4
Raisins	2 tablespoons	0.4

SOURCES OF IRON

Good sources of iron include liver and other meats, whole grains, shellfish, green leafy vegetables, and nuts. Iron is one of the nutrients added to enriched cereals and bread. According to recent research, soybean hulls (not the whole soybean) contain a very absorbable form of iron. In the future, these hulls may fortify other foods with iron.

Cooking in iron pots adds iron to the foods prepared in them. This is especially true of acidic foods such as tomatoes.

Take note that milk is a poor source of iron and should not be relied on to provide iron for infants and children.

DIETARY REQUIREMENTS
FOR IRON

The RDA for iron is 10 mg per day for adult men and postmenopausal women and 15 mg per day for menstruating women. Women who are pregnant or breast-feeding require more iron. Iron requirements are also greater during periods of growth and development.

DEFICIENCY OF IRON

The typical American diet provides about 6 mg of iron for every 1,000 calories. This presents a problem for women who often eat fewer than 2,000 calories a day. Men, on the other hand, who often eat 2,500 calories a day or more, are much more likely to meet their RDA, which is lower anyway. Women have the added problem of losing iron in menstrual flow each month.

Absorption of iron is notoriously poor—only about ten percent of what's eaten. The iron in meat, heme iron, is absorbed better than the non-heme iron found in vegetables. (The soy hulls mentioned earlier are an exception.) Meat, fish, poultry, and vitamin C all increase iron absorption. Any of these at a meal increases the amount of iron absorbed from other foods eaten during that meal. Coffee, tea, whole soybeans, and whole grains, on the other hand, all reduce the amount of iron absorbed from foods eaten at the same meal.

Iron deficiency is the most common cause of anemia. Headache, shortness of breath, weakness, fatigue, heart palpitations, and sore tongue are some of the symptoms. For people who are anemic, even mild exercise can cause chest pain. Mild iron deficiency even without anemia may cause learning problems in school children.

Pica, a desire to eat nonfood substances such as clay, chalk, ashes, or laundry starch (none of which contains iron) sometimes accompanies iron deficiency. This abnormal craving may be an underlying factor contributing to the anemia.

Long-term use of aspirin can cause bleeding in the lining of the stomach. The blood loss may lead to iron deficiency. Aspirin coated with a special material reduces irritation to the stomach lining.

Drinking plenty of water when you take aspirin also helps.

Young children fed mostly milk, with few other foods, can develop a milk-induced anemia. Milk contains little iron and in very large quantities may actually promote irritation and bleeding in the stomach. Anemia can result from this loss of blood.

The normal acidity of the stomach helps promote iron absorption in the intestine. Chronic use of antacids decreases the acidity of the stomach, reducing the amount of iron absorbed. A deficiency may result.

An estimated eight percent of women and one percent of men in the United States exhibit symptoms of iron deficiency. Even more probably have inadequate iron reserves. However, there's been an improvement in the iron status of children due, at least in part, to the greater use of iron-fortified formula.

IRON USE AND MISUSE

To treat an iron deficiency, you need iron supplements in conjunction with an iron-rich diet. Iron in all ferrous forms is better absorbed than as ferric iron. When you read labels of iron supplements, check for the amount of elemental iron. That's what's important. For example, the label may state, "Each tablet provides 200 mg of ferrous fumarate, which yields 67 mg of elemental iron."

Some people don't tolerate iron supplements well and may develop side effects such as heartburn, nausea, stomachache, constipation, or diarrhea. Taking the supplement with food can eliminate or minimize these symptoms. You can also gradually work up to the desired dose or divide the high dose into several small doses. Do not worry if your stool appears dark. It's just some of the unabsorbed iron.

In healthy people, the intestines control the amount of iron that's absorbed. The body increases its rate of iron absorption if reserves are low. And when the body becomes saturated with iron, the rate decreases. If the intestines do not or cannot properly perform this regulatory function—as can happen from excessive and prolonged alcohol intake—the body can absorb toxic quantities.

A certain percentage of the population suffers from *hemochromatosis*, a hereditary disease in which the body absorbs too much iron and deposits it in body tissues. Symptoms of this condition only appear after significant and irreversible damage occurs. They include weakness, weight loss, change in skin color, abdominal pain, loss of sex drive, and the onset of diabetes. Heart, liver, and joints may also become impaired. Men are most often affected by this disease. Because men usually get enough iron, some experts advise that men avoid the extra iron in some supplements and cereals.

Iron poisoning is the most common accidental poisoning in young children. Iron tablets may be coated with sugar to mask their taste, and if allowed access to them, children will eat them like candy. *IRON CAN BE FATAL TO CHILDREN. All supplements should be kept out of the reach of children.*

Iodine

FUNCTIONS OF IODINE

Almost half the body's iodine is in the thyroid gland. Iodine is an important component of thyroid hormones, which control energy metabolism in the body as well as body temperature, reproduction, and growth.

SOURCES OF IODINE

Saltwater seafood is a primary source of iodine. Iodized salt, in use since 1924, is another rich source. One teaspoon of iodized salt provides 260 micrograms (μg) of iodine, nearly twice the RDA. The amount of iodine in vegetables and grains varies according to how much is present in the soil where they are grown. In certain regions of the world, this amount is less than optimal.

In the United States, the need for iodized salt is not as great as it was 50 years ago. Thanks to refrigerated trucks, most of the country gets produce from coastal regions where soil is rich in iodine. Iodine deficiency is a concern only in isolated areas where all the food eaten is locally grown.

Dairy equipment is sometimes disinfected with iodine-containing compounds, and dairy cattle are fed iodine-containing feed. Both contribute to an increasing amount of iodine in milk and dairy products. Iodine is also in dough conditioners used by bakeries, in food colorings, and even in polluted air, providing the lone benefit of air pollution.

DEFICIENCY OF IODINE

A deficiency of iodine causes the thyroid gland to enlarge greatly—a condition known as *goiter*. The thyroid gland, which is normally about the size of a lima bean, can become as large as a person's head! A deficiency of thyroid hormones can result in mental and physical sluggishness, slowed heart rate, weight gain, constipation, and increased sleep needs (14 to 16 hours a day).

In pregnancy, the results of iodine deficiency are more serious. The baby of an iodine-deficient mother may have retarded physical and mental development—a condition known as *cretinism*.

Certain substances known as *goitrogens* induce goiter when iodine intake is low. Cabbage, brussels sprouts, rutabagas, cauliflower, turnips, and peanuts contain these substances. However, since heat destroys goitrogens, the potential dangers exist only if large amounts of these foods are eaten raw.

IODINE USE AND MISUSE

Because Americans get several times the RDA for iodine, they rarely need supplements. Some experts even question whether iodized table salt is still necessary. As salt intake declines, this source becomes less important.

Some people who are overweight mistakenly blame their overweight condition on an underactive thyroid gland. In the hopes of speeding up their metabolism, they may start taking a supplement or eating sea salt or seaweed. But in very large amounts, iodine can be poisonous, so we advise against iodine supplementation.

Some people are sensitive to iodine and break out in a rash if they eat a lot or are exposed to it during X rays involving an injectable contrast medium. The rash, which resembles acne, disappears when the iodine is reduced.

Zinc

FUNCTIONS OF ZINC

Most zinc resides in our bones. The rest of this trace mineral turns up in skin, hair, and nails. In men, the prostate gland contains more zinc than any other organ. Zinc is a part of more than 70 different enzyme systems that aid the metabolism of carbohydrates, fats, and proteins. One of these enzymes, superoxide dismutase, serves as an antioxidant in cells. Zinc is also part of the hormone insulin, and it helps transport vitamin A from its storage site in the liver to where it's used in the body.

SOURCES OF ZINC

Oysters contain much more zinc than any other food. Meat, poultry, eggs, and liver are also rich sources. Two servings of animal protein daily provide most of the zinc a healthy person needs. Whole grains contain fair amounts of zinc, but they also harbor phytates, substances that tie up zinc and prevent its absorption. Yeast counteracts the action of phytates, so eating whole-grain breads still affords good nutrition.

DIETARY REQUIREMENTS
FOR ZINC

The RDA for zinc is 15 mg daily for adult men and 12 mg daily for adult women. Pregnant or breast-feeding women need larger amounts. Experts estimate that the average American diet provides about 10 mg per day. Apparently, our diets are falling short.

DEFICIENCY OF ZINC

Zinc deficiency has serious effects, including:

• retarded growth and sexual development
• delayed wound healing

Zinc Content of Common Foods

Food	Quantity	Milligrams (mg)
Meat-Protein Group		
Oysters, Eastern, raw	6	76.3
Beef, chuck	3 ounces	4.4
Chicken, white meat, no skin	3 ounces	1.4
Peas, split, cooked	½ cup	1.0
Soybeans, cooked	½ cup	1.0
Salmon, steak, broiled	4 ounces	0.8
Peanut butter	2 tablespoons	0.8
Egg, whole	1 large	0.6
Milk-Dairy Group		
Milk, whole	1 cup	0.9
American cheese	1 ounce	0.8
Bread-Cereal/Grain Group		
Bran flakes	1 cup	2.0
Rice, brown	⅔ cup	0.8
Bread, whole-grain	1 slice	0.6
Egg noodles, enriched, cooked	½ cup	0.5
Bread, white, enriched	1 slice	0.2
Fruits-Vegetables Group		
Potato, baked, with skin	1 medium	0.4
Broccoli, cooked	½ cup	0.3
Carrot, raw	1 medium	0.2
Pineapple, fresh or canned	1 cup	0.1
Tomato, raw	1 medium	0.1
Orange	1 medium	0.1

- a low sperm count
- depressed immune system (making infections more likely)
- reduced appetite
- altered sense of taste and smell

Low zinc intakes may be a factor in a condition that sometimes occurs in pregnancy called *toxemia*—a condition that may contribute to a lower birth weight of the baby.

Many experts suspect that marginal zinc intakes are common in the United States. As many as 90 percent of elderly Americans may take in suboptimal amounts of zinc. Why? As we cut back on meat, we cut out an important source of zinc. Low-calorie diets also tend to be low in zinc.

Vegetarian diets, especially vegan diets that do not contain any animal products, may promote a zinc deficit. If vegetarians eat whole-grain breads made with yeast, they absorb zinc better, because yeast breaks down the phytates in whole grains. Un-leavened bread, such as pita and flat bread, contains intact phytates that tie up zinc, preventing its absorption. Strict vegetarians should consult their doctors about the use of a zinc supplement. A multimineral supplement that contains iron might not provide the zinc you think, because iron interferes with zinc absorption.

Infections, injuries, or other physical sources of stress can cause zinc loss in the urine. Pica—eating nonfood substances such as clay, chalk, or ashes—can contribute to reduced zinc absorption.

ZINC USE AND MISUSE

These days, zinc is a popular supplement. Many people suffer a loss of smell and taste due to aging, cancer treatments, or serious infections. In some people, zinc supplements are legitimately useful in restoring these sensations. Zinc also improves healing in people with bedsores and other wounds. Restoring zinc to optimal levels certainly aids these conditions, but whether zinc in excess of needs has any real effect is debatable.

People with sickle-cell disease may lose a lot of zinc in their urine. Zinc supplements can help restore normal blood levels. Zinc supplements may also help reduce perspiration odor and treat acne. The effectiveness of these treatments is still in question.

A rare inherited disease called *acrodermatitis enteropathica* impairs zinc absorption. Zinc supplementation can control the symptoms, which include eczema, hair loss, retarded growth, and emotional problems.

People who suffer from a rare inherited disorder called *Wilson disease* need zinc to treat the abnormally large copper accumulations that occur in their bodies.

Excessive zinc supplementation—more than 50 mg per day—can cause copper deficiency and anemia. Large amounts of zinc can cause vomiting, diarrhea, fever, kidney failure, and even death. In the past, when certain foods and drinks were served in galvanized containers, the zinc coatings leached into the food, poisoning people. However, the chance of such toxicity occurring is low.

Because of high zinc levels in the prostate gland, doctors use zinc therapy as treatment for certain prostate disorders. Whether such zinc therapy is at all beneficial is still unclear. However, there is no hard evidence that a zinc deficiency causes these disorders.

Fluoride

Fluoride is an essential trace mineral found in bones, teeth, and body fluids. If fluoride is available when bones and teeth develop, it's incorporated into their structures, making teeth more resistant to decay and bones more resistant to osteoporosis. Fluoride also maintains the structure of bones and teeth after they are formed.

There is no RDA for fluoride, but there is a suggested safe and adequate range of intake of 1.5 to 4.0 mg daily.

Water is the most common source of fluoride in the diet. Fish and tea are surprisingly good sources as well. A cup of tea provides about 0.2 mg of fluoride.

Research shows that people who live in areas where the drinking water contains less than one part per million of fluoride have more dental decay and osteoporosis. In many areas of the country, water is fluoridated to a level of one part per million—the optimal level. Studies clearly show that children raised in such areas have 50 percent fewer cavities than children who do not drink fluoridated water.

In areas where the natural fluoride concentration in the water is high (two to eight parts per million), the enamel on children's teeth becomes mottled (spotted)—a condition called *fluorosis*. Although unsightly, the condition doesn't seem to be harmful; in fact, mottled teeth are very resistant to decay.

There is strong opposition to fluoridation of drinking water in some areas. Opponents claim that fluoridated water increases the incidence of cancer, birth defects, and other health problems. However, there is no established evidence to indicate that drinking fluoridated water is harmful in any way.

Indeed, fluoridation is one of the most thoroughly studied community health measures in recent history. The U.S. Public Health Service, the World Health Organization, the National Cancer Institute, and the U.S. Centers for Disease Control have all refuted claims linking fluoridation to public health risks. The only effect optimally fluoridated water seems to have on lifelong users is a decreased incidence of tooth decay and osteoporosis.

Copper

Copper helps the body absorb and use iron. It's part of several enzymes that help form hemoglobin (the oxygen-carrying pigment in red blood cells) and collagen (a connective-tissue protein found in skin and tendons).

Some of the sources of copper include shellfish, liver, dried peas and beans, nuts, cocoa, fruits, and vegetables.

There is no RDA for copper, but the suggested safe and adequate range of intake is 1.5 to 3.0 mg. The average American diet provides about 2.0 mg per day.

A dietary deficiency of copper is very rare, but has occurred in severely malnourished children, disrupting their growth and metabolism. It can also occur in infants born prematurely, because copper isn't usually transferred from the mother to the fetus until the last few weeks of pregnancy.

Excessive intake, which has occurred after water was stored in copper tanks, causes headache, dizziness, and vomiting. Children who inherit the gene for *Wilson disease* cannot get rid of excess copper. It accumulates in certain organs in their bodies, especially the eyes, brain, liver, and kidneys. It's treated with a copper-free diet and medication designed to bind with the copper, rendering it harmless.

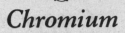

Chromium

Chromium is part of glucose tolerance factor that regulates the actions of insulin—the hormone necessary for glucose metabolism. In chromium-deficient people, insulin doesn't function properly. In such cases, chromium supplements can improve the body's ability to handle glucose. Experts believe a suboptimal chromium deficit is widespread, particularly among older people, and may explain why the incidence of glucose intolerance increases with age.

A diet rich in refined carbohydrates such as sugar increases the need for chromium. And the more refined and processed foods are, the less chromium they contain. Americans' high intake of sugary, processed foods could well be contributing to a minor chromium crisis.

Brewer's yeast and wheat germ are rich in chromium. Other sources include whole grains, meats, cheeses, broccoli, and eggs.

Increasingly popular chromium picolinate supplements may improve some people's chromium nutrition but will not magically melt away pounds as some ads imply.

There is no RDA for chromium. However, a suggested safe and adequate range of intake is 0.05 to 0.2 mg per day. If you have diabetes or glucose intolerance, consult with a physician before taking supplements. Although they might benefit your condition, they might also alter your need for medication.

Manganese

Manganese helps ensure proper bone formation and connective-tissue growth. It activates many enzymes that regulate metabolism. It may also play a role as an antioxidant, as part of the enzyme superoxide dismutase.

Good sources of manganese include nuts, whole grains, and dried peas and beans. There is no RDA for manganese. However, a suggested safe and adequate range of intake is 2.0 to 5.0 mg per day. Deficiencies have not been reported. Miners exposed to large amounts of manganese dust over long periods show symptoms of brain disease.

Selenium

Selenium is found in all body tissues, with the highest concentrations in the kidneys, liver, spleen, pancreas, and testicles.

Selenium functions as an antioxidant as part of the enzyme glutathione peroxidase. It helps prevent cell damage from free radicals that form when oxygen attacks, or oxidizes, fats and other compounds.

Severe deficiency of selenium affects heart function, but a deficiency is hard to detect because vitamin E can substitute for selenium in some of its functions, thus masking the classic symptoms.

A super source of selenium is the Brazil nut. It's so super, in fact, you probably shouldn't eat more than a few at a time. More down-to-earth sources include meat and fish. The amount found in grains depends on the selenium content of the soil in which they were grown.

The RDA for selenium is 55 µg for adult women and 70 µg for adult men. A typical American diet generally provides this amount without the use of supplements.

Some studies suggest that selenium may have anticancer properties, by working as an antioxidant along with vitamin E (see Chapter 5). This idea arose from cancer rates that are high in areas of the world where the soil contains little selenium. A recent Harvard University study, however, found no such protective effect when it looked at six different cancer sites in 1,000 women. In a surprising twist, the study actually found an increased risk for cancer among the women with the highest selenium intakes.

This is certainly of concern, because too much selenium is toxic. This mineral can substitute for sulfur in the proteins of some important enzymes, altering their functions. So if you take selenium supplements, they should contain no more than the RDA. Selenium taken as seleno-amino acids is much less toxic because the selenium substitution has already been made.

Molybdenum

This hard-to-pronounce mineral (muh LIB duh num) functions as part of the enzyme systems involved in carbohydrate, fat, and protein metabolism.

Good sources of molybdenum are liver, wheat germ, whole grains, and dried peas and beans. The molybdenum content of food varies according to what was in the soil from which it came.

No RDA exists for molybdenum, but a safe and adequate range of intake is 0.075 to 0.25 mg daily—easily acquired from the diet.

Reports indicate that excessive intakes of molybdenum trigger goutlike symptoms and other toxic effects. Do not take supplements of this mineral unless advised by a doctor.

Cobalt

As part of vitamin B_{12}, cobalt plays a major role in the body's metabolic processes. There is no RDA for cobalt because it is usually obtained from vitamin B_{12}.

Other Trace Minerals

While we do not yet know enough about some of the trace elements to establish requirements for them, evidence is accumulating that some of them may be essential for humans.

There is a case for a mineral being declared essential when its presence in the diet promotes growth or other responses related to health. Another piece of evidence is when its absence in the diet causes blood levels to decrease. Perhaps the most convincing of all is when the mineral is found in the tissues of newborn infants. The placenta normally serves as a barrier to protect the fetus from environmental contaminants. If a mineral transcends this barrier, it is probably because the fetus needs it.

Evidence is growing that nickel, silicon, arsenic, and boron will soon be classified as essential for humans.

- Nickel is present in all tissues of the body. It is firmly attached to DNA and a protein that binds to it in the blood.
- Silicon stimulates bone growth in animals.
- Boron is involved in human bone growth.
- Even arsenic might be essential, based on its importance for metabolism of the amino acid methionine.

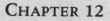

CHAPTER 12

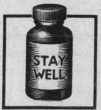

Supplement Product Profiles

Although we make clear throughout this book that there's no substitute for a healthy diet, we also know that nutritional needs can change with time and circumstance. We live in a time when we are unsure of the optimal amounts of vitamins and minerals needed to prevent disease. The levels for some nutrients may be too high to get from diet alone, and so a supplement may be needed.

Keep in mind that the smartest way to use a supplement is as just that—a supplement to your diet. Food should supply the basic levels of nutrients, with supplements providing any additional amounts needed. By relying on food for most of your nutritional needs, you get the benefits of the other components of foods—namely, phyto-chemicals.

Until we know exactly how much of each nutrient is ideal, be sure to keep dosages at reasonable levels to prevent toxicity.

To guide you in your choice of supplements, we've profiled more than 90 of the mainstream vitamin, mineral, and combination products commonly available in the United States. In each profile, you will find the product name, the manufacturer, the dosage form (capsules, tablets, liquid), the ingredients, and their amounts.

The dosage levels are expressed as a percentage of the U.S. RDA, as this is the current labeling regulations for dietary supplements. This may change when new regulations take effect. Specific comments, however, are based on the current 1989 RDAs and not on the older U.S. RDAs.

CONSUMER GUIDE® does not recommend that people who are in good health use supplements as a way to replace a balanced diet. If you're in doubt as to your vitamin or mineral status, check with your doctor or a registered dietitian. After a thorough evaluation of your diet, eating habits, state of health, and other factors that may affect your nutritional needs, he or she can help you determine whether supplements are necessary and which ones might be beneficial.

ALBEE C-800
(multivitamin supplement)

Manufacturer: A.H. Robins Company
Dosage form: Tablets
Ingredients:

vitamin C	800 mg
thiamin (B_1)	15 mg
riboflavin (B_2)	17 mg
niacin	100 mg
vitamin B_6	25 mg
pantothenic acid	25 mg
vitamin E	45 IU
vitamin B_{12}	12 mg

Comments:

• This product contains more than 100 percent of the RDAs for adult men and women for all of the nutrients that it contains.

• This product also has more than three times the upper limit of the recommended intake for pantothenic acid.

• Vitamin C, thiamin, and riboflavin are provided in megadose amounts (ten or more times the RDA).

ALBEE C-800 PLUS IRON
(multivitamin supplement with iron)

Manufacturer: A.H. Robins Company
Dosage form: Tablets

Ingredients:

vitamin C	800 mg
thiamin (B_1)	15 mg
riboflavin (B_2)	17 mg
niacin	100 mg
vitamin B_6	25 mg
pantothenic acid	25 mg
vitamin E	45 IU
folic acid	0.4 mg
vitamin B_{12}	12 mg
iron	27 mg

Comments:

- This product contains more than 100 percent of the RDAs for adult men and women for all of the nutrients that it contains. It is also more than three times the upper limit of the recommended intake for pantothenic acid.
- Vitamin C, thiamin, and riboflavin are provided in megadoses (ten or more times the RDA).
- Iron interacts with antacids and oral tetracycline antibiotics, reducing absorption of these drugs.
- Accidental iron poisoning is a possibility, especially with young children. Be sure to keep all supplements stored out of their reach.

ALBEE WITH C
(vitamin C supplement with B vitamins)

Manufacturer: A.H. Robins Company
Dosage form: Caplets

Ingredients:

vitamin C	300 mg
thiamin (B_1)	15 mg
riboflavin (B_2)	10.2 mg
niacin	50 mg
vitamin B_6	5 mg
pantothenic acid	10 mg

Comment:

• This product contains more than 100 percent of the RDAs for adult men and women for all of the nutrients that it contains.

AVAIL
(calcium supplement plus multivitamins/minerals)

Manufacturer: Menley & James
Dosage form: Tablets
Ingredients:

vitamin A	5,000 IU
vitamin D	400 IU
thiamin (B_1)	2.25 mg
riboflavin (B_2)	2.55 mg
niacin	20 mg
vitamin C	90 mg
vitamin B_6	3 mg
vitamin B_{12}	9 µg
folic acid	0.4 mg
vitamin E	30 IU
iron	18 mg
magnesium	100 mg

calcium	400 mg
zinc	22.5 mg
iodine	150 µg
chromium	15 µg
selenium	15 µg

Comments:

- This product contains more than 100 percent RDA of vitamins C, B_1, B_2, B_6, and B_{12} and the mineral zinc.
- Accidental iron poisoning is a possibility, especially with young children. To avoid accidental poisoning, be sure to keep all supplements stored out of their reach.

BETA-CAROTENE
(vitamin supplement)

Manufacturer: Nature's Bounty, Inc.
Dosage form: Softgels
Ingredient:

beta-carotene (provitamin A)   25,000 IU

Comments:

- Beta-carotene is a precursor of vitamin A. There is currently no RDA for beta-carotene. The recommended intake made by many health professionals is 6 mg (10,000 IU). This product contains 15 mg or 2½ times the recommended amount.
- Ample provitamin A can be provided by beta-carotene-rich deep-yellow or dark-orange vegetables and fruits, and green, leafy vegetables.

BUGS BUNNY COMPLETE
(multivitamin/mineral children's chewable supplement)

Manufacturer: Miles Laboratories, Inc.
Dosage form: Chewable tablets
Ingredients:

vitamin A	5,000 IU
vitamin D	400 IU
vitamin E	30 IU
vitamin C	60 mg
folic acid	0.4 mg
thiamin (B_1)	1.5 mg
riboflavin (B_2)	1.7 mg
niacin	20 mg
vitamin B_6	2 mg
vitamin B_{12}	6 µg
biotin	40 µg
pantothenic acid	10 mg
iron	18 mg
calcium	100 mg
copper	2 mg
phosphorus	100 mg
iodine	150 µg
magnesium	20 mg
zinc	15 mg

Comments:

• Dosage levels for most of the nutrients are at 100 percent of the adult RDAs. Despite the name, the vitamin levels are greater than most RDAs for children.

- Calcium and magnesium levels are well below recommended amounts.
- This product contains no manganese, selenium, chromium, or molybdenum.
- This product contains phenylalanine and should not be used by those with phenylketonuria.
- Iron is well above the level recommended for children.
- Iron interacts with antacids and oral tetracycline antibiotics, reducing absorption of these drugs.
- Accidental iron poisoning is a possibility, especially with young children. Be sure to keep all supplements, especially those that are designed to be attractive to children, stored out of their reach.
- This product is sugar free.

BUGS BUNNY PLUS IRON
(multivitamin children's chewable supplement)

Manufacturer: Miles Laboratories, Inc.
Dosage form: Chewable tablets
Ingredients:

vitamin A	2500 IU
vitamin D	400 IU
vitamin E	15 IU
vitamin C	60 mg
folic acid	0.3 mg
thiamin (B_1)	1.05 mg
riboflavin (B_2)	1.2 mg

niacin	13.5 mg
vitamin B_6	1.05 mg
vitamin B_{12}	4.5 µg
iron	15 mg

Comments:

- Dosage levels are reasonable for most of the nutrients provided.
- Calcium and magnesium are well below recommended amounts.
- This product contains phenylalanine and should not be used by those with phenylketonuria.
- Iron interacts with antacids and oral tetracycline antibiotics, reducing absorption of these drugs.
- Accidental iron poisoning is a possibility, especially with young children. Be sure to keep all supplements, especially those that are designed to be attractive to children, stored out of their reach.
- This product is sugar free.

BUGS BUNNY WITH EXTRA C
(multivitamin children's chewable supplement)

Manufacturer: Miles Laboratories, Inc.
Dosage form: Chewable tablets
Ingredients:

vitamin A	2500 IU
vitamin D	400 IU

vitamin E	15 IU
vitamin C	250 mg
folic acid	0.3 mg
thiamin (B_1)	1.05 mg
riboflavin (B_2)	1.2 mg
niacin	13.5 mg
vitamin B_6	1.05 mg
vitamin B_{12}	4.5 µg

Comments:

• Dosage levels are reasonable for most of the nutrients provided.
• This product is sugar free.

CALTRATE 600
(calcium supplement)

Manufacturer: Lederle Laboratories
Dosage form: Tablets
Ingredient:

elemental calcium	600 mg

Comments:

• The calcium is provided as calcium carbonate.
• This product contains no sugar, salt, or lactose.

CALTRATE 600 + D
(calcium supplement
with vitamin D)

Manufacturer: Lederle Laboratories
Dosage form: Tablets

Ingredients:

elemental calcium	600 mg
vitamin D	200 IU

Comments:

• The calcium is provided as calcium carbonate (1500 mg).

• The vitamin D may not be needed if you are taking a multivitamin supplement that contains vitamin D. The vitamin aids with the process of calcium deposition in bones, but also adds to the cost.

• This product does not contain sugar, salt, or lactose.

CALTRATE PLUS
(multivitamin/mineral supplement)

Manufacturer: Lederle Laboratories
Dosage form: Tablets
Ingredients:

elemental calcium	600 mg
vitamin D	200 IU
magnesium	40 mg
zinc	7.5 mg
copper	1 mg
manganese	1.8 mg
boron	250 µg

Comment:

• The calcium is provided as calcium carbonate (1500 mg).

CENTRUM ADVANCED FORMULA
(multivitamin/mineral supplement)

Manufacturer: Lederle Laboratories
Dosage form: Tablets
Ingredients:

vitamin A	5,000 IU
vitamin E	30 IU
vitamin C	60 mg
folic acid	0.4 mg
thiamin (B_1)	1.5 mg
riboflavin (B_2)	1.7 mg
niacinamide	20 mg
vitamin B_6	2 mg
vitamin B_{12}	6 µg
vitamin D	400 IU
biotin	30 µg
pantothenic acid	10 mg
calcium	162 mg
phosphorus	109 mg
iodine	150 µg
iron	18 mg
magnesium	100 mg
copper	2 mg
manganese	3.5 mg
potassium	80 mg
chloride	72 mg
chromium	65 µg
molybdenum	160 µg

selenium	20 µg
zinc	15 mg
vitamin K	25 µg
nickel	5 µg
tin	10 µg
silicon	2 mg
vanadium	10 µg
boron	150 µg

Comments:

- This product contains more than 100 percent of the adult RDA for vitamin B_{12}, vitamin E, and iron.
- This product has reasonable amounts of vitamins A, C, and B_6 and most minerals.
- The levels of calcium, magnesium, potassium, and selenium, are below recommended intake levels.
- This product also includes trace minerals for which a need has not been demonstrated.
- Accidental iron poisoning is a possibility, especially with young children. Be sure to keep all supplements stored out of their reach.

CENTRUM ADVANCED FORMULA
(multivitamin/mineral supplement)

Manufacturer: Lederle Laboratories
Dosage form: Liquid

Ingredients:

vitamin A	2500 IU
vitamin E	30 IU
vitamin C	60 mg
thiamin (B_1)	1.5 mg
riboflavin (B_2)	1.7 mg
niacinamide	20 mg
vitamin B_6	2 mg
vitamin B_{12}	6 μg
vitamin D	400 IU
biotin	300 μg
pantothenic acid	10 mg
iodine	150 μg
iron	9 mg
manganese	2.5 mg
chromium	25 μg
molybdenum	25 μg
zinc	3 mg

Comments:

- Don't be fooled. Though it has the same name, this liquid form of Centrum Advanced Formula has an entirely different formulation from the tablets.
- This supplement contains more than 100 percent of the adult RDA for both vitamin B_{12} and vitamin E.
- This product has reasonable amounts of vitamins A, C, and B_6.
- It contains no folate, calcium, magnesium, copper, potassium, or selenium. Molybdenum is below recommended intake level.

CENTRUM JR. WITH IRON
(multivitamin/mineral children's chewable supplement)

Manufacturer: Lederle Laboratories
Dosage form: Chewable tablets
Ingredients:

vitamin A	5000 IU
vitamin E	30 IU
vitamin C	60 mg
thiamin (B_1)	1.5 mg
riboflavin (B_2)	1.7 mg
niacinamide	20 mg
folic acid	0.4 mg
vitamin B_6	2 mg
vitamin B_{12}	6 mg
vitamin D	400 IU
biotin	45 mg
pantothenic acid	10 mg
vitamin K	10 µg
iodine	150 mg
iron	18 mg
calcium	108 mg
phosphorus	50 mg
magnesium	40 mg
manganese	1 mg
chromium	20 mg
copper	2 mg
molybdenum	20 mg
zinc	15 mg

Comments:
- For children 2 to 4 years of age, this product contains more than 100 percent of the RDA for all the nutrients it contains, except vitamin D.
- This product contains no potassium or selenium. Molybdenum is below recommended intake level.

CITRACAL
(calcium supplement)

Manufacturer: Mission Pharmaceuticals
Dosage form: Tablets
Ingredient:

calcium	200 mg

Comment:
- The calcium in this supplement is provided as calcium citrate (950 mg).

DAYALETS
(multivitamin supplement)

Manufacturer: Abbott Laboratories
Dosage form: Tablets
Ingredients:

vitamin A	5,000 IU
vitamin D	400 IU
vitamin E	30 IU
vitamin C	60 mg
folic acid	0.4 mg

thiamin (B_1)	1.5 mg
riboflavin (B_2)	1.7 mg
niacin	20 mg
vitamin B_6	2 mg
vitamin B_{12}	6 µg

Comments:
- Levels of vitamins are reasonable.
- This product is sugar free.

DAYALETS PLUS IRON
(multivitamin supplement plus iron)

Manufacturer: Abbott Laboratories
Dosage form: Tablets
Ingredients:

DAYALETS PLUS IRON contains the same ingredients as DAYALETS, plus 18 mg of iron.

Comments:
- Accidental iron poisoning is a possibility, especially with young children. Be sure to keep all supplements stored out of their reach.
- This product is sugar free.

ENER-B
(vitamin B_{12} supplement)

Manufacturer: Nature's Bounty, Inc.
Dosage form: Intranasal gel

Ingredient:

    vitamin B_{12} 400 µg

Comments:

• Each applicator delivers $1/10$ cc of gel into the nose.

• Each application contains a megadose of vitamin B_{12} (ten or more times the U.S. RDA).

• The name is gimmicky. Vitamin B_{12} does NOT provide energy.

FEMIRON
(iron supplement)

Manufacturer: Menley & James
Dosage form: Tablets
Ingredient:

    Iron   20 mg

Comments:

• This supplement contains more than 100 percent of the adult RDA for iron.

• This product is not for alcoholics or those with liver or pancreatic disease.

• This product could irritate the stomach and intestines if not taken with food.

• A darkened stool may result from use of this supplement.

• Iron interacts with antacids and oral tetracycline, reducing absorption of these drugs.

• Accidental iron poisoning is a possibility, especially with young children. Be sure to keep all supplements stored out of their reach.

FEMIRON MULTIVITAMINS AND IRON
(iron supplement plus multivitamins)

Manufacturer: Menley & James
Dosage form: Tablets
Ingredients:

iron	20 mg
vitamin A	5,000 IU
vitamin D	400 IU
thiamin (B_1)	1.5 mg
riboflavin (B_2)	1.7 mg
niacin	20 mg
vitamin C	60 mg
vitamin B_6	2 mg
vitamin B_{12}	6 μg
pantothenic acid	10 mg
folic acid	0.4 mg
vitamin E	15 IU

Comments:

- Amounts of vitamins included in this supplement are at reasonable levels.
- This supplement contains more than 100 percent of the adult RDA for iron.
- This product does not contain vitamin K or biotin.
- This product should not be used by alcoholics or individuals with chronic liver or pancreatic disease.
- This product could depress zinc absorption.

- This product could irritate the linings of the stomach and intestines if not taken with some food.
- A darkened stool may result from use of this supplement.
- Iron interacts with antacids and oral tetracycline antibiotics, reducing absorption and efficacy of these drugs.
- Accidental iron poisoning is a possibility, especially with young children. Be sure to keep all supplements stored out of their reach.

FEOSOL
(iron supplement)

Manufacturer: SmithKline Beecham
Dosage form: Capsules
Ingredient:
    elemental iron   50 mg
Comments:

- The supplement contains 500 percent of the RDA for iron for men and more than 300 percent of the RDA for iron for women.
- Capsules contain FD&C Red No. 40—a food coloring whose safety is in question.
- This product may cause gastrointestinal discomfort and nausea. These side effects may be minimized by taking the supplement with meals.
- Other side effects include constipation or diarrhea.
- This product could depress zinc absorption.

- Iron interacts with antacids and oral tetracycline antibiotics, reducing the absorption of these drugs.
- Accidental iron poisoning is a possibility, especially with young children. Be sure to keep all supplements stored out of their reach.

FEOSOL ELIXIR
(iron supplement)

Manufacturer: SmithKline Beecham
Dosage form: Liquid
Ingredient:
    elemental iron   44 mg
Comments:
- This supplement contains more than 400 percent of the adult RDA for iron.
- This product contains five percent alcohol.
- This product may cause gastrointestinal discomfort and nausea. These side effects may be minimized by taking the supplement along with meals.
- Other side effects include constipation or diarrhea and temporary staining of the teeth.
- The amount of iron in this product might depress zinc absorption.
- Iron interacts with antacids and oral tetracycline antibiotics, reducing absorption of these drugs.
- Accidental iron poisoning is a possibility, especially with young children. Be sure to keep all supplements stored out of their reach.

FERGON
(iron supplement)

Manufacturer: Bayer Corp.

Dosage form: Tablets

Ingredient:

elemental iron   36 mg

Comments:

- The iron in this product provides more than 300 percent of the RDA for iron for men and more than 200 percent for women.
- Iron is provided as ferrous gluconate (320 mg).
- This product may cause nausea, abdominal cramps, constipation, or diarrhea.
- The amount of iron in this product might depress zinc absorption.
- Iron interacts with antacids and oral tetracycline antibiotics, reducing proper absorption of these drugs.
- Accidental iron poisoning is a possibility, especially with young children. Be sure to keep all supplements stored out of their reach.

FERRO-SEQUELS
(iron supplement)

Manufacturer: Lederle Laboratories

Dosage form: Timed-release tablets

Ingredient:

50 mg of elemental iron as 150 mg ferrous fumarate

Comments:

- This product contains an active ingredient (100 mg of docusate sodium) to prevent constipation, which iron can cause.
- This product contains lactose and sodium, but qualifies as "low-sodium."
- It is formulated to release iron slowly.
- Iron interacts with antacids and oral tetracycline antibiotics, reducing the absorption of these drugs.
- Accidental iron poisoning is a possibility, especially with young children. Be sure to keep all supplements stored out of their reach.

FLINTSTONES
(multivitamin children's chewable supplement)

Manufacturer: Bayer Corp.
Dosage form: Chewable tablets
Ingredients:

vitamin A	2,500 IU
vitamin D	400 IU
vitamin E	15 IU
vitamin C	60 mg
folic acid	0.3 mg
thiamin (B_1)	1.05 mg
riboflavin (B_2)	1.2 mg
niacin	13.5 mg
vitamin B_6	1.05 mg
vitamin B_{12}	4.5 µg

Comments:

- For children 2 to 4 years of age, this product contains more than 100 percent of the RDA for vitamins C and E, folic acid, thiamin, riboflavin, niacin, and vitamin B_6. It contains more than 400 percent of the RDA for vitamin B_{12}.
- For children over 4 years of age, this product contains more than 100 percent of the RDA for folic acid and vitamins B_{12}, C, and E.
- This product does not include vitamin K, biotin, and pantothenic acid.
- This product should not be used by children who have phenylketonuria.

FLINTSTONES WITH EXTRA C
(multivitamin children's chewable supplement)

Manufacturer: Bayer Corp.
Dosage form: Chewable tablets
Ingredients:

vitamin A	2,500 IU
vitamin D	400 IU
vitamin E	15 IU
vitamin C	250 mg
folic acid	0.3 mg
thiamin (B_1)	1.05 mg
riboflavin (B_2)	1.2 mg
niacin	13.5 mg

| vitamin B_6 | 1.05 mg |
| vitamin B_{12} | 4.5 µg |

Comments:

- For children 2 to 4 years of age, this product contains more than 100 percent of the RDA for vitamin E, folic acid, thiamin, riboflavin, niacin, and vitamin B_6. It contains more than 500 percent of the RDA for vitamin C and more than 400 percent of the RDA for vitamin B_{12}.
- For children over 4 years of age, this product contains more than 100 percent of the RDA for folic acid, vitamins E and B_{12}. It contains more than 500 percent of the RDA for vitamin C.
- Long-term use of chewable vitamin C tablets has been linked to dental erosion.
- This product does not include vitamin K, biotin, and pantothenic acid.
- This product should not be used by children who have phenylketonuria.

FLINTSTONES WITH IRON
(multivitamin children's chewable supplement with iron)

Manufacturer: Bayer Corp.
Dosage form: Chewable tablets
Ingredients:

vitamin A	2,500 IU
vitamin D	400 IU
vitamin E	15 IU
vitamin C	60 mg

folic acid	0.3 mg
thiamin (B$_1$)	1.05 mg
riboflavin (B$_2$)	1.2 mg
niacin	13.5 mg
vitamin B$_6$	1.05 mg
vitamin B$_{12}$	4.5 μg
iron	15 mg

Comments:

• For children aged 2 to 4, this product contains more than 100 percent of the RDA for vitamin E, vitamin C, folic acid, thiamin, riboflavin, niacin, vitamin B$_6$, and iron. It contains more than 400 percent of the RDA for vitamin B$_{12}$.

• This product does not contain vitamin K, biotin, or pantothenic acid.

• This product contains phenylalanine and should not be used by children who have phenylketonuria.

• Accidental iron poisoning is a possibility, especially with young children. Be sure to keep all supplements stored out of their reach.

FLINTSTONES COMPLETE
(multivitamin/mineral children's chewable supplement)

Manufacturer: Bayer Corp.
Dosage form: Chewable tablets
Ingredients:

vitamin A	5000 IU
vitamin D	400 IU

vitamin E	30 IU
vitamin C	60 mg
folic acid	0.4 mg
thiamin (B_1)	1.5 mg
riboflavin (B_2)	1.7 mg
niacin	20 mg
vitamin B_6	2 mg
vitamin B_{12}	6 µg
biotin	40 µg
pantothenic acid	10 mg
iodine	150 µg
iron	10 mg
calcium	100 mg
phosphorus	100 mg
magnesium	20 mg
copper	2 mg
zinc	15 mg

Comments:

• For children 2 to 4 years of age, this product contains more than 100 percent of the RDA for vitamin C, thiamin, riboflavin, niacin, and vitamin B_6.

• For children 2 to 4 years of age, it contains 500 percent or more of the RDA for folic acid, vitamin E, and vitamin B_{12}.

• For children over 4 years of age, this product contains more than 100 percent of the RDA for vitamin C, folic acid, vitamin E, and vitamin B_{12}.

• This product does not include vitamin K.

• This product contains sorbitol and aspartame.

• This product should not be used by children who have phenylketonuria.

GARFIELD
(multivitamin/mineral children's chewable supplement)

Manufacturer: Menley & James
Dosage form: Chewable tablets
Ingredients:

vitamin A	5000 IU
vitamin D	400 IU
vitamin E	30 IU
vitamin C	60 mg
folic acid	0.4 mg
thiamin (B_1)	1.5 mg
riboflavin (B_2)	1.7 mg
niacin	20 mg
vitamin B_6	2 mg
vitamin B_{12}	6 µg
biotin	40 µg
pantothenic acid	10 mg
iodine	150 µg
iron	18 mg
calcium	100 mg
phosphorus	100 mg
magnesium	20 mg
copper	2 mg
zinc	15 mg

Comments:

- For children 2 to 4 years of age, this product contains more than 100 percent of the RDA for vitamin C, thiamin, riboflavin, niacin, B_6 and iron.
- It contains 500 percent or more of the RDA for folic acid, vitamin E and vitamin B_{12}.

- For children over 4 years of age, this product contains more than 100 percent of the RDA for vitamin C, folic acid, vitamin E, vitamin B_{12} and iron.
- This product does not include vitamin K.
- Contains sorbitol and aspartame. This product should not be used by children who have phenylketonuria.

GERITOL
(iron and multivitamin tonic)

Manufacturer: SmithKline Beecham
Dosage form: Liquid
Ingredients:

iron	18 mg
thiamin (B_1)	2.5 mg
riboflavin (B_2)	2.5 mg
niacin	50 mg
pantothenic acid	2 mg
vitamin B_6	0.5 mg
choline	50 mg
methionine	25 mg

Comments:
- This product contains more than 100 percent of the adult RDA for thiamin, riboflavin and iron. It contains more than 300 times the adult RDA for niacin.
- Vitamin B_6 is at about one third the level of the adult RDA for these vitamins. The level of pantothenic acid is below the recommended range.

- It does not contain vitamin B_{12}.
- The usefulness of added choline and methionine is questionable.
- It contains alcohol, which may accelerate the absorption of iron.
- This supplement should not be used by alcoholics or individuals with chronic liver or pancreatic disease or those with inherited iron storage disease.
- This product may cause darkening of the stool.
- Iron interacts with antacids and oral tetracycline antibiotics, reducing the absorption of these drugs.
- Accidental iron poisoning is a possibility, especially with young children. Be sure to keep all supplements stored out of their reach.

GERITOL EXTEND
(multivitamin/mineral supplement for adults 50+)

Manufacturer: SmithKline Beecham
Dosage form: Caplets
Ingredients:

vitamin A	3,333 IU
vitamin E	15 IU
vitamin C	60 mg
folic acid	0.2 mg
thiamin (B_1)	1.2 mg
riboflavin (B_2)	1.4 mg

niacin	15 mg
vitamin B_6	2 mg
vitamin B_{12}	2 μg
vitamin D	200 IU
vitamin K	80 μg
calcium	130 mg
phosphorus	100 mg
iodine	150 μg
iron	10 mg
magnesium	35 mg
selenium	70 μg
zinc	15 mg

Comments:

• This supplement contains more than 100 percent of the adult RDA for vitamin E and folic acid.

• This product does not contain pantothenic acid or biotin.

• It contains FD&C Red No. 40, whose safety as a food colorant is in question. It also contains yellow dye No. 6—tartrazine—to which some people are allergic.

• Accidental iron poisoning is a possibility, especially with young children. Be sure to keep all supplements stored out of their reach.

GERITOL COMPLETE
(multivitamin/mineral supplement)

Manufacturer: SmithKline Beecham
Dosage form: Tablets

Ingredients:

vitamin A	
(as beta-carotene)	6,000 IU
vitamin E	30 IU
vitamin C	30 mg
folic acid	0.4 mg
thiamin (B_1)	1.5 mg
riboflavin (B_2)	1.7 mg
niacin	20 mg
vitamin B_6	2 mg
vitamin B_{12}	6 µg
vitamin D	400 IU
biotin	45 µg
pantothenic acid	10 mg
vitamin K	25 µg
calcium	162 mg
phosphorus	125 mg
iodine	150 µg
iron	50 mg
magnesium	100 mg
copper	2 mg
manganese	2.5 mg
potassium	37.5 mg
chloride	34.1 mg
chromium	15 µg
molybdenum	15 µg
selenium	15 µg
zinc	15 mg
nickel	5 µg
silicon	80 µg
tin	10 µg
vanadium	10 µg

Comments:

- This product contains more than 400 percent of the adult RDA for iron. It also contains more than 100 percent of the adult RDA for vitamin A, vitamin E, folic acid, vitamin B_{12}, and vitamin D. It also contains more than the recommended intake for pantothenic acid.
- This supplement should not be used by alcoholics or by individuals who have chronic liver or pancreatic disease.
- This product contains FD&C Red No. 40—a food colorant whose safety is in question.
- Accidental iron poisoning is a possibility, especially with young children. Be sure to keep all supplements stored out of their reach.

GEVRABON
(multivitamin/mineral supplement)

Manufacturer: Lederle Laboratories
Dosage form: Liquid
Ingredients:

thiamin (B_1)	5 mg
riboflavin (B_2)	2.5 mg
niacin	50 mg
vitamin B_6	1 mg
vitamin B_{12}	1 µg
pantothenic acid	10 mg
iodine	100 µg
iron	15 mg

magnesium	2 mg
zinc	2 mg
choline	100 mg
manganese	2 mg

Comments:

- This product provides more than 100 percent of the adult RDA for thiamin, riboflavin, and niacin, and above the recommended range of intake for pantothenic acid.
- This product contains most of the B vitamins. Folate is not included.
- Except for iron, this product contains only small amounts of some minerals.
- The usefulness of choline is questionable.
- This supplement contains 18 percent alcohol.
- Accidental iron poisoning is a possibility, especially with young children. Be sure to keep all supplements stored out of their reach.

GOOD SENSE CENTURY
(multivitamin/mineral supplement)

Manufacturer: Perrigo
Dosage form: Tablets
Ingredients:

vitamin A	5,000 IU
vitamin E	30 IU
vitamin C	60 mg
folic acid	0.4 mg
thiamin (B_1)	1.5 mg

riboflavin (B$_2$)	1.7 mg
niacinamide	20 mg
vitamin B$_6$	2 mg
vitamin B$_{12}$	6 μg
vitamin D	400 IU
biotin	30 μg
pantothenic acid	10 mg
calcium	162 mg
phosphorus	109 mg
iodine	150 μg
iron	18 mg
magnesium	100 mg
copper	2 mg
manganese	3.5 mg
potassium	80 mg
chloride	72 mg
chromium	65 μg
molybdenum	160 μg
selenium	20 μg
zinc	15 mg
vitamin K	25 μg

Comments:

- This product contains more than 100 percent of the adult RDA for vitamins B$_{12}$ and E and iron.
- This product has reasonable amounts of vitamins A, C, and B$_6$ and most minerals.
- The levels of calcium, magnesium, potassium, and selenium, are below recommended intake levels.
- Accidental iron poisoning is a possibility, especially with young children. Be sure to keep all supplements stored out of their reach.

HALLS VITAMIN C DROPS
(vitamin C supplement)

Manufacturer: Warner-Lambert
Dosage form: Drops
Ingredient:

vitamin C	60 mg

Comments:
- This product provides 100 percent of the adult RDA for vitamin C.
- This product contains sugar.

ICAPS PLUS
(antioxidant supplement)

Manufacturer: La Haye Laboratories
Dosage form: Tablets
Ingredients:

vitamin A (as beta-carotene)	6,000 IU
vitamin E	60 IU
vitamin C	200 mg
riboflavin (B$_2$)	20 mg
copper	2 mg
manganese	5 mg
selenium	20 µg
zinc	40 mg

Comments:
- Contains more than 100 percent of the RDA for vitamin A, vitamin C, vitamin E, and riboflavin.
- This supplement contains more than 100 percent of the RDA for zinc.

• Copper, manganese, and selenium levels are within recommended levels.

MYADEC PROFESSIONAL FORMULA
(multivitamin/mineral supplement)

Manufacturer: Parke-Davis
Dosage form: Tablets
Ingredients:

vitamin A	5,000 IU
vitamin D	400 IU
vitamin E	30 IU
vitamin C	60 mg
folic acid	0.4 mg
thiamin (B_1)	1.7 mg
riboflavin (B_2)	2.0 mg
niacin	20 mg
vitamin B_6	3 mg
vitamin B_{12}	6 µg
pantothenic acid	10 mg
vitamin K	25 µg
biotin	30 µg
iodine	150 µg
iron	18 mg
magnesium	100 mg
copper	2 mg
zinc	15 mg
manganese	2.5 mg

calcium	162 mg
phosphorus	125 mg
potassium	40 mg
selenium	25 µg
molybdenum	25 µg
chromium	25 µg

Comments:

- This product provides well above 100 percent of the adult RDA for vitamin A, vitamin C, thiamin, riboflavin, B_6, B_{12}, and iron. Amounts of pantothenic acid and copper are above the recommended intakes for these minerals.
- Accidental iron poisoning is a possibility, especially with young children. Be sure to keep all supplements stored out of their reach.

NATALINS
(multivitamin/mineral prenatal supplement)

Manufacturer: Mead-Johnson Nutritional Div.
Dosage form: Tablets
Ingredients:

vitamin A	4,000 IU
vitamin D	400 IU
vitamin E	15 IU
vitamin C	70 mg
folic acid	0.5 mg
thiamin (B_1)	1.5 mg
riboflavin (B_2)	1.6 mg
niacin	17 mg

vitamin B_6	2.6 mg
vitamin B_{12}	2.5 µg
calcium	200 mg
elemental iron	30 mg
zinc	15 mg
copper	1.5 mg

Comments:

- This product provides 100 percent of the RDA for pregnant and breast-feeding women for vitamin D, iron, and zinc.
- This supplement contains more than 100 percent of the RDA for vitamin B_6, vitamin E, and folic acid.
- This product supplies vitamin A, vitamin C, thiamin, riboflavin, and niacin at 100 percent of the RDA for pregnant women but not for breast-feeding women.
- Calcium is supplied at well below the RDAs for both pregnant and breast-feeding women.
- Iron interacts with antacids and oral tetracycline antibiotics, reducing absorption and efficacy of these drugs.
- Accidental iron poisoning is a possibility, especially with young children. Be sure to keep all supplements stored out of their reach.

N'ICE VITAMIN C DROPS
(sugarless vitamin C drops)
Manufacturer: SmithKline Beecham
Dosage form: Capsules

Ingredients:

60 mg of vitamin C (adult flavors: lemon, orange)

45 mg of vitamin C (children's flavor: grape)

Comments:

- This product provides 100 percent of the adult RDA at 60 mg and 100 percent of the RDA for children over 4 years of age at 45 mg.
- This product contains sorbitol.

OCUVITE
(vitamin/mineral supplement)

Manufacturer: Lederle Laboratories
Dosage form: Tablets
Ingredients:

zinc	40 mg
copper	2 mg
vitamin C	60 mg
vitamin E	30 IU
beta-carotene	5,000 IU
selenium	40 µg

Comments:

- This product provides 200 percent or more of the adult RDA for zinc and vitamin E.
- This supplement provides 100 percent of the RDA for vitamin C and is within the recommended range for copper.
- This product provides 8.3 mg of beta-carotene, which is about one third higher than the recommended intake of 6 mg.

⊚

• This product contains lactose. People who are lactose intolerant may wish to avoid it.

OCUVITE EXTRA
(antioxidant supplement plus Z and B)

Manufacturer: Lederle Laboratories
Dosage form: Tablets
Ingredients:

beta-carotene	6,000 IU
riboflavin (B_2)	3 mg
nicacin	40 mg
vitamin C	200 mg
vitamin E	50 IU
zinc	40 mg
copper	2 mg
selenium	40 µg
manganese	5 mg
L-glutathione	5 mg

Comments:

• This product provides 200 percent or greater of the adult RDA for vitamins C and E, niacin, and the mineral zinc.
• This supplement is within the recommended range for copper.
• This product provides about 50 percent more than the recommended daily amount of beta-carotene.
• The usefulness of added L-glutathione is questionable.

• This product contains lactose. People who are lactose intolerant may wish to avoid it.

ONE-A-DAY ESSENTIAL VITAMINS
(multivitamin supplement)

Manufacturer: Miles Laboratories, Inc.
Dosage form: Tablets
Ingredients:

vitamin A	5,000 IU
vitamin C	60 mg
thiamin (B_1)	1.5 mg
riboflavin (B_2)	1.7 mg
niacin	20 mg
vitamin D	400 IU
vitamin E	30 IU
vitamin B_6	2 mg
folic acid	0.4 mg
vitamin B_{12}	6 μg
pantothenic acid	10 mg

Comments:
• Most of the vitamins in this supplement are supplied in amounts that equal 100 percent of the adult RDA.
• It contains more than 100 percent of the adult RDA for vitamin E, vitamin D, folic acid, and vitamin B_{12}.
• The amount of pantothenic acid is above the range of intake recommended for this vitamin.

ONE-A-DAY MAXIMUM FORMULA
(multivitamin/mineral supplement)

Manufacturer: Miles Laboratories, Inc.
Dosage form: Tablets
Ingredients:

vitamin A	5,000 IU
vitamin C	60 mg
thiamin (B_1)	1.5 mg
riboflavin (B_2)	1.7 mg
niacin	20 mg
vitamin D	400 IU
vitamin E	30 IU
vitamin B_6	2 mg
folic acid	0.4 mg
vitamin B_{12}	6 µg
biotin	30 µg
pantothenic acid	10 mg
iron	18 mg
calcium	130 mg
phosphorus	100 mg
iodine	150 µg
magnesium	100 mg
copper	2 mg
zinc	15 mg
chromium	10 µg
selenium	10 µg
molybdenum	10 µg
manganese	2.5 mg

potassium	37.5 mg
chloride	34 mg

Comments:

- This product provides 100 percent of the adult RDA for most nutrients.
- Folic acid and vitamins B_6, B_{12}, D, and E are provided in amounts greater than the upper limits of the recommended ranges of intake for these nutrients.
- Iron, iodine, copper, and zinc are the only minerals supplied in amounts high enough to meet the adult RDAs.
- Accidental iron poisoning is a possibility, especially with young children. Be sure to keep all supplements stored out of their reach.

ONE-A-DAY WOMEN'S
(multivitamin supplement with calcium, iron, and zinc)

Manufacturer: Miles Laboratories, Inc.

Dosage form: Tablets

Ingredients:

vitamin A	5,000 IU
vitamin C	60 mg
thiamin (B_1)	1.5 mg
riboflavin (B_2)	1.7 mg
niacin	20 mg
vitamin D	400 IU
vitamin E	30 IU
vitamin B_6	2 mg

folic acid	0.4 mg
vitamin B_{12}	6 µg
pantothenic acid	10 mg
iron	27 mg
calcium	450 mg
zinc	15 mg

Comments:

- This product provides 100 percent of the adult RDA for most of the nutrients it contains. Folic acid, iron, and vitamins B_6, B_{12}, D, and E are provided in amounts greater than the upper limits of the recommended ranges of intake.
- The only minerals it provides are calcium, iron, and zinc.
- Calcium is higher than in many multivitamins.
- It does not contain biotin.
- Iron interacts with antacids and oral tetracycline antibiotics, reducing the absorption of these drugs.
- Accidental iron poisoning is a possibility, especially with young children. Be sure to keep all supplements stored out of their reach.

ONE-A-DAY MEN'S
(multivitamin supplement)

Manufacturer: Miles Laboratories, Inc.
Dosage form: Tablets
Ingredients:

vitamin A	5,000 IU
vitamin C	200 mg

thiamin (B_1)	2.25 mg
riboflavin (B_2)	2.55 mg
niacin	20 mg
vitamin D	400 IU
vitamin E	45 IU
vitamin B_6	3 mg
folic acid	0.4 mg
vitamin B_{12}	9 µg
pantothenic acid	10 mg

Comments:

• This product provides more than 100 percent of the adult RDA for men for most of the vitamins it contains.

• This product contains no biotin.

• Antioxidant vitamins are provided in larger amounts than recommended levels, however, this product does not provide the entire spectrum of antioxidants.

• This product does not contain iron—an unnecessary supplement for adult men, but neither does it provide any other minerals.

ONE-A-DAY 55 PLUS (multivitamin/mineral supplement)

Manufacturer: Miles Laboratories, Inc.
Dosage form: Tablets
Ingredients:

| vitamin A | 6,000 IU |
| vitamin C | 120 mg |

thiamin (B_1)	4.5 mg
riboflavin (B_2)	3.4 mg
niacin	20 mg
vitamin D	400 IU
vitamin E	60 IU
vitamin B_6	6 mg
folic acid	0.4 mg
vitamin B_{12}	25 µg
biotin	30 µg
pantothenic acid	20 mg
vitamin K	25 µg
calcium	220 mg
iodine	150 µg
magnesium	100 mg
copper	2 mg
zinc	15 mg
chromium	10 µg
selenium	10 µg
molybdenum	10 µg
manganese	2.5 mg
potassium	37.5 mg
chloride	34 mg

Comments:

- This product provides more than 100 percent of the RDAs for most vitamins.
- It provides 200 percent of the RDA or more for vitamins B_1, B_2, C, D, E, B_6, and B_{12} and folic acid.
- Iodine, copper, and zinc are the only minerals supplied in amounts high enough to meet the adult RDAs. There is no iron in this product, as it is not usually a problem in older individuals.

ONE-A-DAY EXTRAS— ANTIOXIDANT
(antioxidant supplement)

Manufacturer: Miles Laboratories, Inc.
Dosage form: Softgels
Ingredients:

beta-carotene	5,000 IU
vitamin C	250 mg
vitamin E	200 IU
zinc	7.5 mg
copper	1 mg
selenium	15 mg
manganese	1.5 mg

Comments:

• This products provides a general array of antioxidant nutrients: Beta-carotene meets the recommended intake for vitamin A; vitamin C level is over 400 percent of the adult RDA; vitamin E level is more than ten times the RDA.

• None of the minerals present meets the recommended levels of intakes.

OPTILETS 500
(multivitamin supplement)

Manufacturer: Abbott Laboratories
Dosage form: Tablets
Ingredients:

vitamin C	500 mg
niacin	100 mg

pantothenic acid	20 mg
thiamin (B_1)	15 mg
riboflavin (B_2)	10 mg
vitamin B_6	5 mg
vitamin A	5,000 IU
vitamin B_{12}	12 µg
vitamin D	400 IU
vitamin E	30 IU

Comments:

- This product provides more than 500 percent of the RDA for vitamin C, niacin, riboflavin, and vitamin B_{12} and 200 percent or more for vitamin B_6, vitamin D, and vitamin E.
- The product also contains well above the upper limit of the recommended range for pantothenic acid.
- Thiamin is provided by this supplement in a megadose amount (ten or more times the adult RDA).

OPTILETS-M-500
(multivitamin/mineral supplement)

Manufacturer: Abbott Laboratories
Dosage form: Tablets
Ingredients:

vitamin C	500 mg
niacin	100 mg
pantothenic acid	20 mg
thiamin (B_1)	15 mg

riboflavin (B_2)	10 mg
vitamin B_6	5 mg
vitamin A	5,000 IU
vitamin B_{12}	12 µg
vitamin D	400 IU
vitamin E	30 IU
magnesium	80 mg
iron	20 mg
copper	2 mg
zinc	1.5 mg
manganese	1 mg
iodine	0.15 mg

Comments:

- This product provides more than 500 percent of the adult RDA for vitamin C, niacin, riboflavin, and vitamin B_{12} and 200 percent or more for vitamin B_6, vitamin D, and vitamin E.
- This product also contains well above the upper limit of the recommended range of intake for pantothenic acid.
- Thiamin is provided by this supplement in a megadose amount (ten or more times the adult RDA).
- Only copper, iodine, and iron are supplied in amounts that meet the adult RDAs for these minerals.
- Ten percent of the zinc, 50 percent of the manganese, and 25 to 30 percent of the magnesium RDAs are provided by this supplement.
- Accidental iron poisoning is a possibility, especially with young children. Be sure to keep all supplements stored out of their reach.

OS-CAL 500 CHEWABLE TABLETS
(calcium supplement)

Manufacturer: SmithKline Beecham
Dosage form: Chewable tablets
Ingredient:

elemental calcium	500 mg

Comments:
- This product supplies about 40 percent of the recommended amount of calcium for teenage girls and boys and adult women.
- Taking one tablet two times daily should supplement the diet for teenagers and adult women. Adult men may only need one supplement tablet depending on their daily intake of dairy products.
- The calcium source for this supplement is calcium carbonate.

OS-CAL 500 TABLETS
(calcium supplement)

Manufacturer: SmithKline Beecham
Dosage form: Tablets
Ingredient:

elemental calcium	500 mg

Comment:
- The calcium source for this supplement is crushed oyster shell powder, which is primarily calcium carbonate.

OS-CAL 500+D TABLETS
(calcium supplement with vitamin D)

Manufacturer: SmithKline Beecham
Dosage form: Tablets
Ingredients:

elemental calcium	500 mg
vitamin D	125 IU

Comments:

- The calcium source is crushed oyster shell powder, which is primarily calcium carbonate.
- The vitamin D is useful for ensuring the optimum use of calcium.

OS-CAL FORTIFIED TABLETS
(multivitamin/mineral supplement)

Manufacturer: SmithKline Beecham
Dosage form: Tablets
Ingredients:

vitamin D	125 IU
thiamin (B_1)	1.7 mg
riboflavin (B_2)	1.7 mg
vitamin B_6	2 mg
vitamin C	50 mg
vitamin E	0.8 IU
niacin	15 mg
calcium	250 mg

iron	5 mg
magnesium	3.0 mg
manganese	0.5 mg
zinc	0.5 mg

Comments:
- This product contains slightly more than 100 percent of the adult RDAs for thiamin and vitamin C. It contains about one third of the adult women's requirement for iron and calcium. Manganese levels do not meet the adult minimum recommended level. Magnesium and zinc levels are way below the adult RDAs.
- The calcium source of this supplemental product is crushed oyster shell powder, which is primarily calcium carbonate.
- This level of calcium inake is not sufficient for teenagers and adult women who may need additional calcium.

OS-CAL 250+D TABLETS
(calcium supplement with vitamin D)

Manufacturer: SmithKline Beecham
Dosage form: Tablets
Ingredients:

elemental calcium	250 mg
vitamin D	125 IU

Comments:
- The calcium source is crushed oyster shell powder, which is primarily calcium carbonate.

- The added vitamin D is not necessary if a multivitamin supplement containing this vitamin is also being taken; it only adds to the cost.
- Teenagers and adult women would have to take more than three tablets a day if they need to supplement their diets.
- This supplement's dosage is more suitable for adult men.

POLY-VI-SOL
(multivitamin children's supplement)

Manufacturer: Mead Johnson Nutritional Division

Dosage form: Liquid

Ingredients:

vitamin A	1,500 IU
vitamin D	400 IU
vitamin E	5 IU
vitamin C	35 mg
thiamin (B_1)	0.5 mg
riboflavin (B_2)	0.6 mg
niacin	8 mg
vitamin B_6	0.4 mg
vitamin B_{12}	2 µg

Comments:

- This supplement provides at least 100 percent of the RDA for infants for most nutrients. Niacin, vitamin D, and vitamin B_{12} are provided in

greater amounts. Only vitamins D and B_{12} would meet the RDAs for older children.
• This product is alcohol free.

POLY-VI-SOL
(multivitamin children's supplement)

Manufacturer: Mead Johnson Nutritional Division
Dosage forms: Chewable tablets
Ingredients:

vitamin A	2,500 IU
vitamin D	400 IU
vitamin E	15 IU
vitamin C	60 mg
folic acid	0.3 mg
thiamin (B_1)	1.05 mg
riboflavin (B_2)	1.2 mg
niacin	13.5 mg
vitamin B_6	1.05 mg
vitamin B_{12}	4.5 μg

Comments:
• This supplement provides 100 percent or greater of the RDAs for vitamin E, vitamin D, vitamin C, folic acid, thiamin, riboflavin, niacin, vitamin B_6, and vitamin B_{12} for children under age 4. For children over age 4, the RDA is provided for all nutrients except vitamin B_6.
• This product contains sugar.

POLY-VI-SOL WITH IRON
(multivitamin children's supplement with iron)

Manufacturer: Mead Johnson Nutritional Division

Dosage form: Liquid

Ingredients:

vitamin A	1,500 IU
vitamin D	400 IU
vitamin E	5 IU
vitamin C	35 mg
thiamin (B_1)	0.5 mg
riboflavin (B_2)	0.6 mg
niacin	8 mg
vitamin B_6	0.4 mg
iron	10 mg

Comments:

• This supplement provides at least 100 percent of the RDA for infants for most nutrients.

• Niacin, vitamin D, and vitamin B_{12} are provided in amounts greater than the RDA for infants.

• Only vitamins D and B_{12} would meet the RDAs for older children.

• This product may cause a temporary symptom of darkened stools or temporary discoloration of the gums.

• Accidental iron poisoning is a possibility, especially with young children. Be sure to keep all supplements stored out of their reach.

• This product is alcohol free.

POLY-VI-SOL WITH IRON
(multivitamin children's supplement with iron)

Manufacturer: Mead Johnson Nutritional Division

Dosage form: Chewable tablets

Ingredients:

vitamin A	2,500 IU
vitamin D	400 IU
vitamin E	15 IU
vitamin C	60 mg
folic acid	0.3 mg
thiamin (B_1)	1.05 mg
riboflavin (B_2)	1.2 mg
niacin	13.5 mg
vitamin B_6	1.05 mg
vitamin B_{12}	4.5 mg
iron	12 mg
copper	0.8 mg
zinc	8 mg

Comments:

- This supplement provides 100 percent or more of the RDAs for vitamin E, vitamin D, vitamin C, folic acid, thiamin, riboflavin, niacin, vitamin B_6, and vitamin B_{12} for children under 4 years of age.
- For children over age 4, the RDA is provided for all nutrients except vitamin B_6.
- This product may cause a temporary symptom of darkened stools or temporary discoloration of the gums.

• Accidental iron poisoning is a possibility, especially with young children. To avoid accidental poisoning, be sure to keep all supplements stored out of their reach.
• This product contains sugar.

POSTURE
(calcium supplement)

Manufacturer: Whitehall Laboratories
Dosage form: Tablets
Ingredient:
  elemental calcium   600 mg
Comment:
• The calcium source is tricalcium phosphate (1,565 mg).

POSTURE-D
(calcium supplement plus vitamin D)

Manufacturer: Whitehall Laboratories
Dosage form: Tablets
Ingredients:
  elemental calcium   600 mg
  vitamin D   125 IU
Comment:
• The calcium source is tricalcium phosphate (1,565 mg).

PROTEGRA
(antioxidant multivitamin/ mineral supplement)

Manufacturer: Lederle Laboratories
Dosage form: Softgels
Ingredients:

vitamin E	200 IU
vitamin C	250 mg
beta-carotene	3 mg
zinc	7.5 mg
copper	1 mg
selenium	15 µg
manganese	1.5 mg

Comments:

- This product provides the complete range of antioxidant vitamins and minerals.
- This product provides a megadose amount of vitamin E and over 400 percent of the RDA for vitamin D. These levels are used in studies examining antioxidant functions of vitamins.
- Beta-carotene and the minerals are provided in amounts less than the recommended intakes.

SESAME STREET COMPLETE
(multivitamin/mineral children's chewable supplement)

Manufacturer: Johnson & Johnson
Dosage form: Chewable tablets

Ingredients:

vitamin A	2,250 IU
beta-carotene	500 IU
vitamin D	200 IU
thiamin	0.75 mg
riboflavin	0.85 mg
niacin	10 mg
pantothenic acid	5 mg
vitamin B_6	0.7 mg
vitamin B_{12}	3 µg
vitamin C	40 mg
vitamin E	10 IU
folic acid	0.2 mg
biotin	15 µg
iron	10 mg
iodine	75 µg
zinc	8 mg
copper	1 mg
calcium	80 mg
magnesium	20 mg

Comments:

• This product provides much more than 100 percent of the children's RDA for vitamin B_{12} and folic acid.

SLO-NIACIN
(niacin supplement)
Manufacturer: Upsher-Smith Labs
Dosage form: polygel controlled-release capsules

Ingredient:

nicotinic acid   250 mg

Comments:

- This is an effective megadose treatment for extremely high blood cholesterol levels.
- This product may cause side effects such as flushing and tingling of the skin.
- This slow-release form can cause liver damage and should only be used if liver enzymes are monitored by a physician.

SLOW FE
(iron supplement)

Manufacturer: Ciba Consumer
Dosage form: Wax matrix tablets
Ingredient:

50 mg of elemental iron as 160 mg of ferrous sulfate

Comments:

- This product contains more than 300 percent of the RDA for adult women.
- Wax matrix tablets are designed to release iron in the intestines.
- Slow release of iron makes abdominal discomfort, constipation, and diarrhea less of a problem.
- Iron interacts with antacids and oral tetracycline antibiotics, reducing absorption of these drugs.
- Accidental iron poisoning is a possibility, especially with young children. Be sure to keep all supplements stored out of their reach.

STRESSTABS
(multivitamin supplement)

Manufacturer: Lederle Laboratories
Dosage form: Tablets
Ingredients:

vitamin E	30 IU
vitamin C	500 mg
folic acid	0.4 mg
thiamin (B_1)	10 mg
riboflavin (B_2)	10 mg
niacin	100 mg
vitamin B_6	5 mg
vitamin B_{12}	12 µg
biotin	45 µg
pantothenic acid	20 mg

Comments:

- This product provides more than 100 percent of the adult RDA for riboflavin and vitamin B_6.
- This product provides a megadose (ten or more times the RDA) of vitamin C and thiamin.
- This supplement also provides about 500 percent, or five times, the adult RDA for niacin and vitamin B_{12}.

STRESSTABS + IRON
(multivitamin supplement with iron)

Manufacturer: Lederle Laboratories
Dosage form: Tablets

Ingredients:

vitamin E	30 IU
vitamin C	500 mg
folic acid	0.4 mg
thiamin (B_1)	10 mg
riboflavin (B_2)	10 mg
niacin	100 mg
vitamin B_6	5 mg
vitamin B_{12}	12 µg
biotin	45 µg
pantothenic acid	20 mg
iron	18 mg

Comments:

• This product provides more than 100 percent of the adult RDA for riboflavin and vitamin B_6.

• This supplemental product provides a megadose (ten or more times the adult RDA) of two nutrients—vitamin C and thiamin.

• This supplement provides about five times the adult RDA for niacin and vitamin B_{12}.

• Accidental iron poisoning is a possibility, especially with young children. To avoid accidental poisoning, be sure to keep all supplements stored out of their reach.

STRESSTABS+ ZINC
(multivitamin/mineral supplement)

Manufacturer: Lederle Laboratories
Dosage form: Tablets

Ingredients:

vitamin E	30 IU
vitamin C	500 mg
folic acid	0.4 mg
thiamin (B_1)	10 mg
riboflavin (B_2)	10 mg
niacin	100 mg
vitamin B_6	5 mg
vitamin B_{12}	12 µg
biotin	45 µg
pantothenic acid	20 mg
copper	3 mg
zinc	23.9 mg

Comments:

- This product provides more than 100 percent of the adult RDA for riboflavin, vitamin B_6, and zinc and more than the recommended range of intake for pantothenic acid.
- This product provides a megadose (ten or more times the U.S. RDA) of vitamin C and thiamin.
- It provides about 500 percent, or five times, the adult RDA for niacin and vitamin B_{12}.
- Copper is supplied at the upper limit of the recommended range of intake.

STUART FORMULA, THE
(multivitamin/mineral supplement)

Manufacturer: J & J Merck
Dosage form: Tablets

Ingredients:

vitamin A	5,000 IU
vitamin D	400 IU
vitamin E	10 IU
vitamin C	50 mg
folic acid	0.1 mg
thiamin (B_1)	1.5 mg
riboflavin (B_2)	1.7 mg
niacin	20 mg
vitamin B_6	1 mg
vitamin B_{12}	3 μg
calcium	125 mg
iodine	150 μg
elemental iron	5 mg
copper	1 mg

Comments:

- Most nutrients present are provided at reasonable levels—that is, at or near the recommended daily intake levels.
- The vitamin B_{12} level of this supplement exceeds the adult RDA.
- Calcium is supplied in a relatively insignificant amount.
- Vitamins B_6 and C, folic acid, and iron are present in amounts below the RDA.
- The copper level is below the recommended range of intake.
- This supplement does not provide biotin, pantothenic acid, or most minerals, including zinc and selenium.
- This supplement contains sugar.

STUART PRENATAL
(multivitamin/mineral prenatal supplement)

Manufacturer: Wyeth-Ayerst Labs
Dosage form: Tablets
Ingredients:

vitamin A	4,000 IU
vitamin D	400 IU
vitamin E	11 IU
vitamin C	100 mg
folic acid	0.8 mg
thiamin (B_1)	1.84 mg
riboflavin (B_2)	1.7 mg
niacin	18 mg
vitamin B_6	2.6 mg
vitamin B_{12}	4 μg
calcium	200 mg
elemental iron	60 mg
zinc	25 mg

Comments:

- This product provides 100 percent of the RDA for pregnant and breast-feeding women for vitamin D, vitamin E, vitamin C, thiamin, riboflavin, and niacin.
- It provides more than 100 percent of the RDA for vitamin B_6, iron, folic acid, vitamin B_{12}, and zinc.
- This product supplies vitamin A at 100 percent of the RDA for pregnant women but not for breast-feeding women.
- Calcium is supplied at well below the RDAs for both pregnant and breast-feeding women.

332

- This supplement contains FD&C Red No. 3— a food colorant whose safety is in question.
- This product could depress zinc absorption.
- Iron interacts with antacids and oral tetracycline antibiotics, reducing the absorption of these drugs.
- Accidental iron poisoning is a possibility, especially with young children. Be sure to keep all supplements stored out of their reach.

SUNKIST MULTIVITAMINS
(children's chewable multivitamin supplement)

Manufacturer: CIBA Consumer Pharmaceuticals
Dosage forms: Chewable tablets
Ingredients:

vitamin A	2500 IU
folic acid	0.3 mg
thiamin (B_1)	1.05 mg
riboflavin (B_2)	1.2 mg
niacinamide	13.5 mg
vitamin B_6	1.05 mg
vitamin B_{12}	4.5 µg
vitamin C	60 mg
vitamin D	400 IU
vitamin E	15 IU
vitamin K_1	5 µg

Comments:
- Levels are reasonable for most nutrients.

- This product contains phenylalanine and should not be used by those with phenylketonuria.
- This product is sugar free and contains sorbitol and aspartame.

SUNKIST MULTIVITAMINS + EXTRA C
(children's chewable multivitamin supplement with extra C)

Manufacturer: CIBA Consumer Pharmaceuticals

Dosage forms: Chewable tablets

Ingredients:

vitamin A	2500 IU
folic acid	0.3 mg
thiamin (B_1)	1.05 mg
riboflavin (B_2)	1.2 mg
niacinamide	13.5 mg
vitamin B_6	1.05 mg
vitamin B_{12}	4.5 µg
vitamin C	250 mg
vitamin D	400 IU
vitamin E	15 IU
vitamin K_1	5 µg

Comments:

- Dosage levels are reasonable for most of the nutrients provided.
- Vitamin C is present at 500 percent of the RDA for children.

- This product contains phenylalanine and should not be used by children who have phenylketonuria.
- This product is sugar free and contains sorbitol and aspartame.

SUNKIST MULTIVITAMINS + IRON
(children's chewable multivitamin supplement with iron)

Manufacturer: CIBA Consumer Pharmaceuticals

Dosage forms: Chewable tablets

Ingredients:

vitamin A	2500 IU
folic acid	0.3 mg
thiamin (B_1)	1.05 mg
riboflavin (B_2)	1.2 mg
niacinamide	13.5 mg
vitamin B_6	1.05 mg
vitamin B_{12}	4.5 µg
vitamin C	60 mg
vitamin D	400 IU
vitamin E	15 IU
vitamin K_1	5 µg
iron	15 mg

Comments:
- Dosage levels are reasonable for most of the nutrients provided.

- Vitamin C is present at 500 percent of the RDA for children.
- Iron is present at 150 percent of the RDA for children.
- This product contains phenylalanine and should not be used by children who have phenylketonuria.
- Accidental iron poisoning is a possibility, especially with young children. Be sure to keep all supplements, especially those designed to be attractive to children, stored out of their reach.
- This product is sugar free and contains sorbitol and aspartame.

SUNKIST COMPLETE
(children's chewable multivitamin/mineral supplement)

Manufacturer: CIBA Consumer Pharmaceuticals
Dosage forms: Chewable tablets
Ingredients:

vitamin A	5,000 IU
vitamin D	400 IU
vitamin E	30 IU
vitamin C	60 mg
folic acid	0.4 mg
thiamin (B_1)	1.5 mg
riboflavin (B_2)	1.7 mg

niacin	20 mg
vitamin B_6	2 mg
vitamin B_{12}	6 µg
vitamin K_1	10 µg
biotin	40 µg
pantothenic acid	10 mg
iron	18 mg
calcium	100 mg
copper	2 mg
phosphorus	78 mg
iodine	150 µg
magnesium	20 mg
manganese	1 mg
zinc	10 mg

Comments:

• Dosage levels for most of the nutrients are at 100 percent of the adult RDAs—more than most of the RDAs for children.

• Calcium and magnesium are well below recommended amounts.

• Iron level is well above recommended level for children.

• This product contains phenylalanine and should not be used by those with phenylketonuria.

• Iron interacts with antacids and oral tetracycline antibiotics, reducing absorption of these drugs.

• Accidental iron poisoning is a possibility, especially with young children. Be sure to keep all supplements, especially those that are designed to be attractive to children, stored out of their reach.

• This product is sugar free and contains sorbitol and aspartame.

SUNKIST VITAMIN C
(vitamin C supplement)

Manufacturer: CIBA Consumer
Pharmaceuticals
Dosage forms: Chewable tablets or caplets
Ingredient:
vitamin C

chewable tablet (sold in rolls)	60 mg
chewable tablet	250 mg
chewable tablet	500 mg
caplet	500 mg

Comments:
• The 60-mg tablet provides 100 percent of the adult RDA.
• The 250-mg tablet provides more than 100 percent of the adult RDA for vitamin C.
• The 500-mg tablet and caplet both provide well above 100 percent of the adult RDA for vitamin C—almost ten times the RDA.
• Long-term use of high-dose chewable vitamin C tablets has been linked to erosion of dental enamel.
• This product contains sugar, sorbitol, and lactose.

SURBEX
(B-complex supplement)

Manufacturer: Abbott Laboratories
Dosage form: Tablets

Ingredients:

niacin	30 mg
pantothenic acid	10 mg
thiamin (B_1)	6 mg
riboflavin (B_2)	6 mg
vitamin B_6	2.5 mg
vitamin B_{12}	5 μg

Comment:

• This supplement provides more than 100 percent of the adult RDA for niacin, thiamin, riboflavin, and vitamin B_6.

SURBEX WITH C
(vitamin C and B-complex supplement)

Manufacturer: Abbott Laboratories
Dosage form: Tablets
Ingredients:

niacin	30 mg
pantothenic acid	10 mg
thiamin (B_1)	6 mg
riboflavin (B_2)	6 mg
vitamin B_6	2.5 mg
vitamin B_{12}	5 μg
vitamin C	250 mg

Comment:

• This supplement provides over 400 percent of the adult RDA for vitamin C and over 100 percent of the adult RDA for niacin, thiamin, riboflavin, and vitamin B_6.

SURBEX-T
(vitamin C and B-complex supplement)

Manufacturer: Abbott Laboratories
Dosage form: Tablets
Ingredients:

vitamin C	500 mg
niacin	100 mg
pantothenic acid	20 mg
thiamin (B$_1$)	15 mg
riboflavin (B$_2$)	10 mg
vitamin B$_6$	5 mg
vitamin B$_{12}$	10 µg

Comments:

- This product provides over 500 percent of the RDA for vitamin C.
- This supplement provides over 100 percent of the RDA for niacin, riboflavin, vitamin B$_6$, and vitamin B$_{12}$ and above the recommended safe and sufficient range of intake for pantothenic acid.
- This product provides a megadose (ten or more times the adult RDA) of the B vitamin thiamin.

SURBEX-750 WITH IRON
(vitamin C, B-complex and E supplement plus iron)

Manufacturer: Abbott Laboratories
Dosage form: Tablets

Ingredients:

vitamin C	750 mg
niacin	100 mg
vitamin B_6	25 mg
pantothenic acid	20 mg
thiamin (B_1)	15 mg
riboflavin (B_2)	15 mg
vitamin B_{12}	12 µg
folic acid	0.4 mg
vitamin E	30 IU
elemental iron	27 mg

Comments:

• This product provides well above 100 percent of the adult RDA for niacin, riboflavin, vitamin B_{12}, and iron and the recommended range of intake for pantothenic acid.

• This product provides a megadose (ten times the RDA) of vitamin C, vitamin B_6, and thiamin.

• Accidental iron poisoning is a possibility, especially with young children. Be sure to keep all supplements stored out of their reach.

SURBEX-750 WITH ZINC
(vitamin C, B-complex and E supplement plus zinc)

Manufacturer: Abbott Laboratories
Dosage form: Tablets
Ingredients:

vitamin C	750 mg
niacin	100 mg

vitamin B$_6$	20 mg
pantothenic acid	20 mg
thiamin (B$_1$)	15 mg
riboflavin (B$_2$)	15 mg
vitamin B$_{12}$	12 µg
folic acid	0.4 mg
vitamin E	30 IU
zinc	22.5 mg

Comments:
• This product provides well above 100 percent of the adult RDA for riboflavin, niacin, and vitmain B$_{12}$ and above the recommended range of intake for pantothenic acid.
• This product provides a megadose ten times the RDA) of vitamin C, thiamin, and vitmain B$_6$.

THERAGRAN LIQUID
(multivitamin supplement)

Manufacturer: Bristol-Myers Squibb
Dosage form: Liquid
Ingredients:

beta-carotene	5,000 IU
vitamin D	400 IU
vitamin C	200 mg
thiamin (B$_1$)	10 mg
riboflavin (B$_2$)	10 mg
niacin	100 mg
vitamin B$_6$	4.1 mg
vitamin B$_{12}$	5 µg
pantothenic acid	21.4 mg

Comment:
- This product provides well above the adult RDA for vitamin C, vitamin D, thiamin, riboflavin, niacin, vitamin B_6, and vitamin B_{12} and above the recommended range of intake for pantothenic acid.

THERAGRAN-M ADVANCED FORMULA
(multivitamin/mineral supplement)

Manufacturer: Bristol-Myers Squibb
Dosage form: Tablets
Ingredients:

vitamin A	5,000 IU
vitamin C	90 mg
thiamin (B_1)	3 mg
riboflavin (B_2)	3.4 mg
niacin	20 mg
vitamin B_6	3 mg
vitamin B_{12}	9 µg
vitamin D	400 IU
vitamin E	30 IU
pantothenic acid	10 mg
folic acid	0.4 mg
biotin	30 µg
calcium	40 mg
iodine	150 µg
iron	27 mg

magnesium	100 mg
copper	2 mg
zinc	15 mg
chromium	15 µg
selenium	10 µg
molybdenum	15 µg
phosphorus	31 mg
potassium	7.5 mg
chloride	7.5 mg

Comments:

- This product provides more than 100 percent of the adult RDA for vitamin C, vitamin D, thiamin, riboflavin, niacin, vitamin B_6, and iron. The amount of vitamin B_{12} is more than 400 percent of the adult RDA.
- This product contains insignificant amounts of calcium, potassium, and chloride. The amounts of magnesium, selenium, and chromium are well below recommended intakes.
- Accidental iron poisoning is a possibility, especially with young children. Be sure to keep all supplements stored out of their reach.

THERAGRAN STRESS FORMULA
(multivitamin supplement with iron)

Manufacturer: Bristol-Myers Squibb
Dosage form: Tablets

Ingredients:

vitamin E	30 IU
vitamin C	600 mg
folic acid	0.4 mg
thiamin (B_1)	15 mg
riboflavin (B_2)	15 mg
niacin	100 mg
vitamin B_6	25 mg
vitamin B_{12}	12 µg
biotin	45 µg
pantothenic acid	20 mg
iron	27 mg

Comments:

- This product provides more than the adult RDA for vitamins E, riboflavin, niacin, folic acid, and vitamin B_{12} and for the mineral iron.
- This product provides megadoses (10 or more times the RDA) of vitamin C, thiamin, and vitamin B_6.
- Accidental iron poisoning is a possibility, especially with young children. To avoid accidental poisoning, be sure to keep all supplements stored out of their reach.

THERAGRAN ANTIOXIDANT
(antioxidant supplement)

Manufacturer: Bristol-Myers Squibb
Dosage form: Tablets

Ingredients:

beta-carotene	5,000 IU
vitamin C	250 mg
vitamin E	200 IU
copper	1 mg
manganese	1.5 mg
selenium	15 mg
zinc	7.5 mg

Comments:

• Beta-carotene provides 100 percent of the RDA for vitamin A.
• This product provides over 400 percent of the RDA for vitamin C.
• Vitamin E is present in a megadose.
• The minerals are all present in amounts below the RDAs or recommended intake levels.

TRI-VI-SOL
(multivitamin children's supplement)

Manufacturer: Mead Johnson Nutritional Division

Dosage form: Liquid

Ingredients:

vitamin A	1,500 IU
vitamin D	400 IU
vitamin C	35 mg

Comment:

• This product provides 100 percent of the RDA for infants over 6 months for each nutrient.

TRI-VI-SOL WITH IRON
(multivitamin children's supplement with iron)

Manufacturer: Mead Johnson Nutritional
Division

Dosage form: Liquid

Ingredients:

vitamin A	1,500 IU
vitamin D	400 IU
vitamin C	35 mg
iron	10 mg

Comments:

• This product provides 100 percent of the RDA for infants over 6 months of age for each nutrient. The amounts are only slightly higher than the RDA for infants under 6 months of age.

• Accidental iron poisoning is a possibility, especially with young children. Be sure to keep all supplements stored out of their reach.

UNICAP
(multivitamin supplement)

Manufacturer: The Upjohn Company

Dosage forms: Tablets, capsules

Ingredients:

vitamin A	5,000 IU
vitamin D	400 IU
vitamin E	30 IU
vitamin C	60 mg

folic acid	0.4 mg
thiamin (B_1)	1.5 mg
riboflavin (B_2)	1.7 mg
niacin	20 mg
vitamin B_6	2 mg
vitamin B_{12}	6 µg

Comments:

• This product provides 100 percent of the adult RDA for most nutrients, but more than 100 percent for vitamin E, vitamin D, folic acid, and vitamin B_{12}.

• This supplement is sugar and sodium free.

UNICAP JUNIOR
(multivitamin children's supplement)

Manufacturer: The Upjohn Company
Dosage form: Chewable tablets
Ingredients:

vitamin A	5,000 IU
vitamin D	400 IU
vitamin E	30 IU
vitamin C	60 mg
folic acid	0.4 mg
thiamin (B_1)	1.5 mg
riboflavin (B_2)	1.7 mg
niacin	20 mg
vitamin B_6	2 mg
vitamin B_{12}	6 µg
vitamin E	15 IU

Comments:

- This product provides 100 percent or more of the adult RDA for all nutrients. All the nutrients except vitamin D are present at levels greater than 100 percent of the RDAs.
- This supplement contains sugar, mannitol, and lactose.

UNICAP M
(multivitamin/mineral supplement)

Manufacturer: The Upjohn Company
Dosage form: Tablets
Ingredients:

vitamin A	5,000 IU
vitamin D	400 IU
vitamin E	30 IU
vitamin C	60 mg
folic acid	0.4 mg
thiamin (B_1)	1.5 mg
riboflavin (B_2)	1.7 mg
niacin	20 mg
vitamin B_6	2 mg
vitamin B_{12}	6 µg
pantothenic acid	10 mg
iodine	150 µg
iron	18 mg
copper	2 mg
zinc	15 mg
calcium	60 mg

phosphorus	45 mg
manganese	1 mg
potassium	5 mg

Comments:

- This supplemental product provides 100 percent of the adult RDA for all nutrients, except vitamin E, folic acid, and vitamin B_{12}, which are provided in larger doses.
- The supplement provides insignificant amounts of the minerals calcium, phosphorus, manganese, and potassium.
- This product is sugar- and sodium free.

UNICAP PLUS IRON
(multivitamin supplement with iron)

Manufacturer: The Upjohn Company
Dosage form: Tablets
Ingredients:

vitamin A	5,000 IU
vitamin D	400 IU
vitamin E	30 IU
vitamin C	60 mg
folic acid	0.4 mg
thiamin (B_1)	1.5 mg
riboflavin (B_2)	1.7 mg
niacin	20 mg
vitamin B_6	2 mg
vitamin B_{12}	6 µg
iron	22.5 mg

calcium	100 mg
pantothenic acid	10 mg

Comments:

- This product provides 100 percent of the adult RDA for all nutrients except vitamin E, folic acid, and vitamin B_{12}, which are provided in larger doses.
- Accidental iron poisoning is a possibility, especially with young children. Be sure to keep all supplements stored out of their reach.
- This supplement contains sugar.

UNICAP SENIOR
(multivitamin/mineral supplement)

Manufacturer: The Upjohn Company
Dosage form: Tablets
Ingredients:

vitamin A	5,000 IU
vitamin D	200 IU
vitamin E	15 IU
vitamin C	60 mg
folic acid	0.4 mg
thiamin (B_1)	1.2 mg
riboflavin (B_2)	1.4 mg
niacin	16 mg
vitamin B_6	2.2 mg
vitamin B_{12}	3 μg
pantothenic acid	10 mg
iodine	150 mg

iron	10 mg
copper	2 mg
zinc	15 mg
calcium	100 mg
phosphorus	77 mg
magnesium	30 mg
manganese	1 mg
potassium	5 mg

Comments:

• Amounts of all vitamins are reasonable.
• This product contains insignificant amounts of magnesium and potassium.
• Calcium is supplied in a small amount.
• Accidental iron poisoning is a possibility, especially with young children. Be sure to keep all supplements stored out of their reach.
• This supplement is sugar- and sodium free.

UNICAP T
(multivitamin/mineral supplement)

Manufacturer: The Upjohn Company
Dosage form: Tablets
Ingredients:

vitamin A	5,000 IU
vitamin D	400 IU
vitamin E	30 IU
vitamin C	500 mg
folic acid	0.4 mg
thiamin (B_1)	10 mg

riboflavin (B$_2$)	10 mg
niacin	100 mg
vitamin B$_6$	6 mg
vitamin B$_{12}$	18 μg
pantothenic acid	25 mg
iodine	150 μg
iron	18 mg
copper	2 mg
zinc	15 mg
manganese	1 mg
potassium	5 mg
selenium	10 μg

Comments:

- This product provides more than 100 percent of the adult RDA for vitamin C, vitamin E, thiamin, riboflavin, niacin, folic acid, and vitamin B$_6$.
- This supplement product provides above the recommended range of intake for pantothenic acid.
- This product contains 900 percent of the adult requirement for vitamin B$_{12}$.
- The amounts of manganese and potassium are insignificant.
- This supplement is sugar- and sodium free.

Z-BEC
(vitamin C, B-complex and E supplement with zinc)

Manufacturer: A. H. Robins Company
Dosage form: Tablets

Ingredients:

vitamin C	600 mg
thiamin	15 mg
riboflavin	10.2 mg
niacin	100 mg
vitamin B_6	10 mg
vitamin B_{12}	6 μg
pantothenic acid	25 mg
vitamin E	45 IU
zinc	22.5 mg

Comments:

- This product provides more than 100 percent of the adult RDA for zinc and vitamin B_6, and more than twice the upper limit of the recommended range of intake for pantothenic acid.
- This product provides 500 percent or more of the adult RDA for niacin and riboflavin.
- This product provides a megadose (ten times the RDA) of vitamin C and thiamin.

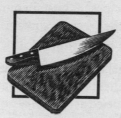

Recipes for Healthier Living

The recipes that follow provide healthy doses of vitamins and minerals, as well as other nutrients that your body needs. They are designed to fit within the American Heart Association's guidelines for fat intake (which recommend that your daily total fat intake not exceed 30 percent of total calories and your saturated fat intake not exceed 10 percent of total calories). They also tend to be low in sodium and cholesterol.

The nutritional chart that follows each recipe shows number of calories (kc); grams (g) of protein, carbohydrate, and fat; and milligrams (mg) of cholesterol and sodium in a serving. There is also a listing of the vitamin and mineral content in one serving; units of measure used for these include retinol equivalents (RE) and micrograms (μg), as well as milligrams (mg). You'll notice that different vitamins and minerals are listed under

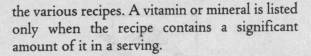

the various recipes. A vitamin or mineral is listed only when the recipe contains a significant amount of it in a serving.

The nutritional information in the chart includes all the ingredients listed in the recipe, *except* ingredients labeled as "optional" or "for garnish." If a range is given in the yield of a recipe ("Makes 6 to 8 servings," for example), the *higher* yield was used to calculate the per serving information. If a range is offered for an ingredient (¼ to ⅛ teaspoon, for example), the *first* amount given was used to calculate the nutritional information. If an ingredient is presented with an option ("2 tablespoons margarine or oil"), the *first* ingredient given was used to calculate the nutritional information. Foods offered as "serve with" suggestions at the end of a recipe are *not* included in the chart unless it is stated in the per serving line. Because numerous variables account for a wide range of values for certain foods, all nutritional information that appears in this book should be considered approximate.

The recipes in this book are NOT intended as a medically therapeutic program, nor as a substitute for medically approved diet plans for people on fat-, cholesterol-, or sodium-restricted diets. Consult your physician before beginning any diet plan.

CREAMY CARROT SOUP

- 3 cups water
- 4 cups sliced carrots
- ½ cup chopped onion
- 2 tablespoons packed brown sugar
- 2 teaspoons curry powder
- 2 garlic cloves, minced
- ⅛ teaspoon ground ginger
- ½ cube chicken bouillon
  Dash ground cinnamon
- ½ cup skim milk

In large saucepan, bring water to a boil. Add all
remaining ingredients except milk. Reduce heat to
low; simmer 40 minutes or until carrots and onion
are very tender. Remove from heat; pour mixture in
batches into food processor or blender. Process until
smooth. Return mixture to saucepan. Over low heat,
stir in milk, heating until warm but not boiling.
Serve warm.   Makes 6 servings

NUTRITIONAL INFORMATION PER SERVING

Calories	69.46	kc	Niacin (B_3)	0.96	mg
Protein	1.92	g	Pantothenic Acid	0.23	mg
Fat	0.63	g	Phosphorus	67.72	mg
% of Calories			Potassium	338.30	mg
from Fat:	8		Pyridoxine (B_6)	0.15	mg
Saturated Fat	0.08	g	Riboflavin (B_2)	0.08	mg
Cholesterol	0.33	mg	Thiamin (B_1)	0.09	mg
Dietary Fiber	2.80	g	Vitamin A	2,075	RE
Sodium	156.90	mg	Vitamin C	8.24	mg
Beta-Carotene	12,377	RE	Copper	0.09	mg
Calcium	56.71	mg	Folate	14.29	µg
Cobalamin (B_{12})	0.10	µg	Vitamin D	0.22	µg
Iron	0.78	mg	Vitamin E	0.45	mg
Magnesium	17.75	mg	Zinc	0.33	mg

GAZPACHO

- 1 cucumber
- ½ red bell pepper, seeded
- 2 carrots
- 1 medium tomato
- 2 cups spicy tomato juice
- ½ cup water
- ½ cup tomato sauce
- ¼ cup chopped green onions
- 3 tablespoons vinegar
- 2 teaspoons sugar
- 1 garlic clove, minced
- 1 (15-ounce) can navy beans, drained and rinsed

Cut cucumber, bell pepper, carrots and tomato into large chunks. Place all ingredients except beans in food processor; process until almost puréed but still chunky. Transfer to large bowl. Stir in beans; cover and refrigerate until serving.   Makes 6 servings

NUTRITIONAL INFORMATION PER SERVING

Calories	129.90	kc	Pantothenic Acid	0.64	mg
Protein	7.04	g	Phosphorus	144.60	mg
Fat	0.59	g	Potassium	674.10	mg
% of Calories			Pyridoxine (B$_6$)	0.29	mg
from Fat:	4		Riboflavin (B$_2$)	0.12	mg
Saturated Fat	0.13	g	Thiamin (B$_1$)	0.21	mg
Dietary Fiber	2.55	g	Vitamin A	774.80	RE
Sodium	737.10	mg	Vitamin C	23.72	mg
Beta-Carotene	4220	RE	Copper	.32	mg
Calcium	61.52	mg	Folate	76.96	µg
Iron	2.42	mg	Vitamin E	0.68	mg
Magnesium	58.39	mg	Zinc	0.92	mg
Niacin (B$_3$)	1.65	mg			

APRICOT AND RICOTTA STUFFED CELERY

2½ cups (1½-inch) celery pieces
3 tablespoons coarsely chopped dried apricots
½ cup part-skim ricotta cheese
1½ teaspoons sugar
¼ teaspoon grated orange peel
⅛ teaspoon salt

Cut a thin lengthwise slice from bottom of each
celery piece to prevent tipping; set aside. In food
processor or blender, process apricots until finely
chopped. Set aside 1 tablespoon for garnish. Add
ricotta cheese, sugar, orange peel, and salt to food
processor or blender; process until cheese is smooth.
Fill celery pieces with cheese mixture. Cover and
refrigerate up to 3 hours before serving. Just before
serving, sprinkle with reserved chopped apricots.

Makes about 25 appetizers

NUTRITIONAL INFORMATION PER SERVING

Calories	10.27	kc	Niacin (B$_3$)	0.07	mg
Protein	0.54	g	Pantothenic Acid	0.03	mg
Fat	0.33	g	Phosphorus	4.14	mg
% of Calories			Potassium	47.88	mg
from Fat:	27		Pyridoxine (B$_6$)	0.01	mg
Saturated Fat	0.01	g	Riboflavin (B$_2$)	0.01	mg
Cholesterol	1.65	mg	Thiamin (B$_1$)	0.01	mg
Dietary Fiber	0.27	g	Vitamin A	10.80	RE
Sodium	25.50	mg	Vitamin C	0.89	mg
Beta-Carotene	51.71	RE	Copper	0.01	mg
Calcium	13.54	mg	Folate	3.47	µg
Iron	0.10	mg	Vitamin E	0.09	mg
Magnesium	1.78	mg	Zinc	0.02	mg

APPLE SLICES WITH CITRUS-YOGURT DIP

- 2 to 3 Empire apples, cored and sliced
- ¼ cup lemon juice
- 1 cup plain low fat yogurt
- 2 tablespoons honey
- 1 tablespoon frozen orange juice concentrate, thawed
- 1 teaspoon grated orange peel
- ½ teaspoon grated lemon peel

Dip apple slices in lemon juice to prevent browning; set aside. Combine remaining ingredients in small bowl. Cover; refrigerate until chilled. Arrange apple slices on platter; serve with dip.

Makes 20 (1 tablespoon) servings

NUTRITIONAL INFORMATION PER SERVING

Calories	24.10	kc	Niacin (B₃)	0.04	mg
Protein	0.66	g	Pantothenic Acid	0.09	mg
Fat	0.23	g	Phosphorus	18.11	mg
% of Calories			Potassium	53.62	mg
from Fat:	8		Pyridoxine (B₆)	0.01	mg
Saturated Fat	0.12	g	Riboflavin (B₂)	0.03	mg
Cholesterol	0.70	mg	Thiamin (B₁)	0.01	mg
Dietary Fiber	0.33	g	Vitamin A	3.35	RE
Sodium	8.21	mg	Vitamin C	3.83	mg
Beta-Carotene	5.09	RE	Copper	0.01	mg
Calcium	22.58	mg	Folate	3.44	µg
Cobalamin (B₁₂)	0.06	µg	Vitamin E	0.10	mg
Iron	0.05	mg	Zinc	0.11	mg
Magnesium	3.17	mg			

ZUCCHINI WITH PIMIENTO

2 **cups thin zucchini slices
      (about 2 medium zucchini)**
1 **small onion, chopped**
1 **jar (2 ounces) pimiento, drained and diced**
½ **teaspoon salt (optional)**
½ **teaspoon dried oregano leaves, crushed**
⅛ **teaspoon garlic powder**
⅛ **teaspoon ground red pepper**

In 2-quart microwavable casserole, combine all
ingredients; cover. Microwave at HIGH (100%
power) 6 to 7 minutes or until fork-tender, stirring
halfway through cooking time.

Makes 4 servings

NUTRITIONAL INFORMATION PER SERVING

Calories	21.68	kc	Pantothenic Acid	0.08	mg
Protein	1.16	g	Phosphorus	30.69	mg
Fat	0.23	g	Potassium	236.60	mg
% of Calories			Pyridoxine (B$_6$)	0.11	mg
from Fat:	8		Riboflavin (B$_2$)	0.03	mg
Saturated Fat	0.04	g	Thiamin (B$_1$)	0.06	mg
Dietary Fiber	1.65	g	Vitamin A	58.36	RE
Sodium	273.50	mg	Vitamin C	20.59	mg
Beta-Carotene	180.50	RE	Copper	0.07	mg
Calcium	19.66	mg	Folate	19.89	µg
Iron	0.62	mg	Vitamin E	0.31	mg
Magnesium	17.65	mg	Zinc	0.21	mg
Niacin (B$_3$)	0.37	mg			

COUNTRY BEAN SOUP

½ pound (1¼ cups) dried navy beans or lima
  beans
2½ cups water
 4 ounces salt pork or fully cooked ham,
  chopped
¼ cup chopped onion
½ teaspoon dried oregano, crushed
¼ teaspoon salt
¼ teaspoon ground ginger
¼ teaspoon dried sage, crushed
¼ teaspoon black pepper
 2 cups skim milk
 2 tablespoons butter

Rinse navy beans. Place beans in large saucepan;
add enough water to cover. Bring to a boil; reduce
heat and simmer 2 minutes. Remove from heat;
cover and let stand for 1 hour.*

Drain; return beans to saucepan. Stir in 2½ cups
water, salt pork, chopped onion, oregano, salt,
ground ginger, sage, and pepper. Bring to a boil;
reduce heat. Cover and simmer for 2 to 2½ hours
or until beans are tender. (If necessary, add more
water during cooking time.)

Add milk and butter, stirring until mixture is heated through and butter is melted. Season to taste with additional salt and pepper.   Makes 6 servings

*Or, cover beans with water and let soak 8 hours or overnight.

NUTRITIONAL INFORMATION PER SERVING

Calories	229.70	kc	Pantothenic Acid	0.59	mg
Protein	15.12	g	Phosphorus	259.90	mg
Fat	6.93	g	Potassium	519.80	mg
% of Calories			Pyridoxine (B_6)	0.27	mg
from Fat:	27		Riboflavin (B_2)	0.24	mg
Saturated Fat	3.82	g	Selenium	0.01	mg
Cholesterol	26.63	mg	Thiamin (B_1)	0.34	mg
Dietary Fiber	0.13	g	Vitamin A	86.07	RE
Sodium	420.10	mg	Vitamin C	2.16	mg
Beta-Carotene	10.21	RE	Copper	0.29	mg
Calcium	166.80	mg	Folate	127.20	mc
Cobalamin (B_{12})	0.43	µg	Vitamin D	0.89	µg
Iron	2.49	mg	Vitamin E	0.29	mg
Magnesium	67.71	mg	Zinc	1.75	mg
Niacin (B_3)	1.51	mg			

CRISPY VEGETABLES WITH ORANGE FLAVOR

    1   tablespoon vegetable oil
    2   cups diagonally sliced celery
    1   cup broccoli florets
  3/4   cup red bell pepper chunks
  1/2   cup sliced green onions
    4   strips (2 × 1/2-inch) orange peel
 1 1/2 teaspoons ground ginger
 1 1/2 cups (about 8 ounces) firm tofu, cut into
          1-inch pieces
    1   tablespoon soy sauce
    1   packet low-sodium vegetable bouillon dis-
          solved in 1 1/2 cups water *or*
 1 1/2 cups no-salt-added tomato juice
    2   tablespoons cornstarch
    6   ounces thin spaghetti, cooked
        Orange slices (optional)

Heat oil in large nonstick skillet or wok until hot.
Add celery, broccoli, red pepper, green onions,
orange peel, and ginger; cook and stir until
vegetables are crisp-tender, 4 to 5 minutes.

Meanwhile, in small bowl, toss tofu with soy sauce
until well coated; set aside. In measuring cup,
combine bouillon and cornstarch. When vegetables
are cooked, add cornstarch mixture to skillet; bring
to a boil, stirring constantly until mixture is slightly

thickened, about 1 minute. Gently stir in tofu mixture; cook until heated through, about 1 minute. Serve over cooked spaghetti. Garnish with orange slices, if desired.

Makes 4 servings

Tip: Tofu, or soybean curd, is sometimes fortified with calcium. It is very perishable and should be used within one week of purchasing. Store tofu covered with water in the refrigerator. For maximum freshness, change the water every day, making sure to recover tofu each time.

NUTRITIONAL INFORMATION PER SERVING

Calories	341.10	kc	Pantothenic Acid	0.56	mg
Protein	17.20	g	Phosphorus	219.30	mg
Fat	9.65	g	Potassium	533.20	mg
% of Calories			Pyridoxine (B_6)	0.31	mg
from Fat:	25		Riboflavin (B_2)	0.28	mg
Saturated Fat	1.32	g	Thiamin (B_1)	0.42	mg
Dietary Fiber	3.74	g	Vitamin A	106.40	RE
Sodium	342.10	mg	Vitamin C	73.14	mg
Beta-Carotene	484.30	RE	Copper	0.41	mg
Calcium	181.50	mg	Folate	69.93	µg
Iron	8.72	mg	Vitamin E	3.87	mg
Magnesium	95.95	mg	Zinc	1.83	mg
Niacin (B_3)	3.58	mg			

RATATOUILLE

- ½ pound eggplant, cut into ½-inch cubes
- 1 small onion, sliced and separated into rings
- 1 small zucchini, thinly sliced
- ½ medium green bell pepper, chopped
- 1 medium tomato, cut into wedges
- 1 stalk celery, chopped
- 1 tablespoon grated Parmesan cheese
- ¼ teaspoon salt (optional)
- ¼ teaspoon dried chervil, crushed
- ¼ teaspoon dried oregano, crushed
- ⅛ teaspoon instant minced garlic
- ⅛ teaspoon dried thyme, crushed
- Dash black pepper

Combine all ingredients in 2-quart microwavable casserole; cover. Microwave at HIGH (100% power) 7 to 10 minutes or until eggplant is translucent, stirring every 3 minutes.

Makes 6 servings

NUTRITIONAL INFORMATION PER SERVING

Calories	28.98	kc	Niacin (B_3)	0.48	mg
Protein	1.40	g	Pantothenic Acid	0.13	mg
Fat	0.53	g	Phosphorus	34.79	mg
% of Calories			Potassium	230.20	mg
from Fat:	15		Pyridoxine (B_6)	0.10	mg
Saturated Fat	0.24	g	Riboflavin (B_2)	0.03	mg
Cholesterol	0.82	mg	Thiamin (B_1)	0.06	mg
Dietary Fiber	1.97	g	Vitamin A	29.41	RE
Sodium	29.20	mg	Vitamin C	13.09	mg
Beta-Carotene	81.71	RE	Copper	0.08	mg
Calcium	28.25	mg	Folate	18.11	µg
Cobalamin (B_{12})	0.02	µg	Vitamin E	0.30	mg
Iron	0.46	mg	Zinc	0.19	mg
Magnesium	14.52	mg			

ORANGE-SPIKED ZUCCHINI AND CARROTS

1   pound zucchini, cut into ¼-inch slices
1   (10-ounce) package frozen sliced carrots, thawed
1   cup unsweetened orange juice
1   stalk celery, finely chopped
2   tablespoons chopped onion
    Salt and pepper to taste (optional)

Combine all ingredients in large nonstick saucepan. Simmer, covered, 10 to 12 minutes or until zucchini is tender. Uncover and continue to simmer, stirring occasionally, until most of the liquid has evaporated.

Makes 7 servings

NUTRITIONAL INFORMATION PER SERVING

Calories	40.84	kc	Pantothenic Acid	0.21	mg
Protein	1.14	g	Phosphorus	39.89	mg
Fat	0.16	g	Potassium	288.60	mg
% of Calories			Pyridoxine (B_6)	0.12	mg
from Fat:	3		Riboflavin (B_2)	0.05	mg
Saturated Fat	0.03	g	Thiamin (B_1)	0.07	mg
Dietary Fiber	2.70	g	Vitamin A	737.20	RE
Sodium	30.80	mg	Vitamin C	21.84	mg
Beta-Carotene	4,368	RE	Copper	0.09	mg
Calcium	24.88	mg	Folate	34.76	µg
Iron	0.48	mg	Vitamin E	0.40	mg
Magnesium	20.35	mg	Zinc	0.22	mg
Niacin (B_3)	0.57	mg			

FRUIT SOUP

5 fresh California nectarines, diced
1 cup plain low-fat yogurt
½ cup low-fat milk
1 tablespoon sugar
1 teaspoon almond extract
¼ teaspoon curry powder
½ cup strawberries, diced
Mint leaves (optional)

Reserve ½ cup nectarines. Place remaining nectarines, yogurt, milk, sugar, almond extract, and curry powder in blender; cover. Blend until smooth. Pour into bowl. Stir in reserved nectarines and strawberries. Chill; garnish with mint leaves.

Makes 6 servings

NUTRITIONAL INFORMATION PER SERVING

Calories	103.40	kc	Niacin (B₃)	1.22	mg
Protein	3.81	g	Pantothenic Acid	0.51	mg
Fat	1.56	g	Phosphorus	94.48	mg
% of Calories			Potassium	381.80	mg
from Fat:	13		Pyridoxine (B₆)	0.06	mg
Saturated Fat	0.68	g	Riboflavin (B₂)	0.17	mg
Cholesterol	3.83	mg	Thiamin (B₁)	0.05	mg
Dietary Fiber	2.17	g	Vitamin A	103.80	RE
Sodium	36.85	mg	Vitamin C	13.66	mg
Beta-Carotene	86.72	RE	Copper	0.10	mg
Calcium	101.70	mg	Folate	11.56	µg
Cobalamin (B₁₂)	0.29	µg	Vitamin D	0.21	µg
Iron	0.28	mg	Vitamin E	1.26	mg
Magnesium	19.95	mg	Zinc	0.54	mg

VEGETABLES
CELERY AND CHICKPEA CURRY WITH APPLE

- 1 tablespoon vegetable oil
- 2 cups diagonally sliced celery
- 1 cup tart apple slices
- ½ cup chopped onion
- 2 teaspoons curry powder
- 1 teaspoon minced garlic
- 1 can (10½ ounces) chickpeas, rinsed and drained
- 1 can (8 ounces) stewed tomatoes, broken up
- 3 cups cooked brown rice

Heat oil in large skillet until hot. Add celery, apple, onion, curry powder, and garlic; cook and stir until vegetables are crisp-tender, 8 minutes. Stir in chickpeas and tomatoes. Bring to a boil; reduce heat and simmer, uncovered, until flavors are blended, about 5 minutes. Serve over cooked rice.

Makes 4 servings

NUTRITIONAL INFORMATION PER SERVING

Calories	318.40	kc	Pantothenic Acid	0.63	mg
Protein	8.72	g	Phosphorus	241.10	mg
Fat	6.50	g	Potassium	599.40	mg
% of Calories			Pyridoxine (B_6)	0.31	mg
from Fat:	18		Riboflavin (B_2)	0.12	mg
Saturated Fat	0.94	g	Selenium	0.06	mg
Dietary Fiber	8.98	g	Thiamin (B_1)	0.22	mg
Sodium	500.20	mg	Vitamin A	42.89	RE
Beta-Carotene	143.10	RE	Vitamin C	18.42	mg
Calcium	98.29	mg	Copper	0.42	mg
Iron	3.54	mg	Folate	30.44	µg
Magnesium	106.50	mg	Vitamin E	9.28	mg
Niacin (B_3)	3.15	mg	Zinc	1.89	mg

DELICIOUS APPLE COMPOTE

- 2 **Red or Golden Delicious apples**
- 2 **cups seeded watermelon cubes**
- 1 **cup seedless grapes**
- 1 **orange, peeled, sliced, and seeded**
- 1 **banana, peeled and sliced**
- 2 **cups chilled ginger ale**
- 2 **tablespoons lime juice**

Core apples; cut into bite-sized pieces. Toss with watermelon, grapes, orange, and banana. Combine ginger ale and lime juice. Pour over fruit. Serve immediately.   Makes 6 servings

NUTRITIONAL INFORMATION PER SERVING

Calories	120.00	kc	Pantothenic Acid	0.26	mg
Protein	1.02	g	Phosphorus	18.68	mg
Fat	0.67	g	Potassium	285.40	mg
% of Calories			Pyridoxine (B$_6$)	0.25	mg
from Fat:	5		Riboflavin (B$_2$)	0.06	mg
Saturated Fat	0.12	g	Thiamin (B$_1$)	0.10	mg
Dietary Fiber	2.37	g	Vitamin A	29.90	RE
Sodium	7.86	mg	Vitamin C	25.45	mg
Beta-Carotene	179.30	RE	Copper	0.11	mg
Calcium	23.33	mg	Folate	14.18	µg
Iron	0.46	mg	Vitamin E	0.65	mg
Magnesium	18.27	mg	Zinc	0.17	mg
Niacin (B$_3$)	0.39	mg			

SPICED PEAR-CRANBERRY SOUP

2   fresh California Bartlett pears, peeled and chopped

2   thin slices fresh ginger (optional)

¼   teaspoon ground cinnamon

⅛   teaspoon ground cloves

1½ cups low-calorie cranberry juice cocktail
Plain low-fat yogurt (optional)

Combine pears, ginger, cinnamon, and cloves in food processor or blender; cover. Process until smooth. With machine running, slowly add cranberry juice until mixture is well blended. Garnish each serving with dollop of yogurt, if desired. Soup may be served warm or cold.

Makes 4 servings

NUTRITIONAL INFORMATION PER SERVING

Calories	75.23	kc	Pantothenic Acid	0.13	mg
Protein	0.33	g	Phosphorus	9.74	mg
Fat	0.35	g	Potassium	112.00	mg
% of Calories			Pyridoxine (B$_6$)	0.02	mg
from Fat:	4		Riboflavin (B$_2$)	0.04	mg
Saturated Fat	0.02	g	Thiamin (B$_1$)	0.02	mg
Dietary Fiber	2.16	g	Vitamin A	2.19	RE
Sodium	1.60	mg	Vitamin C	13.09	mg
Beta-Carotene	10.33	RE	Copper	0.10	mg
Calcium	13.68	mg	Folate	6.05	µg
Iron	0.31	mg	Vitamin E	0.55	mg
Magnesium	6.17	mg	Zinc	0.12	mg
Niacin (B$_3$)	0.09	mg			

DILLED GREEN BEANS

- 1 (10-ounce) package frozen cut green beans
- ½ cup *plus* 2 tablespoons water
- 2 green onions, finely chopped
- 2 teaspoons cornstarch
- 1 teaspoon instant chicken bouillon granules
- 1 teaspoon cider vinegar
- ¼ teaspoon grated lime peel
- ¼ teaspoon dill weed
- Dash pepper

Place beans and 2 tablespoons water in 1-quart microwavable casserole; cover. Microwave at HIGH (100% power) 4 to 7 minutes or until beans are tender, stirring after 3 minutes. Drain. Cover; set aside. In small microwavable bowl, blend remaining ingredients. Microwave at HIGH (100% power) 1½ to 2 minutes or until clear and thickened. Pour over beans. Toss to coat.   Makes 4 servings

Tip: For low-salt diets, substitute low-salt bouillon.

NUTRITIONAL INFORMATION PER SERVING

Calories	75.23	kc	Pantothenic Acid	0.13	mg
Protein	0.33	g	Phosphorus	9.74	mg
Fat	0.35	g	Potassium	112.00	mg
% of Calories			Pyridoxine (B_6)	0.02	mg
from Fat:	4		Riboflavin (B_2)	0.04	mg
Saturated Fat	0.02	g	Thiamin (B_1)	0.02	mg
Dietary Fiber	2.16	g	Vitamin A	2.19	RE
Sodium	1.60	mg	Vitamin C	13.09	mg
Beta-Carotene	10.33	RE	Copper	0.10	mg
Calcium	13.68	mg	Folate	6.05	µg
Iron	0.31	mg	Vitamin E	0.55	mg
Magnesium	6.17	mg	Zinc	0.12	mg
Niacin (B_3)	0.09	mg			

VEGETABLES
TODAY'S SLIM TUNA
STUFFED TOMATOES

    6   medium tomatoes
    1   cup dry curd cottage cheese
    ½   cup plain low-fat yogurt
    ¼   cup chopped cucumber
    ¼   cup chopped green bell pepper
    ¼   cup thinly sliced radishes
    ¼   cup chopped green onion
    ½   teaspoon dried basil, crushed
    ⅛   teaspoon garlic powder
    1   (6½-ounce) can tuna, packed in water, drained
        and flaked
        Lettuce leaves

Cut each tomato into 6 wedges, cutting to, but not
through, each base. Refrigerate. Just before serving,
in medium bowl, combine cottage cheese and yogurt;
mix well. Stir in remaining ingredients except lettuce leaves. Place tomatoes on lettuce-lined plates;
spread wedges apart. Spoon cottage cheese mixture
into center of each tomato.   Makes 6 servings

NUTRITIONAL INFORMATION PER SERVING

Calories	98.48	kc	Pantothenic Acid	0.51	mg
Protein	14.00	g	Phosphorus	131.80	mg
Fat	1.39	g	Potassium	414.40	mg
% of Calories			Pyridoxine (B_6)	0.19	mg
from Fat:	12		Riboflavin (B_2)	0.18	mg
Saturated Fat	0.39	g	Selenium	0.01	mg
Cholesterol	8.36	mg	Thiamin (B_1)	0.11	mg
Dietary Fiber	1.97	g	Vitamin A	113.30	RE
Sodium	47.66	mg	Vitamin C	34.53	mg
Beta-Carotene	250.70	RE	Copper	0.12	mg
Calcium	58.71	mg	Folate	29.47	µg
Cobalamin (B_{12})	1.12	µg	Vitamin D	0.01	µg
Iron	1.19	mg	Vitamin E	1.11	mg
Magnesium	29.61	mg	Zinc	0.58	mg
Niacin (B_3)	4.72	mg			

GLAZED FRUIT KABOBS

- 2 **fresh California nectarines, each cut into 6 wedges**
- 3 **fresh California plums, quartered**
- ½ **fresh pineapple, peeled and cut into 2-inch cubes**
- ¼ **cup firmly packed brown sugar**
- 2 **tablespoons water**
- 1½ **teaspoons cornstarch**
- ¾ **teaspoon rum extract**

Alternately thread fruit onto skewers. Combine sugar, water, cornstarch and rum extract in small saucepan. Bring to a boil, stirring constantly, until thickened and clear. Place fruit kabobs in shallow pan. Brush with glaze mixture.* Grill kabobs about 4 to 5 inches from heat, 6 to 8 minutes or until hot, turning once, brushing occasionally with glaze mixture.   Makes 4 servings

*Kabobs may be prepared early and refrigerated until grilling time.

NUTRITIONAL INFORMATION PER SERVING

Calories	163.00	kc	Pantothenic Acid	0.33	mg
Protein	1.10	g	Phosphorus	25.58	mg
Fat	0.81	g	Potassium	358.60	mg
% of Calories			Pyridoxine (B_6)	0.14	mg
from Fat:	4		Riboflavin (B_2)	0.08	mg
Saturated Fat	0.07	g	Thiamin (B_1)	0.13	mg
Dietary Fiber	2.94	g	Vitamin A	58.63	RE
Sodium	5.37	mg	Vitamin C	22.34	mg
Beta-Carotene	102.30	RE	Copper	0.23	mg
Calcium	25.53	mg	Folate	15.28	µg
Iron	1.08	mg	Vitamin E	1.04	mg
Magnesium	25.97	mg	Zinc	0.21	mg
Niacin (B_3)	1.26	mg			

FETA POCKETS

- 2 cups bean sprouts
- 1 small cucumber, chopped
- ½ cup (2 ounces) crumbled Wisconsin Feta cheese
- ¼ cup plain yogurt
- 1 tablespoon sesame seed, toasted
- ¼ teaspoon black pepper
- 2 pita bread rounds, halved
- 1 medium tomato, cut into 4 slices

In medium bowl, stir together sprouts, cucumber, cheese, yogurt, sesame seed, and pepper. Spoon mixture into pita bread halves. Place tomato slice on filling in each bread half.   Makes 4 servings

NUTRITIONAL INFORMATION PER SERVING

Calories	145.10	kc	Niacin (B$_3$)	1.77	mg
Protein	7.46	g	Pantothenic Acid	0.69	mg
Fat	5.04	g	Phosphorus	151.50	mg
% of Calories			Potassium	334.50	mg
from Fat:	30		Pyridoxine (B$_6$)	0.22	mg
Saturated Fat	2.58	g	Riboflavin (B$_2$)	0.29	mg
Cholesterol	13.90	mg	Thiamin (B$_1$)	0.22	mg
Dietary Fiber	2.61	g	Vitamin A	45.53	RE
Sodium	288.70	mg	Vitamin C	16.56	mg
Beta-Carotene	41.52	RE	Copper	0.27	mg
Calcium	154.90	mg	Folate	66.02	µg
Cobalamin (B$_{12}$)	0.33	µg	Vitamin E	2.01	mg
Iron	1.75	mg	Zinc	1.27	mg
Magnesium	40.00	mg			

CRUNCHY APPLE STIR-FRY

  1 cup thinly sliced carrots (2 medium carrots)
 ½ cup onion slices
  1 teaspoon dried basil, crushed
1½ teaspoons vegetable oil
  1 cup fresh or thawed frozen snow peas
  1 tablespoon water
  1 medium Washington Golden Delicious or
       Criterion apple, cored and thinly sliced

Stir-fry carrots, onion, and basil in oil in nonstick skillet until carrots are tender. Stir in snow peas and water; stir-fry 2 minutes. Remove from heat; stir in apple slices. Serve hot.   Makes 4 servings

NUTRITIONAL INFORMATION PER SERVING

Calories	70.95	kc	Pantothenic Acid	0.37	mg
Protein	1.65	g	Phosphorus	42.18	mg
Fat	2.00	g	Potassium	244.40	mg
% of Calories			Pyridoxine (B$_6$)	0.14	mg
from Fat:	24		Riboflavin (B$_2$)	0.06	mg
Saturated Fat	0.26	g	Thiamin (B$_1$)	0.10	mg
Dietary Fiber	2.90	g	Vitamin A	783.70	RE
Sodium	12.04	mg	Vitamin C	27.74	mg
Beta-Carotene	4,693	RE	Copper	0.07	mg
Calcium	37.03	mg	Folate	23.75	µg
Iron	1.15	mg	Vitamin E	2.84	mg
Magnesium	17.82	mg	Zinc	0.22	mg
Niacin (B$_3$)	0.56	mg			

VEGETABLES
APPLE AND CARROT CASSEROLE

- 6 large carrots, sliced
- 4 large apples, peeled and sliced
- 5 tablespoons all-purpose flour
- 1 tablespoon firmly packed brown sugar
- ½ teaspoon ground nutmeg
- 1 tablespoon margarine
- ½ cup orange juice

Preheat oven to 350°F. Cook carrots in large saucepan in boiling water for 5 minutes; drain. Layer carrots and apples in large casserole. In small bowl, mix flour, sugar, and nutmeg; sprinkle over carrots and apples. Dot with margarine; pour orange juice over flour mixture. Bake 30 minutes or until carrots are tender.

Makes 6 servings

NUTRITIONAL INFORMATION PER SERVING

Calories	144.30	kc	Pantothenic Acid	0.27	mg
Protein	1.77	g	Phosphorus	50.59	mg
Fat	2.52	g	Potassium	396.90	mg
% of Calories			Pyridoxine (B$_6$)	0.16	mg
from Fat:	15		Riboflavin (B$_2$)	0.10	mg
Saturated Fat	0.51	g	Thiamin (B$_1$)	0.16	mg
Dietary Fiber	4.67	g	Vitamin A	2,057	RE
Sodium	48.65	mg	Vitamin C	22.24	mg
Beta-Carotene	12,206	RE	Copper	0.10	mg
Calcium	31.83	mg	Folate	25.78	µg
Iron	0.96	mg	Vitamin D	0.19	µg
Magnesium	19.51	mg	Vitamin E	2.38	mg
Niacin (B$_3$)	1.21	mg	Zinc	0.24	mg

MINT-GLAZED CARROTS AND SNOW PEAS

- 1 **tablespoon margarine**
- 3 **medium carrots, thinly sliced diagonally**
- ½ **pound fresh snow peas, trimmed**
- 2 **tablespoons sugar**
- 1 **tablespoon fresh lemon juice**
- 1 **tablespoon chopped fresh mint leaves** *or*
  1 **teaspoon dried mint, crushed**

In large nonstick skillet, melt margarine over medium heat. Cook and stir carrots 3 to 4 minutes. Add snow peas, sugar, lemon juice, and mint. Cook and stir an additional 1 to 2 minutes until vegetables are glazed and crisp-tender.   Makes 4 servings

NUTRITIONAL INFORMATION PER SERVING

Calories	94.39	kc	Pantothenic Acid	0.47	mg
Protein	2.34	g	Phosphorus	54.39	mg
Fat	3.05	g	Potassium	309.20	mg
% of Calories			Pyridoxine (B_6)	0.16	mg
from Fat:	28		Riboflavin (B_2)	0.07	mg
Saturated Fat	0.59	g	Thiamin (B_1)	0.12	mg
Dietary Fiber	3.24	g	Vitamin A	1,561	RE
Sodium	54.01	mg	Vitamin C	32.52	mg
Beta-Carotene	9,132	RE	Copper	0.07	mg
Calcium	38.38	mg	Folate	23.59	µg
Iron	1.33	mg	Vitamin D	0.28	µg
Magnesium	22.43	mg	Vitamin E	2.95	mg
Niacin (B_3)	0.80	mg	Zinc	0.31	mg

VEGETABLES
FRENCH CARROT MEDLEY

- 2 **cups fresh or thawed frozen carrot slices**
- ³/₄ **cup unsweetened orange juice**
- 1 **(4-ounce) can sliced mushrooms, undrained**
- 4 **stalks celery, sliced**
- 2 **tablespoons chopped onion**
- ½ **teaspoon dillweed**
  Salt and pepper to taste (optional)
- 2 **teaspoons cornstarch or arrowroot**
- ¼ **cup cold water**

Combine all ingredients except cornstarch and water in medium saucepan. Simmer, covered, 12 to 15 minutes or until carrots are tender. Combine cornstarch and water in small bowl. Stir into vegetable mixture; cook and stir until mixture thickens and bubbles.　　　　Makes 6 servings

NUTRITIONAL INFORMATION PER SERVING

Calories	42.49	kc	Pantothenic Acid	0.33	mg
Protein	1.17	g	Phosphorus	41.43	mg
Fat	0.22	g	Potassium	281.90	mg
% of Calories			Pyridoxine (B_6)	0.12	mg
from Fat:	4		Riboflavin (B_2)	0.05	mg
Saturated Fat	0.04	g	Thiamin (B_1)	0.08	mg
Dietary Fiber	2.22	g	Vitamin A	1,040	RE
Sodium	117.60	mg	Vitamin C	16.48	mg
Beta-Carotene	6,240	RE	Copper	0.09	mg
Calcium	27.46	mg	Folate	32.56	µg
Iron	0.63	mg	Vitamin E	0.48	mg
Magnesium	15.42	mg	Zinc	0.28	mg
Niacin (B_3)	0.83	mg			

INDONESIAN CHICKEN AND PEAR SALAD

Curry Dressing (page 395)

1½ cups cold cooked chicken, cubed

3 fresh California Bartlett pears, halved, cored, divided

½ cup macadamia nuts or peanuts, coarsely chopped (optional)

½ cup cucumber, sliced

3 tablespoons crystallized ginger, slivered (optional)

2 tablespoons green onion, thinly sliced

Lemon juice

Iceberg lettuce cups

Toasted shredded coconut (optional)

Prepare Curry Dressing; set aside. Place chicken in large bowl. Cube 2 pear halves; add to chicken along with nuts, cucumber, ginger and onion. Add Curry Dressing; mix gently.

Dip remaining 4 pear halves in lemon juice and arrange in lettuce cup on salad plate. Spoon salad over pear halves. Sprinkle with toasted coconut, if desired.   Makes 4 servings

Curry Dressing: Combine ½ cup plain low fat yogurt, ½ teaspoon curry powder and ¼ teaspoon *each* dry mustard, ground allspice, and garlic powder; mix well. Prepare dressing about 20 minutes before using to allow flavors to blend. Makes about ⅔ cup.

Tip: Chicken is an excellent source of high-quality protein and B vitamins, yet is low in saturated fat. As a rule, one broiler-fryer chicken (about 3 pounds) yields about 2½ cups of chopped, cooked chicken.

NUTRITIONAL INFORMATION PER SERVING

Calories	179.80	kc	Niacin (B₃)	5.62	mg
Protein	14.86	g	Pantothenic Acid	0.71	mg
Fat	4.37	g	Phosphorus	150.60	mg
% of Calories			Potassium	360.10	mg
from Fat:	21		Pyridoxine (B₆)	0.28	mg
Saturated Fat	1.25	g	Riboflavin (B₂)	0.17	mg
Cholesterol	37.77	mg	Selenium	0.01	mg
Dietary Fiber	3.52	g	Thiamin (B₁)	0.07	mg
Sodium	50.45	mg	Vitamin A	33.48	RE
Beta-Carotene	92.00	RE	Vitamin C	7.03	mg
Calcium	77.69	mg	Copper	0.18	mg
Cobalamin (B₁₂)	0.30	µg	Folate	15.66	µg
Iron	0.97		Vitamin E	1.02	mg
Magnesium	27.05	mg			

Sun Country Chicken Salad

   1 large cantaloupe
   2 cups cooked chicken chunks
   1 cup cucumber chunks
   1 cup green grapes
   ½ cup chopped green onions
   2 tablespoons chopped parsley
   1 cup plain nonfat yogurt
   3 tablespoons prepared chutney
   ¼ teaspoon grated lemon peel
   1 tablespoon lemon juice
   ¼ cup whole blanched California almonds, toasted*
   1 large bunch watercress

Cut cantaloupe into 12 wedges, removing seeds and peel. In large bowl, combine chicken, cucumber, grapes, onions, and parsley. In small bowl, blend together yogurt, chutney, lemon peel, and juice. Toss lightly with chicken mixture. Fold in almonds.

Arrange watercress on 4 salad plates. Place 3 wedges of cantaloupe on each plate. Spoon chicken salad mixture over cantaloupe.

Makes 4 servings

*To toast almonds, spread almonds in single layer on baking sheet. Bake at 350°F, 5 to 8 minutes, stirring occasionally, until lightly browned. Cool.

———— ⊚ ————

Tip: Cantaloupe is a very good source of vitamins A and C, and potassium. Look for well-shaped melons with a smoothly rounded, depressed area at stem end. A fragrant aroma is a good sign of ripeness.

NUTRITIONAL INFORMATION PER SERVING

Calories	355.50	kc	Niacin (B_3)	10.37	mg
Protein	25.23	g	Pantothenic Acid	1.55	mg
Fat	9.42	g	Phosphorus	325.00	mg
% of Calories			Potassium	1,259	mg
from Fat:	23		Pyridoxine (B_6)	0.75	mg
Saturated Fat	1.80	g	Riboflavin (B_2)	0.32	mg
Cholesterol	49.02	mg	Selenium	0.02	mg
Dietary Fiber	5.78	g	Thiamin (B_1)	0.23	mg
Sodium	153.70	mg	Vitamin A	1,283	RE
Beta-Carotene	517.40	RE	Vitamin C	131.90	mg
Calcium	206.10	mg	Copper	0.31	mg
Cobalamin (B_{12})	0.53	µg	Folate	25.49	µg
Iron	2.16	mg	Vitamin E	2.93	mg
Magnesium	99.80	mg	Zinc	2.09	mg

APPLESAUCE BERRY SALAD

- 1 (3-ounce) package sugar-free strawberry gelatin
- 1 cup boiling water
- 1 (10-ounce) package frozen strawberries, thawed
- 1 cup applesauce
- 1 cup plain low-fat yogurt or low-fat sour cream

Dissolve gelatin in boiling water. Stir in strawberries and applesauce; pour into 10 × 6-inch dish. Chill until set. Spread yogurt on top of gelatin mixture. Cover and chill 2 hours. Cut into squares.

Makes 6 to 8 servings

NUTRITIONAL INFORMATION PER SERVING

Calories	77.56	kc	Magnesium	9.82	mg
Protein	7.54	g	Niacin (B$_3$)	0.25	mg
Fat	0.49	g	Pantothenic Acid	0.24	mg
% of Calories			Phosphorus	184.60	mg
from Fat:	6		Potassium	142.90	mg
Saturated Fat	0.29	g	Pyridoxine (B$_6$)	0.03	mg
Cholesterol	1.75	mg	Riboflavin (B$_2$)	0.08	mg
Dietary Fiber	1.39	g	Thiamin (B$_1$)	0.02	mg
Sodium	250.80	mg	Vitamin A	8.07	RE
Beta-Carotene	6.67	RE	Vitamin C	15.20	mg
Soluble Fiber	0.28	g	Copper	0.03	mg
Calcium	58.45	mg	Folate	9.25	µg
Cobalamin (B$_{12}$)	0.16	µg	Vitamin E	0.18	mg
Iron	0.33	mg	Zinc	0.31	mg

SALADS
ARTICHOKE WILD RICE SALAD

Salad:
- 2 cups cooked wild rice
- 1 cup frozen peas, thawed
- 1 (8-ounce) can sliced water chestnuts, drained
- 1 (6-ounce) jar marinated artichoke hearts
- 4 ounces shredded mozzarella cheese (optional)
- 1 (2-ounce) jar diced pimiento, drained

Dressing:
- 2 tablespoons canola oil
- 2 tablespoons reserved liquid from artichokes
- 1 tablespoon balsamic vinegar
- ½ teaspoon dried tarragon leaves, crumbled
- ½ teaspoon Dijon mustard
- 2 to 3 drops hot pepper sauce (or to taste)

Drain artichokes, reserving liquid. In large bowl, combine salad ingredients. In small bowl, mix dressing ingredients; pour over salad and toss. Chill 4 hours or overnight to allow flavors to blend.

Makes 6 to 8 servings

NUTRITIONAL INFORMATION PER SERVING

Calories	129.00	kc	Niacin (B$_3$)	1.20	mg
Protein	3.80	g	Pantothenic Acid	0.23	mg
Fat	3.83	g	Phosphorus	80.65	mg
% of Calories			Potassium	201.90	mg
from Fat:	22		Pyridoxine (B$_6$)	0.16	mg
Saturated Fat	0.30	g	Riboflavin (B$_2$)	0.08	mg
Dietary Fiber	2.85	g	Thiamin (B$_1$)	0.10	mg
Sodium	48.17	mg	Vitamin A	36.89	RE
Soluble Fiber	0.40	g	Vitamin C	11.12	mg
Beta-Carotene	132.30	RE	Copper	0.13	mg
Calcium	20.75	mg	Folate	36.90	µg
Iron	1.34	mg	Vitamin E	0.28	mg
Magnesium	34.86	mg	Zinc	0.97	mg

SALADS

CALIFORNIA APRICOT FRUIT SALAD

- **2** cups sliced fresh California apricots (about 1 pound)
- **1½** cups sliced fresh strawberries
- **1½** cups peeled and sliced kiwifruit
- **¼** cup California apricot nectar
- **¼** cup flake coconut, lightly toasted
- **1** tablespoon finely chopped fresh mint

In medium bowl, combine all ingredients. Refrigerate until chilled. Serve as salad or arrange on wooden skewers for fresh fruit kabobs.

Makes 5 servings

NUTRITIONAL INFORMATION PER SERVING

Calories	114.70	kc	Pantothenic Acid	0.42	mg
Protein	2.18	g	Phosphorus	50.02	mg
Fat	2.38	g	Potassium	523.80	mg
% of Calories			Pyridoxine (B_6)	0.13	mg
from Fat:	17		Riboflavin (B_2)	0.09	mg
Saturated Fat	1.50	g	Thiamin (B_1)	0.05	mg
Dietary Fiber	4.71	g	Vitamin A	266.70	RE
Sodium	16.48	mg	Vitamin C	83.18	mg
Calcium	33.23	mg	Copper	0.20	mg
Iron	1.03	mg	Folate	34.73	µg
Magnesium	28.46	mg	Vitamin E	1.76	mg
Niacin (B_3)	0.94	mg	Zinc	0.47	mg

CALIFORNIA BROWN RICE SALAD

- 1 (16-ounce) can California fruit cocktail in juice or extra light syrup
- 1 cup brown rice
- 1 medium tomato, diced
- 1 cup celery slices
- ½ cup green onion slices
- 2 tablespoons red wine vinegar
- 1 tablespoon vegetable oil
- 1 tablespoon Dijon-style mustard
- ½ teaspoon dried tarragon, crumbled
- ⅛ teaspoon garlic powder

Drain fruit cocktail, reserving ¼ cup liquid; save remainder for other uses. Cook rice according to package directions; chill thoroughly. In large bowl, toss rice with fruit cocktail, tomato, celery, and green onions. In small bowl, combine reserved fruit cocktail liquid, vinegar, oil, mustard, tarragon, and garlic powder. Stir into rice mixture; chill to allow flavors to blend.   Makes 6 servings

NUTRITIONAL INFORMATION PER SERVING

Calories	181.70	kc	Pantothenic Acid	0.65	mg
Protein	3.43	g	Phosphorus	133.50	mg
Fat	3.46	g	Potassium	269.40	mg
% of Calories			Pyridoxine (B_6)	0.23	mg
from Fat:	17		Riboflavin (B_2)	0.07	mg
Saturated Fat	0.51	g	Thiamin (B_1)	0.16	mg
Dietary Fiber	3.01	g	Vitamin A	72.28	RE
Sodium	58.28	mg	Vitamin C	10.36	mg
Beta-Carotene	265.60	RE	Copper	0.16	mg
Calcium	31.18	mg	Folate	17.60	µg
Iron	1.03	mg	Vitamin E	2.71	mg
Magnesium	56.26	mg	Zinc	0.78	mg
Niacin (B_3)	2.08	mg			

GRILLED CHICKEN AND FLORIDA GRAPEFRUIT SALAD

- ½ cup frozen Florida grapefruit juice concentrate, thawed
- 1 ripe banana, mashed
- 1 tablespoon olive oil
- 2 teaspoons red wine vinegar
- ¼ cup finely minced green onions
- 2 tablespoons chopped dill
- 2 cloves garlic, minced
- 1 teaspoon brown sugar
- ½ teaspoon salt
- ¼ teaspoon pepper
- 4 skinless, boneless chicken breast halves
- 4 cups mixed salad greens (Boston, romaine, red leaf)
- 1 pint cherry tomatoes, halved
- 1 green bell pepper, cut into strips
- 2 Florida grapefruit, peeled and cut into ½-inch-thick wheels

Preheat grill or broiler. In medium bowl, combine grapefruit juice concentrate, banana, oil, vinegar, green onions, dill, garlic, sugar, salt, and pepper; stir to combine. Place chicken in shallow, nonmetallic bowl. Divide marinade mixture; pour half over chicken. Marinate in refrigerator 30 minutes, turning chicken over once.

Place chicken on grill or broiler, 4 inches from heat; discard marinade. Cook 5 to 7 minutes on each side, or until chicken is cooked through. Remove to plate and allow to cool for 5 minutes.

Divide and arrange salad greens, tomatoes, pepper, and grapefruit wheels on serving plates. Slice each chicken breast in half diagonally; place on serving plate.

Drizzle juices and remaining dressing over chicken and salad greens. Garnish with additional dill and green onions, if desired. Makes 4 servings

Tip: When selecting grapefruits, choose ones that feel heavy for their size as these will be the juiciest. Grapefruit is an excellent source of vitamin C and is also high in antioxidants.

NUTRITIONAL INFORMATION PER SERVING

Calories	296.00	kc	Niacin (B_3)	12.74	mg
Protein	29.48	g	Pantothenic Acid	1.59	mg
Fat	7.01	g	Phosphorus	260.00	mg
% of Calories			Potassium	837.50	mg
from Fat:	21		Pyridoxine (B_6)	0.83	mg
Saturated Fat	1.46	g	Riboflavin (B_2)	0.24	mg
Cholesterol	73.00	mg	Selenium	0.03	mg
Dietary Fiber	3.19	g	Thiamin (B_1)	0.23	mg
Sodium	337.50	mg	Vitamin A	211.50	RE
Beta-Carotene	378.70	RE	Vitamin C	98.33	mg
Calcium	83.28	mg	Copper	0.20	mg
Cobalamin (B_{12})	0.29	µg	Folate	100.40	µg
Iron	2.48	mg	Vitamin E	1.79	mg
Magnesium	62.90	mg	Zinc	1.26	mg

SPICY BEEF AND RICE SALAD

- 1 **pound boneless beef top sirloin steak, 1 inch thick**
- 2 **teaspoons Spicy Seasoning Mix (page 405), divided**
   Salt to taste
- 2 **cups Spicy Cooked Rice (page 405)**
- 1 **medium red apple, cut into small chunks**
- 2 **to 3 green onions, thinly sliced**
- ¼ **cup coarsely chopped walnuts, toasted***
   Leaf lettuce (optional)
   Additional apple chunks (optional)

Prepare Spicy Seasoning Mix; set aside. Heat large nonstick skillet over medium heat 5 minutes. Meanwhile, rub 1 teaspoon Spicy Seasoning into sides of steak. Place steak in skillet and cook 12 to 14 minutes for rare (140°F) to medium (160°F), turning once. Season with salt, if desired.

Meanwhile, combine Spicy Cooked Rice, apple, onions and walnuts. Cut steak into thin slices; arrange over rice mixture. Garnish with leaf lettuce and apple, if desired.   Makes 4 servings

*To toast walnuts, spread walnuts in single layer on baking sheet. Bake at 350°F, 5 to 8 minutes, stirring occasionally, until lightly browned. Cool.

SPICY SEASONING MIX

   3 **tablespoons chili powder**
   2 **teaspoons ground cumin**
1½ **teaspoons garlic powder**
   ¾ **teaspoon dried oregano leaves**
   ½ **teaspoon ground red pepper**

Combine chili powder, cumin, garlic powder, oregano, and red pepper. Store, covered, in airtight container. Shake before using to blend. Makes about ⅓ cup.

Spicy Cooked Rice: Cook ⅔ cup rice according to package directions, adding 1 teaspoon Spicy Seasoning Mix to water before cooking.

NUTRITIONAL INFORMATION PER SERVING

Calories	378.50	kc	Niacin (B₃)	5.82	mg
Protein	34.85	g	Pantothenic Acid	0.88	mg
Fat	10.39	g	Phosphorus	328.80	mg
% of Calories			Potassium	525.40	mg
from Fat:	25		Pyridoxine (B₆)	0.60	mg
Saturated Fat	2.54	g	Riboflavin (B₂)	0.32	mg
Cholesterol	71.62	mg	Selenium	0.02	mg
Dietary Fiber	2.39	g	Thiamin (B₁)	0.32	mg
Sodium	67.81	mg	Vitamin A	16.66	RE
Beta-Carotene	87.04	RE	Vitamin C	3.33	mg
Calcium	30.90	mg	Copper	0.30	mg
Cobalamin (B₁₂)	2.82	µg	Folate	19.82	µg
Iron	4.81	mg	Vitamin E	2.34	mg
Magnesium	62.44	mg	Zinc	7.23	mg

HEARTY HEALTHY CHICKEN SALAD

- 1 broiler-fryer chicken, cooked, skinned, boned, and cut into chunks
- 1 cup small macaroni, cooked
- 3 tomatoes, cubed
- 1 cup sliced celery
- ½ cup chopped red bell pepper
- 3 tablespoons chopped green onion
- 1 teaspoon salt
- ½ teaspoon ground black pepper
- ¼ teaspoon oregano
- 1 cup chicken broth
- 1 clove garlic, split
- ¼ cup wine vinegar

In large bowl, mix warm chicken, macaroni, tomatoes, celery, bell pepper, and onion. Sprinkle with salt, black pepper, and oregano. Place broth and garlic in small saucepan; bring to a boil over high heat and boil 10 minutes or until broth is reduced to ½ cup. Add vinegar; pour over salad, mixing well. Chill until cold.   Makes 6 servings

NUTRITIONAL INFORMATION PER SERVING

Calories	249.10	kc	Niacin	10.13	mg
Protein	30.07	g	Pantothenic Acid	1.31	mg
Fat	8.18	g	Phosphorus	236.70	mg
% of Calories			Potassium	512.80	mg
from Fat:	30		Pyridoxine (B_6)	0.58	mg
Saturated Fat	2.08	g	Riboflavin (B_2)	0.29	mg
Cholesterol	85.34	mg	Thiamin (B_1)	0.18	mg
Dietary Fiber	1.96	g	Vitamin A	80.95	RE
Sodium	698.50	mg	Vitamin C	31.49	mg
Beta-Carotene	172.80	RE	Copper	0.18	mg
Calcium	35.86	mg	Folate	27.52	µg
Cobalamin (B_{12})	0.35	µg	Vitamin E	1.22	mg
Iron	2.19	mg	Zinc	2.30	mg
Magnesium	40.47	mg			

SALADS
FRUIT AND GREEN SALAD

2   tablespoons plain yogurt
1   teaspoon lemon juice
1   teaspoon sugar
1½ cups torn lettuce
1   orange, cubed
1   apple, cubed
1   teaspoon walnuts

In small bowl, mix yogurt, lemon juice, and sugar.
In salad bowl, toss lettuce, orange, and apple. Pour
dressing over salad and top with nuts.

Makes 2 servings

NUTRITIONAL INFORMATION PER SERVING

Calories	101.70	kc	Niacin (B_3)	0.34	mg
Protein	2.24	g	Pantothenic Acid	0.32	mg
Fat	1.36	g	Phosphorus	48.97	mg
% of Calories			Potassium	306.30	mg
from Fat:	11		Pyridoxine (B_6)	0.10	mg
Saturated Fat	0.25	g	Riboflavin (B_2)	0.08	mg
Cholesterol	0.88	mg	Thiamin (B_1)	0.10	mg
Dietary Fiber	3.59	g	Vitamin A	34.05	RE
Sodium	14.22	mg	Vitamin C	41.68	mg
Beta-Carotene	116.70	RE	Copper	0.09	mg
Calcium	65.94	mg	Folate	47.64	µg
Cobalamin (B_{12})	0.08	µg	Vitamin E	1.21	mg
Iron	0.45	mg	Zinc	0.33	mg
Magnesium	18.54	mg			

FRUITED SLAW

- 1 (8¼-ounce) can pineapple chunks in syrup
- 1 (8-ounce) carton orange-flavored yogurt
- 1 tablespoon lemon juice
- 3 cups finely shredded cabbage
- 1 (11-ounce) can mandarin orange sections, drained
- 1 cup thin celery slices
- ½ cup chopped walnuts
- ¼ cup raisins
- 1 medium banana, sliced

Drain pineapple, reserving 2 tablespoons syrup. In small bowl, combine reserved syrup, yogurt, and lemon juice. In large bowl, combine pineapple, cabbage, oranges, celery, nuts, and raisins; fold in yogurt mixture. Gently fold in banana. Cover; chill.

Makes 8 servings

Preparation time: 20 minutes plus chilling time

NUTRITIONAL INFORMATION PER SERVING

Calories	140.60	kc	Niacin (B_3)	0.51	mg
Protein	4.52	g	Pantothenic Acid	0.33	mg
Fat	5.04	g	Phosphorus	96.71	mg
% of Calories			Potassium	383.60	mg
from Fat:	30		Pyridoxine (B_6)	0.24	mg
Saturated Fat	0.54	g	Riboflavin (B_2)	0.13	mg
Cholesterol	1.25	mg	Thiamin (B_1)	0.12	mg
Dietary Fiber	2.49	g	Vitamin A	27.10	RE
Sodium	37.97	mg	Vitamin C	32.96	mg
Beta-Carotene	103.00	RE	Copper	0.19	mg
Calcium	84.12	mg	Folate	43.54	µg
Cobalamin (B_{12})	0.13	µg	Vitamin E	2.55	mg
Iron	0.84	mg	Zinc	0.72	mg
Magnesium	42.26	mg			

SALADS
PASTA AND WALNUT FRUIT SALAD

- 8 ounces medium pasta shells, uncooked
- 1 (8-ounce) container nonfat plain yogurt
- ¼ cup frozen orange juice concentrate, thawed
- 1 (15-ounce) can juice-packed mandarin oranges, drained
- 1 cup seedless red grapes, halved
- 1 cup seedless green grapes, halved
- 1 apple, cored and chopped
- ½ cup sliced celery
- ½ cup walnut halves

Cook shells according to package directions; drain. In small bowl, blend yogurt and orange juice concentrate. In large bowl, combine shells and remaining ingredients. Add yogurt mixture; toss to coat. Cover and chill thoroughly.

Makes 6 to 8 servings

NUTRITIONAL INFORMATION PER SERVING

Calories	231.00	kc	Niacin (B$_3$)	1.13	mg
Protein	8.44	g	Pantothenic Acid	0.45	mg
Fat	5.66	g	Phosphorus	148.40	mg
% of Calories			Potassium	334.50	mg
from Fat:	21		Pyridoxine (B$_6$)	0.18	mg
Saturated Fat	0.51	g	Riboflavin (B$_2$)	0.25	mg
Cholesterol	24.98	mg	Thiamin (B$_1$)	0.29	mg
Dietary Fiber	2.93	g	Vitamin A	31.88	RE
Sodium	35.47	mg	Vitamin C	33.07	mg
Beta-Carotene	137.90	RE	Copper	0.22	mg
Calcium	85.95	mg	Folate	42.25	µg
Cobalamin (B$_{12}$)	0.28	µg	Vitamin E	2.27	mg
Iron	1.39	mg	Zinc	1.13	mg
Magnesium	47.29	mg			

FRUITED LAMB SALAD

- 3 cups cooked American lamb cubes or slices
- 3 cups cooked brown and wild rice, chilled
- 1½ cups sliced strawberries
- 1½ cups orange cubes
- ¾ cup green grapes
- ½ cup banana slices
- ¼ cup walnuts
- 2 tablespoons honey
- 2 tablespoons lemon juice
- 12 large Romaine lettuce leaves

In large bowl, combine lamb, rice, fruit, and nuts. In small bowl, mix together honey, and lemon juice; toss with lamb mixture. Chill. Serve on lettuce leaves.   Makes 12 servings

NUTRITIONAL INFORMATION PER SERVING

Calories	167.40	kc	Niacin (B$_3$)	2.99	mg
Protein	12.90	g	Pantothenic Acid	0.47	mg
Fat	5.15	g	Phosphorus	133.40	mg
% of Calories			Potassium	311.30	mg
from Fat:	27		Pyridoxine (B$_6$)	0.20	mg
Saturated Fat	1.35	g	Riboflavin (B$_2$)	0.18	mg
Cholesterol	32.52	mg	Thiamin (B$_1$)	0.10	mg
Dietary Fiber	2.19	g	Vitamin A	12.65	RE
Sodium	30.70	mg	Vitamin C	25.08	mg
Beta-Carotene	20.38	RE	Copper	0.16	mg
Calcium	24.29	mg	Folate	43.29	µg
Cobalamin (B$_{12}$)	0.93	µg	Vitamin E	1.01	mg
Iron	1.30	mg	Zinc	2.60	mg
Magnesium	35.41	mg			

TURKEY, MANDARIN AND POPPY SEED SALAD

- 5 **cups red leaf lettuce, torn**
- 2 **cups spinach leaves, torn**
- ½ **pound honey roasted turkey, cut into ½-inch julienne strips**
- 1 **can (10½ ounces) mandarin oranges, drained**
- ¼ **cup orange juice**
- 1½ **tablespoons red wine vinegar**
- 1½ **teaspoons poppy seed**
- 1½ **teaspoons olive oil**
- 1 **teaspoon Dijon-style mustard**
- ⅛ **teaspoon pepper**

In large bowl, combine lettuce, spinach, turkey, and oranges. In small bowl, combine orange juice, vinegar, poppy seed, oil, mustard, and pepper. Pour dressing over turkey mixture. Serve immediately.

Makes 4 servings

NUTRITIONAL INFORMATION PER SERVING

Calories	142.80	kc	Niacin (B_3)	4.26	mg
Protein	14.87	g	Pantothenic Acid	0.19	mg
Fat	3.20	g	Phosphorus	174.80	mg
% of Calories			Potassium	600.30	mg
from Fat:	20		Pyridoxine (B_6)	0.42	mg
Saturated Fat	1.69	g	Riboflavin (B_2)	0.24	mg
Cholesterol	42.92	mg	Thiamin (B_1)	0.17	mg
Dietary Fiber	2.28	g	Vitamin A	347.00	RE
Sodium	726.50	mg	Vitamin C	48.94	mg
Beta-Carotene	1,318	RE	Copper	0.15	mg
Calcium	119.10	mg	Folate	115.40	µg
Cobalamin (B_{12})	0.20	µg	Vitamin E	2.04	mg
Iron	2.88	mg	Zinc	1.80	mg
Magnesium	58.68	mg			

SALADS

CONFETTI APPLESLAW

2 tablespoons orange or apple juice concentrate, thawed
1 unpeeled red apple, cored and diced
4 cups shredded cabbage
2 small red onions, finely shredded
1 red or green bell pepper, thinly sliced
3 tablespoons raisins
1 tablespoon reduced-calorie mayonnaise
½ cup plain low-fat yogurt
½ teaspoon dry mustard
Paprika to taste
Freshly ground black pepper to taste

In large bowl, combine juice concentrate and diced apple. Add cabbage, onions, bell pepper, and raisins. In small bowl, stir together mayonnaise, yogurt, mustard, paprika, and black pepper. Add to vegetable mixture. Cover tightly and refrigerate until ready to serve.   Makes 7 servings

NUTRITIONAL INFORMATION PER SERVING

Calories	69.78	kc	Niacin (B_3)	0.34	mg
Protein	2.11	g	Pantothenic Acid	0.24	mg
Fat	1.08	g	Phosphorus	52.28	mg
% of Calories			Potassium	298.40	mg
from Fat:	13		Pyridoxine (B_6)	0.14	mg
Saturated Fat	0.27	g	Riboflavin (B_2)	0.07	mg
Cholesterol	1.71	mg	Thiamin (B_1)	0.07	mg
Dietary Fiber	2.24	g	Vitamin A	18.71	RE
Sodium	24.46	mg	Vitamin C	42.21	mg
Beta-Carotene	26.57	RE	Copper	0.06	mg
Calcium	64.11	mg	Folate	44.62	µg
Cobalamin (B_{12})	0.09	µg	Vitamin D	0.02	µg
Iron	0.53	mg	Vitamin E	2.52	mg
Magnesium	17.44	mg	Zinc	0.32	mg

SALADS
GOLDEN FRUIT SALAD

1 **Golden Delicious or Crispin apple, cored and sliced**

1 **Red Delicious or Empire apple, cored and sliced**

1 **banana, peeled and sliced**

½ **cup red or green grapes**

Lettuce

Orange Yogurt Dressing (recipe follows)

Combine fruit; mix well. Serve on lettuce-lined salad plates with Orange Yogurt Dressing.

Makes 3 servings

Orange Yogurt Dressing: Combine ½ cup plain low-fat yogurt, 2 to 3 tablespoons orange juice and dash nutmeg; mix well.

NUTRITIONAL INFORMATION PER SERVING

Calories	136.60	kc	Niacin (B_3)	0.44	mg
Protein	2.81	g	Pantothenic Acid	0.40	mg
Fat	1.27	g	Phosphorus	73.55	mg
% of Calories			Potassium	414.80	mg
from Fat:	8		Pyridoxine (B_6)	0.32	mg
Saturated Fat	0.56	g	Riboflavin (B_2)	0.15	mg
Cholesterol	2.33	mg	Thiamin (B_1)	0.08	mg
Dietary Fiber	3.04	g	Vitamin A	19.43	RE
Sodium	28.12	mg	Vitamin C	16.99	mg
Beta-Carotene	71.62	RE	Copper	0.11	mg
Calcium	82.23	mg	Folate	20.74	µg
Cobalamin (B_{12})	0.21	µg	Vitamin E	0.97	mg
Iron	0.40	mg	Zinc	0.45	mg
Magnesium	24.39	mg			

CURRY RICE SALAD
WITH APPLES

- ⅓ cup plain or vanilla yogurt
- 1½ tablespoons dry sherry or cider vinegar
- 1 to 2 teaspoons curry powder
- ⅛ teaspoon ground cloves
  Salt and pepper to taste
- ¾ cup finely diced celery
- ¼ to ½ cup currants or raisins
- 2 Empire, McIntosh, or Cortland apples,
  unpeeled and cubed *
- 4 cups cooked brown rice .

In large bowl, combine yogurt, sherry, curry
powder, cloves, salt, and pepper. Mix well. Add
celery, currants, and apples. Mix well. Add rice; mix
well. Salad keeps well for a few days in the refrigerator.

Makes 6 servings

*Mix apples with a small amount of lemon juice to
prevent browning.

NUTRITIONAL INFORMATION PER SERVING

Calories	226.10	kc	Niacin (B₃)	2.15	mg
Protein	4.99	g	Pantothenic Acid	0.70	mg
Fat	0.93	g	Phosphorus	101.30	mg
% of Calories			Potassium	214.70	mg
from Fat:	4		Pyridoxine (B₆)	0.18	mg
Saturated Fat	0.33	g	Riboflavin (B₂)	0.08	mg
Cholesterol	1.17	mg	Selenium	0.03	mg
Dietary Fiber	2.99	g	Thiamin (B₁)	0.25	mg
Sodium	29.69	mg	Vitamin A	9.07	RE
Beta-Carotene	29.20	RE	Vitamin C	5.79	mg
Calcium	63.05	mg	Copper	0.12	mg
Soluble Fiber	0.60	g	Folate	12.66	µg
Cobalamin (B₁₂)	0.11	µg	Vitamin E	0.95	mg
Iron	1.82	mg	Zinc	0.86	mg
Magnesium	26.21	mg			

WILD RICE SEAFOOD SALAD

- ⅓ cup low-fat mayonnaise
- ⅓ cup nonfat sour cream
- ¼ cup low-sodium chili sauce
- 1 tablespoon lemon juice
- 1 teaspoon Dijon-style mustard
- 3 cups cooked wild rice
- ½ cup thin green onion slices
- 1 large tomato, peeled, seeded and diced
- 1 cup thin slices celery
- ½ pound imitation crabmeat
- Salt and pepper (optional)
- Lettuce cups (optional)
- Chopped parsley (optional)

For dressing, in medium bowl, blend mayonnaise, sour cream, chili sauce, lemon juice, and mustard. Refrigerate. Combine wild rice, onions, tomato, celery, and crabmeat. Season with salt and pepper to taste, if desired. Place salad in individual lettuce cups and garnish with parsley, if desired. Serve with dressing.   Makes 6 servings

NUTRITIONAL INFORMATION PER SERVING

Calories	186.40	kc	Pantothenic Acid	0.30	mg
Protein	9.20	g	Phosphorus	187.10	mg
Fat	4.49	g	Potassium	242.40	mg
% of Calories			Pyridoxine (B₆)	0.16	mg
from Fat:	21		Riboflavin (B₂)	0.11	mg
Saturated Fat	0.58	g	Selenium	0.01	mg
Cholesterol	12.00	mg	Thiamin (B₁)	0.08	mg
Dietary Fiber	2.08	g	Vitamin A	57.26	RE
Sodium	372.00	mg	Vitamin C	9.48	mg
Beta-Carotene	245.00	RE	Copper	0.14	mg
Calcium	21.70	mg	Folate	32.31	µg
Cobalamin (B₁₂)	0.61	µg	Vitamin D	0.12	µg
Iron	0.96	mg	Vitamin E	7.78	mg
Magnesium	48.87	mg	Zinc	1.32	mg
Niacin (B₃)	1.32	mg			

SPINACH CHICKPEA SALAD

- 2 tablespoons red wine vinegar
- 2 tablespoons water
- 1 teaspoon sesame oil
- 1 teaspoon lite soy sauce
- 1 teaspoon sugar
- 3 cups spinach
- 2 carrots, sliced
- 1 cup canned chickpeas, drained and rinsed
- 1½ tablespoons sesame seeds

In small bowl, mix vinegar, water, oil, soy sauce, and sugar to make dressing. In salad bowl, toss dressing with spinach, carrots, and chickpeas. Sprinkle with sesame seeds.   Makes 4 servings

NUTRITIONAL INFORMATION PER SERVING

Calories	114.20	kc	Pantothenic Acid	0.10	mg
Protein	4.83	g	Phosphorus	119.90	mg
Fat	4.05	g	Potassium	479.00	mg
% of Calories			Pyridoxine (B$_6$)	0.16	mg
from Fat	30		Riboflavin (B$_2$)	0.13	mg
Saturated Fat	0.57	g	Thiamin (B$_1$)	0.10	mg
Dietary Fiber	5.55	g	Vitamin A	1,295	RE
Sodium	323.60	mg	Vitamin C	17.96	mg
Beta-Carotene	7,773	RE	Copper	0.33	mg
Calcium	107.20	mg	Folate	89.49	µg
Iron	3.30	mg	Vitamin E	4.26	mg
Magnesium	69.60	mg	Zinc	1.09	mg
Niacin (B$_3$)	0.96	mg			

Today's Slim Noodles Romanov

- **8 ounces uncooked noodles**
- **1 cup low-fat yogurt**
- **1 cup low-fat (1%) cottage cheese**
- **¼ cup finely chopped onion**
- **¼ cup chopped fresh parsley**
- **2 tablespoons Worcestershire sauce**
- **½ teaspoon salt**
- **3 drops hot pepper sauce**
- **2 tablespoons grated Wisconsin Parmesan cheese**

Cook and drain noodles. Preheat oven to 350°F. In large bowl, combine all remaining ingredients except Parmesan cheese. Fold in cooked noodles. Spoon into 1½-quart buttered casserole; sprinkle with Parmesan cheese. Bake 30 minutes or until hot.

Makes 6 to 8 servings

NUTRITIONAL INFORMATION PER SERVING

Calories	149.90	kc	Pantothenic Acid	0.36	mg
Protein	9.34	g	Phosphorus	147.00	mg
Fat	2.31	g	Potassium	161.50	mg
% of Calories			Pyridoxine (B_6)	0.07	mg
from Fat:	14		Riboflavin (B_2)	0.19	mg
Saturated Fat	1.00	g	Selenium	0.01	mg
Cholesterol	28.71	mg	Thiamin (B_1)	0.16	mg
Dietary Fiber	0.17	g	Vitamin A	28.22	RE
Sodium	340.00	mg	Vitamin C	9.12	mg
Beta-Carotene	63.06	RE	Copper	0.09	mg
Calcium	107.80	mg	Folate	16.56	µg
Cobalamin (B_{12})	0.43	µg	Vitamin D	0.02	µg
Iron	1.62	mg	Vitamin E	0.30	mg
Magnesium	23.28	mg	Zinc	0.90	mg
Niacin (B_3)	1.21	mg			

NOT FRIED ASIAN RICE

- 2 teaspoons sesame oil
- ¾ cup chopped green onions
- ½ cup chopped red bell pepper
- 2 cloves garlic, minced
- 2 cups water
- 1 cup uncooked converted rice
- 2 egg whites
- 1 tablespoon lite soy sauce
- 2 teaspoons sugar

In large nonstick skillet, heat oil over medium-high heat. Add onions, bell pepper, and garlic; cook and stir 1 minute. Add water; bring to a boil. Reduce heat to low; stir in rice and egg whites. Simmer, stirring frequently, 20 minutes or until rice is tender. Stir in soy sauce and sugar. Cook and stir for 3 to 5 minutes or until sugar caramelizes.

Makes 6 servings

NUTRITIONAL INFORMATION PER SERVING

Calories	147.40	kc	Pantothenic Acid	0.47	mg
Protein	3.78	g	Phosphorus	54.35	mg
Fat	1.79	g	Potassium	120.30	mg
% of Calories			Pyridoxine (B_6)	0.18	mg
from Fat:	11		Riboflavin (B_2)	0.09	mg
Saturated Fat	0.27	g	Selenium	0.01	mg
Dietary Fiber	1.17	g	Thiamin (B_1)	0.21	mg
Sodium	124.60	mg	Vitamin A	61.92	RE
Beta-Carotene	310.00	RE	Vitamin C	21.65	mg
Calcium	30.14	mg	Copper	0.08	mg
Cobalamin (B_{12})	0.02	µg	Folate	11.42	µg
Iron	1.45	mg	Vitamin E	0.75	mg
Magnesium	15.77	mg	Zinc	0.38	mg
Niacin (B_3)	1.24	mg			

PASTA
TOMATO ZUCCHINI PESTO

- 6 ounces uncooked pasta
- 1 cup fresh basil leaves, chopped
- 1 teaspoon sugar
- 1 teaspoon vegetable oil
- 2 cloves garlic, minced
- 1 tablespoon grated Parmesan cheese
- ¼ cup part-skim ricotta cheese
- 1 medium zucchini, sliced
- 2 teaspoons water
- 1 cup quartered cherry tomatoes
- ½ teaspoon salt (optional)

Prepare pasta according to package directions. Rinse
and drain; cover. In food processor or blender
container, process basil, sugar, oil, and garlic until
blended. Add Parmesan and ricotta cheeses; process
until blended. Set aside. Place zucchini in large
casserole dish; add water. Cover; microwave on
HIGH (100% power) 4 minutes. Drain. Stir in
pasta and cheese mixture. Garnish with tomatoes.
Sprinkle with salt, if desired.   Makes 4 servings

NUTRITIONAL INFORMATION PER SERVING

Calories	211.70	kc	Niacin (B₃)	1.82	mg
Protein	9.43	g	Pantothenic Acid	0.47	mg
Fat	4.35	g	Phosphorus	143.30	mg
% of Calories			Potassium	342.20	mg
from Fat:	18		Pyridoxine (B₆)	0.15	mg
Saturated Fat	1.42	g	Riboflavin (B₂)	0.26	mg
Cholesterol	42.70	mg	Thiamin (B₁)	0.31	mg
Dietary Fiber	3.56	g	Vitamin A	158.40	RE
Sodium	67.41	mg	Vitamin C	28.34	mg
Beta-Carotene	631.00	RE	Copper	0.19	mg
Calcium	101.10	mg	Folate	54.71	µg
Cobalamin (B₁₂)	0.22	µg	Vitamin E	1.95	mg
Iron	2.75	mg	Zinc	1.13	mg
Magnesium	43.73	mg			

PASTA

TODAY'S SLIM RICOTTA SPINACH ROLLS

  8 **lasagna noodles, cooked and drained**

Sauce:

  1 **medium onion, finely chopped**
  2 **cloves garlic, minced**
  1 **tablespoon butter**
  3 **cups no-salt-added tomato sauce**
  1 **teaspoon dried oregano, crushed**
  ½ **teaspoon dried thyme, crushed**
  ½ **teaspoon dried basil, crushed**
  ¼ **teaspoon dried marjoram leaves, crushed**

Filling:

  1 **(10-ounce) package frozen chopped spinach**
  1 **cup (8 ounces) Wisconsin part-skim Ricotta cheese**
  2 **tablespoons grated Wisconsin Parmesan cheese**
  ¼ **teaspoon ground nutmeg**
     Dash pepper

For sauce, cook and stir onion and garlic in butter in large skillet over medium heat until tender. Add tomato sauce, oregano, thyme, basil, and marjoram. Reduce heat; simmer 30 minutes, stirring occasionally.

For filling, cook spinach according to package directions. Drain and squeeze out excess water.

Preheat oven to 350°F. In medium bowl, combine spinach, Ricotta cheese, Parmesan cheese, nutmeg, and pepper until thoroughly mixed. Spread mixture evenly along entire length of each noodle. Roll up each noodle lengthwise and place on its side in buttered shallow baking dish. Pour sauce over rolls. Bake 20 to 30 minutes or until hot.

Makes 4 servings

NUTRITIONAL INFORMATION PER SERVING

Calories	498.60	·kc	Niacin (B$_3$)	4.57	mg
Protein	23.74	g	Pantothenic Acid	0.53	mg
Fat	10.24	g	Phosphorus	209.00	mg
% of Calories			Potassium	963.90	mg
from Fat:	18		Pyridoxine (B$_6$)	0.51	mg
Saturated Fat	2.78	g	Riboflavin (B$_2$)	0.66	mg
Cholesterol	104.10	mg	Thiamin (B$_1$)	0.65	mg
Dietary Fiber	7.92	g	Vitamin A	796.10	RE
Sodium	265.80	mg	Vitamin C	33.37	mg
Beta-Carotene	4,343	RE	Copper	0.68	mg
Calcium	309.20	mg	Folate	112.80	µg
Cobalamin (B$_{12}$)	0.36	µg	Vitamin D	0.03	µg
Iron	5.58	mg	Vitamin E	5.33	mg
Magnesium	1,28.50	mg	Zinc	2.39	mg

LINGUINE AND FRESH FRUIT COOLER

- 1 **cup fresh berries**
- 1 **cup (1-inch) honeydew or cantaloupe chunks**
- 1 **cup kiwifruit or plum slices**
- 1/4 **cup lemon juice**
- 1 **teaspoon finely grated orange peel**
- 2 **tablespoons cornstarch**
- 1 1/2 **cups apricot nectar**
- 1 **stick cinnamon**
- 4 **whole cloves**
- 4 **whole allspice berries**
- 1/4 **cup dry white wine**
- 1/2 **pound linguine, vermicelli or angel hair pasta, cooked and drained**
- 1/2 **cup fresh mint leaves**

In large bowl, combine berries, honeydew chunks, kiwifruit slices, lemon juice, and orange peel; set aside. Place cornstarch in 2-quart saucepan. Slowly add apricot nectar, over high heat, stirring until well blended. Add cinnamon stick, cloves, and allspice berries. Bring to a boil, stirring frequently. Reduce heat; simmer, uncovered, 15 minutes or until thick.

Remove cinnamon stick, cloves and allspice berries. Stir apricot mixture into fruit mixture. Add wine and linguine; garnish with mint leaves.

Makes 4 lunch or 8 dessert servings

Tip: The tangy-sweet flavor of kiwifruit has been described as a combination of pineapple, melon, and strawberry. It's high in vitamin C and the little black seeds inside make it a good source of fiber.

NUTRITIONAL INFORMATION PER SERVING

Calories	346.40	kc	Niacin (B_3)	3.17	mg
Protein	8.97	g	Pantothenic Acid	0.54	mg
Fat	2.82	g	Phosphorus	149.30	mg
% of Calories			Potassium	575.00	mg
from Fat:	7		Pyridoxine (B_6)	0.18	mg
Saturated Fat	0.47	g	Riboflavin (B_2)	0.21	mg
Cholesterol	48.96	mg	Thiamin (B_1)	0.37	mg
Dietary Fiber	4.09	g	Vitamin A	226.40	RE
Sodium	23.49	mg	Vitamin C	144.30	mg
Beta-Carotene	1,255	RE	Copper	0.33	mg
Calcium	81.03	mg	Folate	42.04	µg
Cobalamin (B_{12})	0.13	µg	Vitamin E	1.10	mg
Iron	3.69	mg	Zinc	1.17	mg
Magnesium	59.28	mg			

RADIATORE SALAD WITH SALMON AND PAPAYA

1. pound uncooked radiatore or other medium-size pasta
2. tablespoons vegetable oil
   Freshly ground black pepper to taste
1. pound skinless, boneless fresh or frozen salmon fillets, cooked and chopped *or* 2 (7½-ounce) cans salmon, drained and flaked
1. papaya, peeled, seeded, and chopped *or* 1 mango or 2 peaches or 2 nectarines, peeled, seeded, and chopped *or* 1 (15-ounce) can papaya or other fruit in light syrup, drained and chopped
1. cup cherry tomatoes
1. bunch green onions, thinly sliced
1. yellow bell pepper, seeded and chopped
1. medium cucumber, quartered lengthwise and sliced
1. small jalapeño, seeded and finely minced
2. tablespoons chopped fresh cilantro
3. tablespoons rice wine vinegar
3. tablespoons white wine vinegar
3. drops hot pepper sauce

Prepare pasta according to package directions; transfer to medium bowl. Toss warm pasta with oil; season with black pepper. Set aside until cool. Add salmon, papaya, tomatoes, green onions, yellow bell pepper, and cucumber; toss until well mixed.

In small bowl, combine jalapeño, cilantro, vinegars, and hot pepper sauce. Pour over pasta mixture; toss until well coated. Cover; refrigerate until chilled.

Makes 6 to 8 servings

Tip: One serving or more of seafood each week is linked to a lower risk of heart disease. All seafood is low in saturated fat and most is low in cholesterol.

NUTRITIONAL INFORMATION PER SERVING

Calories	343.30	kc	Niacin (B$_3$)	5.66	mg
Protein	21.08	g	Pantothenic Acid	0.92	mg
Fat	8.59	g	Phosphorus	251.80	mg
% of Calories			Potassium	544.60	mg
from Fat:	23		Pyridoxine (B$_6$)	0.34	mg
Saturated Fat	1.32	g	Riboflavin (B$_2$)	0.40	mg
Cholesterol	71.37	mg	Selenium	0.02	mg
Dietary Fiber	3.54	g	Thiamin (B$_1$)	0.46	mg
Sodium	92.51	mg	Vitamin A	215.30	RE
Beta-Carotene	1,098	RE	Vitamin C	41.35	mg
Calcium	54.90	mg	Copper	0.23	mg
Cobalamin (B$_{12}$)	1.84	µg	Folate	27.90	µg
Iron	2.98	mg	Vitamin E	4.24	mg
Magnesium	54.96	mg	Zinc	1.25	mg

PASTA

PASTA PRIMAVERA

- ⅓ cup broccoli flowerettes
- ⅓ cup cauliflower flowerettes
- 1 baby carrot, peeled and cut into julienne strips
- 1 tablespoon premium olive oil
- ⅓ cup *each* red and yellow bell peppers, peeled and cut into julienne strips
- ⅓ cup snow peas
- ¼ cup shiitake, morel, or chanterelle mushrooms
- 1 clove garlic, minced
- 1 (16-ounce) package linguine or other long pasta, cooked and drained
- 4 leaves minced fresh basil *or* 2 teaspoons minced fresh chervil

Steam broccoli, cauliflower, and carrot until crisp-tender, about 3 minutes. Heat olive oil in large skillet over medium heat. Add steamed vegetables, peppers, snow peas, mushrooms, and garlic. Cook and stir for 3 minutes. Toss with hot linguine. Sprinkle with basil; serve immediately.

Makes 4 servings

NUTRITIONAL INFORMATION PER SERVING

Calories	438.70	kc	Niacin (B$_3$)	3.36	mg
Protein	16.15	g	Pantothenic Acid	0.64	mg
Fat	6.62	g	Phosphorus	207.50	mg
% of Calories			Potassium	204.50	mg
from Fat:	14		Pyridoxine (B$_6$)	0.21	mg
Saturated Fat	0.94	g	Riboflavin (B$_2$)	0.48	mg
Cholesterol	97.91	mg	Thiamin (B$_1$)	0.66	mg
Dietary Fiber	5.59	g	Vitamin A	287.90	RE
Sodium	24.05	mg	Vitamin C	28.26	mg
Beta-Carotene	1,563	RE	Copper	0.35	mg
Calcium	32.82	mg	Folate	36.31	µg
Cobalamin (B$_{12}$)	0.42	µg	Vitamin E	1.32	mg
Iron	3.82	mg	Zinc	1.85	mg
Magnesium	61.41	mg			

SEAFOOD

FISH STEAKS WITH PEAR JARDINIÈRE

- 2 teaspoons vegetable oil
- 1 cup thin onion slices
- 1 cup julienne carrot strips
- ½ teaspoon dry mustard
- ¼ teaspoon *each* dried basil leaves, crushed, and dill weed
- 2 fresh California Bartlett pears, cored and quartered
- 1½ pounds firm fish fillets, such as sea bass, haddock, salmon
- 2 tomatoes, sliced
- 1 lemon, thinly sliced

Heat oil in large nonstick skillet. Add onion and carrots; stir to mix well. Cover and cook over medium heat 5 to 10 minutes. Mix mustard, basil, and dill weed in large bowl. Add pears; toss lightly. Add fish, tomatoes, lemon slices, and pear mixture to skillet. Cover; simmer 10 minutes or until fish flakes easily with fork.   Makes 4 servings

NUTRITIONAL INFORMATION PER SERVING

Calories	278.00	kc	Niacin (B₃)	3.91	mg
Protein	33.27	g	Pantothenic Acid	0.33	mg
Fat	6.38	g	Phosphorus	382.50	mg
% of Calories			Potassium	849.80	mg
from Fat:	20		Pyridoxine (B₆)	0.90	mg
Saturated Fat	1.23	g	Riboflavin (B₂)	0.33	mg
Cholesterol	70.55	mg	Thiamin (B₁)	0.31	mg
Dietary Fiber	4.63	g	Vitamin A	898.90	RE
Sodium	132.60	mg	Vitamin C	31.52	mg
Beta-Carotene	4,728	RE	Copper	0.21	mg
Calcium	48.70	mg	Folate	38.60	µg
Cobalamin (B₁₂)	0.60	µg	Vitamin D	0.03	µg
Iron	1.30	mg	Vitamin E	5.34	mg
Magnesium	91.56	mg	Zinc	0.98	mg

BAKED SOLE PACIFICA

- 1 can (16 ounces) California cling peach slices in juice or extra light syrup
- 4 sole fillets (about 1 pound)
- ½ teaspoon dill weed
- 1 tablespoon olive oil
- 2 onions, cut into wedges
- 4 cups julienned zucchini strips
- 2 cups red pepper strips
- ½ teaspoon herb pepper seasoning

Preheat broiler. Drain peaches, reserving liquid. Place fish on broiler pan. Brush both sides of fillets with peach liquid; sprinkle with dill. Broil about 4 inches from heat 10 minutes, or until fish flakes easily with fork, turning halfway through cooking. Heat oil over medium-high heat in large skillet. Add onions; cook and stir until crisp-tender. Stir in zucchini; cook and stir 2 minutes. Add red peppers and peach slices. Cook until heated through. Stir in seasoning. Place peach mixture on serving plate; top with fish. Makes 4 servings

NUTRITIONAL INFORMATION PER SERVING

Calories	240.50	kc	Niacin (B_3)	3.80	mg
Protein	22.55	g	Pantothenic Acid	0.77	mg
Fat	5.18	g	Phosphorus	321.40	mg
% of Calories			Potassium	969.70	mg
from Fat:	18		Pyridoxine (B_6)	0.68	mg
Saturated Fat	0.86	g	Riboflavin (B_2)	0.20	mg
Cholesterol	53.20	mg	Selenium	0.01	mg
Dietary Fiber	6.19	g	Thiamin (B_1)	0.28	mg
Sodium	95.65	mg	Vitamin A	155.10	RE
Beta-Carotene	364.70	RE	Vitamin C	119.90	mg
Calcium	61.28	mg	Copper	0.26	mg
Cobalamin (B_{12})	1.96	µg	Folate	75.96	µg
Iron	1.82	mg	Vitamin E	2.98	mg
Magnesium	96.87	mg	Zinc	1.11	mg

SEAFOOD
CHINESE STEAMED FISH

- 12 ounces firm white fish fillets, such as swordfish
  Pepper
- 2 teaspoons cornstarch
- 2 teaspoons low-sodium soy sauce
- 2 teaspoons dry sherry
- 1 tablespoon finely chopped green onion
- ¼ teaspoon minced ginger root
- 1 garlic clove, minced
- 1½ fresh California peaches, sliced (1½ cups)

Cut fish lengthwise into 2-inch-wide strips. Sprinkle with pepper to taste. Combine cornstarch, soy sauce, and sherry in small bowl. Add fish to cornstarch mixture; turn fish to coat. Arrange fish strips in spirals in small, shallow baking dish and sprinkle with onion, ginger, garlic, and peaches. Place low rack in large skillet. Pour hot water into bottom of skillet, under rack; bring to a boil. Place baking dish on rack. Cover. Steam 10 to 15 minutes or just until fish flakes easily with fork. Transfer fish and peaches to serving dish using wide spatula. Spoon sauce over fish, if desired. Makes 4 servings

NUTRITIONAL INFORMATION PER SERVING

Calories	128.60	kc	Niacin (B$_3$)	8.25	mg
Protein	17.29	g	Pantothenic Acid	0.08	mg
Fat	3.45	g	Phosphorus	233.20	mg
% of Calories	from Fat:	25	Potassium	323.10	mg
Saturated Fat	0.94	g	Pyridoxine (B$_6$)	0.28	mg
Cholesterol	33.52	mg	Riboflavin (B$_2$)	0.10	mg
Dietary Fiber	0.58	g	Thiamin (B$_1$)	0.04	mg
Sodium	176.70	mg	Vitamin A	51.08	RE
Beta-Carotene	145.50	RE	Vitamin C	3.66	mg
Calcium	8.38	mg	Copper	0.14	mg
Cobalamin (B$_{12}$)	1.34	µg	Folate	4.21	µg
Iron	0.84	mg	Vitamin E	1.23	mg
Magnesium	26.68	mg	Zinc	1.05	mg

Seafood

Dilled Tuna Sandwiches

- 1 can (12½ ounces) chunk light tuna in water, drained
- ¼ cup thinly sliced green onion with tops
- ¼ cup chopped seeded cucumber
- 3 tablespoons reduced-calorie mayonnaise
- 1½ teaspoons drained capers
- 1 teaspoon Dijon-style mustard
- ½ to 1 teaspoon lemon juice
- ¾ teaspoon dried dill weed
  White pepper
- 4 slices multigrain bread, toasted
- 8 slices cucumber
- 2 slices tomato, cut into halves

Break tuna into chunks in small bowl; add green onion and cucumber. Stir in mayonnaise, capers, mustard, lemon juice, and dill weed; season with pepper to taste. Spread tuna mixture on toasted bread slices (open-faced); garnish with cucumber and tomato slices.   Makes 4 servings

NUTRITIONAL INFORMATION PER SERVING

Calories	200.00	kc	Niacin (B₃)	12.07	mg
Protein	24.58	g	Pantothenic Acid	0.22	mg
Fat	5.57	g	Phosphorus	187.40	mg
% of Calories			Potassium	213.70	mg
from Fat:	24		Pyridoxine (B₆)	0.13	mg
Saturated Fat	0.58	g	Riboflavin (B₂)	0.21	mg
Cholesterol	19.69	mg	Selenium	0.01	mg
Dietary Fiber	1.07	g	Thiamin (B₁)	0.12	mg
Sodium	179.90	mg	Vitamin A	46.49	RE
Beta-Carotene	155.10	RE	Vitamin C	2.85	mg
Calcium	41.98	mg	Copper	0.09	mg
Cobalamin (B₁₂)	2.35	µg	Folate	22.57	µg
Iron	2.08	mg	Vitamin D	0.11	µg
Magnesium	39.99	mg	Vitamin E	7.02	mg

LOBSTER WILD RICE BISQUE

- 2 tablespoons light margarine
- 1 cup chopped onion
- 1 can (4 ounces) sliced mushrooms, drained
- 1 tablespoon all-purpose flour
- 2 teaspoons rosemary leaves, crushed
- ½ teaspoon salt
- ½ teaspoon pepper
- 4 cups low-sodium chicken broth
- 1 cup skim milk
- ¼ cup cooking sherry
- 2 cups cooked wild rice
- 1 cup chopped canned tomatoes
- 6 ounces imitation lobster, in 1-inch chunks
- 1 cup shredded low fat Cheddar cheese

Heat margarine in large skillet until melted. Add onion and mushrooms; cook and stir until tender. Stir in flour, rosemary, salt, and pepper. Cook until bubbly. Gradually stir in broth; bring to a boil, stirring often. Stir in milk and sherry. Add rice, tomatoes, and lobster. Cook until heated through. Fold in cheese.   Makes 10 servings

NUTRITIONAL INFORMATION PER SERVING

Calories	134.50	kc	Pantothenic Acid	0.28	mg
Protein	9.07	g	Phosphorus	125.20	mg
Fat	3.97	g	Potassium	199.10	mg
% of Calories			Pyridoxine (B$_6$)	0.11	mg
from Fat:	26		Riboflavin (B$_2$)	0.12	mg
Saturated Fat	1.46	g	Selenium	0.01	mg
Cholesterol	14.59	mg	Thiamin (B$_1$)	0.08	mg
Dietary Fiber	1.20	g	Vitamin A	62.43	RE
Sodium	436.00	mg	Vitamin C	4.89	mg
Beta-Carotene	86.86	RE	Copper	0.12	mg
Calcium	132.30	mg	Folate	18.52	µg
Cobalamin (B$_{12}$)	0.19	µg	Vitamin D	0.56	µg
Iron	0.94	mg	Vitamin E	0.55	mg
Magnesium	23.38	mg	Zinc	1.05	mg
Niacin (B$_3$)	1.83	mg			

SNAPPER FILLETS WITH ORANGE-SHALLOT SAUCE

- 2 Florida oranges
- 6 red snapper* fillets (about 2¼ pounds)
- 1 tablespoon olive oil
- 1 cup finely chopped shallots
- 2 cloves garlic, minced
- 3 tablespoons all-purpose flour
- 1 cup chicken broth
- 1 cup Florida orange juice
- 1 tablespoon grated orange peel
- 2 tablespoons cooking sherry
- 1½ teaspoons dried oregano leaves, crushed
  Salt and pepper to taste
- 2 tablespoons chopped parsley for garnish

Preheat broiler. Thinly slice oranges; set aside. Place fillets, skin side down, on nonstick jelly-roll pan. Broil about 4 inches from heat source 5 to 8 minutes until fish flakes easily with fork. Remove from broiler; set aside.

Meanwhile, in large nonstick skillet, heat oil over medium-high heat until hot. Add shallots and garlic; cook and stir 3 to 4 minutes until shallots begin to brown. Add flour; cook and stir about 30 seconds or until well blended. Stir in broth, orange juice, orange peel, sherry, oregano, salt, and pepper. Bring to a boil, stirring constantly, until slightly thickened. Add orange slices and fish fillets, skin side up. Cook

1 to 2 minutes until fish is heated through and orange slices are slightly softened. Garnish with parsley, if desired. Serve immediately.

Makes 6 servings

*You may substitute any lightly textured fish, such as tuna, flounder, grouper, swordfish, or scrod, for red snapper.

Tip: While fish broils, prepare the sauce, then assemble. Total preparation and cooking time is 15 minutes.

NUTRITIONAL INFORMATION PER SERVING

Calories	282.00	kc	Niacin (B_3)	1.53	mg
Protein	37.09	g	Pantothenic Acid	0.29	mg
Fat	5.48	g	Phosphorus	313.70	mg
% of Calories			Potassium	990.90	mg
from Fat:	18		Pyridoxine (B_6)	0.15	mg
Saturated Fat	0.91	g	Riboflavin (B_2)	0.07	mg
Cholesterol	62.42	mg	Thiamin (B_1)	0.20	mg
Dietary Fiber	1.54	g	Vitamin A	353.40	RE
Sodium	316.00	mg	Vitamin C	44.14	mg
Beta-Carotene	2,074	RE	Copper	0.16	mg
Calcium	96.75	mg	Folate	41.51	µg
Cobalamin (B_{12})	0.04	µg	Vitamin E	0.58	mg
Iron	1.15	mg	Zinc	0.84	mg
Magnesium	66.07	mg			

SEAFOOD

FLORIDA GRAPEFRUIT MARINATED SHRIMP

- 1 cup frozen Florida grapefruit juice concentrate, thawed
- 2 cloves garlic, minced
- 3 tablespoons chopped cilantro or parsley
- 1 tablespoon honey
- 2 teaspoons ketchup
- ½ teaspoon salt
- ¼ teaspoon red pepper flakes
- 1 pound medium shrimp, shelled and deveined
- 2 teaspoons cornstarch
- 1 cup uncooked long-grain white rice
- 1 tablespoon olive oil
- 1 large red bell pepper, cut into strips
- 2 ribs celery, sliced diagonally into ¼-inch-thick slices
- 2 Florida grapefruit, peeled and sectioned

Combine grapefruit juice concentrate, garlic, cilantro, honey, ketchup, salt, and red pepper flakes in medium bowl. Stir in shrimp. Marinate 20 minutes, turning shrimp once. Drain shrimp, reserving marinade; set shrimp aside. Combine reserved marinade and cornstarch. Meanwhile, prepare rice according to package directions.

Heat oil over medium-high heat in large nonstick skillet; add shrimp. Cook and stir 2 to 3 minutes until shrimp turn orange and just begin to caramelize. Add red bell pepper, celery, and reserved marinade. Bring to a boil over high heat until shrimp turn opaque and marinade thickens slightly, stirring constantly. Add grapefruit and heat 30 seconds. Garnish with fresh sprigs of cilantro. Serve over rice.   Makes 4 servings

NUTRITIONAL INFORMATION PER SERVING

Calories	441.60	kc	Niacin (B_3)	5.20	mg
Protein	24.29	g	Pantothenic Acid	1.28	mg
Fat	5.14	g	Phosphorus	226.90	mg
% of Calories			Potassium	772.40	mg
from Fat:	10		Pyridoxine (B_6)	0.42	mg
Saturated Fat	0.90	g	Riboflavin (B_2)	0.14	mg
Cholesterol	174.20	mg	Selenium	0.07	mg
Dietary Fiber	3.02	g	Thiamin (B_1)	0.46	mg
Sodium	518.90	mg	Vitamin A	138.50	RE
Beta-Carotene	322.50	RE	Vitamin C	137.10	mg
Calcium	99.68	mg	Copper	0.43	mg
Cobalamin (B_{12})	1.33	µg	Folate	41.37	µg
Iron	5.61	mg	Vitamin E	6.51	mg
Magnesium	79.79	mg	Zinc	2.19	mg

ORIENTAL BAKED SEAFOOD

- ¼ cup chopped California almonds
- 2 cups water
- ½ teaspoon salt
- 1 cup uncooked long-grain white rice
- 1 tablespoon sesame oil
- 1 tablespoon grated ginger root
- 1 teaspoon grated lemon peel
- 1 pound halibut
- ½ pound large scallops
- ¼ pound medium shrimp, shelled and deveined
- 1 clove garlic, minced
- 1 tablespoon light soy sauce
- ½ cup slivered green onions

Preheat oven to 350°F. Spread almonds in shallow baking pan. Toast in oven 5 to 8 minutes until lightly browned, stirring occasionally; cool. Bring water and salt to a boil in medium saucepan. Stir in rice, sesame oil, ginger root, and lemon peel. Bring to a boil; cover and reduce heat to low. Simmer 20 to 25 minutes until water is absorbed. Meanwhile, preheat oven to 400°F or preheat broiler or grill. Remove skin and bones from halibut; cut into large pieces. Cut 4 (12-inch) squares of foil. Divide halibut, scallops, and shrimp among foil squares. Sprinkle seafood with garlic and soy sauce; seal squares tightly. Bake 12 minutes or broil or grill 4 inches from heat 15 minutes, turning once. Stir almonds into rice. Pour seafood mixture and juices over rice. Sprinkle with green onions.

Makes 4 servings

Microwave Directions: Spread almonds in shallow pan. Microwave on HIGH (100%) power 2 minutes, stirring often; cool. Combine water, salt, rice, sesame oil, ginger root, and lemon peel in 3-quart microwave-safe dish. Cover with plastic wrap. Microwave on HIGH 12 minutes, stirring halfway through. Let stand 10 minutes. Prepare fish packets as directed on parchment paper instead of foil. Bring edges up and seal with rubber band. Place packets in microwave-safe baking dish halfway through. Microwave on HIGH 5 minutes, rotating dish, halfway through. Serve as directed.

NUTRITIONAL INFORMATION PER SERVING

Calories	417.20	kc	Niacin (B₃)	9.77	mg
Protein	43.13	g	Pantothenic Acid	0.69	mg
Fat	7.84	g	Phosphorus	510.30	mg
% of Calories			Potassium	887.40	mg
from Fat:	17		Pyridoxine (B₆)	0.57	mg
Saturated Fat	0.97	g	Riboflavin (B₂)	0.23	mg
Cholesterol	98.69	mg	Selenium	0.12	mg
Dietary Fiber	1.49	g	Thiamin (B₁)	0.37	mg
Sodium	628.80	mg	Vitamin A	124.20	RE
Beta-Carotene	300.10	RE	Vitamin C	7.76	mg
Calcium	121.90	mg	Copper	0.30	mg
Cobalamin (B₁₂)	2.41	µg	Folate	20.71	µg
Iron	4.37	mg	Vitamin E	3.49	mg
Magnesium	173.60	mg	Zinc	2.17	mg

CALIFORNIA BLACKENED SNAPPER

- 1 can (16 ounces) California cling peach halves in juice or extra light syrup
- 1 tablespoon sweet paprika
- 1 teaspoon onion powder
- 1 teaspoon garlic powder
- ¾ teaspoon white pepper
- ¾ teaspoon black pepper
- ½ teaspoon ground red pepper (cayenne)
- ½ teaspoon dried thyme leaves, crushed
- ½ teaspoon dried oregano leaves, crushed
- 6 red snapper fillets (about 1½ pounds)
- 2 tablespoons soft tub margarine

Drain peaches, reserving liquid; set aside. Combine paprika, onion powder, garlic powder, white pepper, black pepper, and red pepper, thyme and oregano; mix well. Dip fish fillet in reserved peach liquid. Sprinkle both sides of each fish fillet with paprika mixture.

Heat 10-inch skillet on high heat for 5 minutes. Carefully place half the fish fillets in skillet. Cut margarine into small pieces; add half to skillet. (Skillet will smoke as margarine pieces are added.) Cook about 1½ to 2 minutes on each side or until fish flakes easily with fork. Repeat with remaining fish fillets and margarine. Fan peach halves over fish fillets to serve.   Makes 6 servings

Tip: There are over 250 species of snapper. The fish used in this recipe, red snapper, is by far the most popular. Red snapper's firm-textured flesh contains very little fat and is suitable for virtually any type of cooking.

NUTRITIONAL INFORMATION PER SERVING

Calories	187.30	kc	Pantothenic Acid	0.04	mg
Protein	24.02	g	Phosphorus	196.10	mg
Fat	5.63	g	Potassium	567.90	mg
% of Calories			Pyridoxine (B_6)	0.02	mg
from Fat:	27		Riboflavin (B_2)	0.05	mg
Saturated Fat	1.11	g	Thiamin (B_1)	0.08	mg
Cholesterol	41.61	mg	Vitamin A	156.60	RE
Dietary Fiber	0.77	g	Vitamin C	3.53	mg
Sodium	98.54	mg	Copper	0.09	mg
Beta-Carotene	422.90	RE	Folate	2.67	µg
Calcium	49.28	mg	Vitamin D	0.37	µg
Iron	0.96	mg	Vitamin E	3.50	mg
Magnesium	40.46	mg	Zinc	0.54	mg
Niacin (B_3)	1.15	mg			

POULTRY
TURKEY WILD RICE CHILI

- 1 tablespoon canola oil
- 1 medium onion, chopped
- 1 garlic clove, minced
- 1¼ pounds turkey breast slices, cut into ½-inch pieces
- 2 cups cooked wild rice
- 1 can (15 ounces) great northern white beans, drained
- 1 can (11 ounces) white corn (optional)
- 2 cans (4 ounces) diced green chilies
- 1 can (14½ ounces) low-sodium chicken broth
- 1 teaspoon ground cumin
  Hot pepper sauce (optional)
- 4 ounces low-fat Monterey Jack cheese, shredded

Heat oil in large pan over medium heat; add onion and garlic. Cook until tender. Add turkey, wild rice, beans, corn, chilies, broth, and cumin. Cover and simmer over low heat 30 minutes or until turkey is tender. Stir hot pepper sauce into chili to taste. Serve with shredded cheese.   Makes 8 servings

NUTRITIONAL INFORMATION PER SERVING

Calories	272.00	kc	Magnesium	67.11	mg
Protein	26.00	g	Niacin (B$_3$)	4.95	mg
Fat	5.75	g	Pantothenic Acid	0.79	mg
% of Calories			Phosphorus	315.30	mg
from Fat:	19		Potassium	529.70	mg
Saturated Fat	1.36	g	Pyridoxine (B$_6$)	0.40	mg
Cholesterol	35.96	mg	Riboflavin (B$_2$)	0.25	mg
Dietary Fiber	1.88	g	Thiamin (B$_1$)	0.16	mg
Sodium	199.10	mg	Vitamin A	40.64	RE
Beta-Carotene	64.92	RE	Vitamin C	27.51	mg
Soluble Fiber	0.31	g	Copper	0.19	mg
Calcium	202.10	mg	Folate	80.88	µg
Cobalamin (B$_{12}$)	0.28	µg	Vitamin E	0.47	mg
Iron	2.58	mg	Zinc	2.44	mg

TURKEY PISTACHIO SANDWICH

- ½ **cup plain yogurt**
- ¼ **cup salted pistachio nuts, chopped**
- 1 **teaspoon dried dill weed**
- 4 **lettuce leaves**
- 8 **slices whole wheat bread**
- 8 **ounces cooked turkey breast, sliced**

In small bowl, combine yogurt, pistachio nuts, and dill weed. Cover and refrigerate at least 1 hour or overnight to allow flavors to blend.

To serve, place 1 lettuce leaf on bread slice; top with ¼ of turkey. Spoon 2 tablespoons yogurt mixture over turkey; top with bread slice. If desired, repeat with remaining ingredients. Turkey mixture will keep up to four days in refrigerator.

Makes 4 servings

NUTRITIONAL INFORMATION PER SERVING

Calories	283.90	kc	Niacin (B₃)	6.03	mg
Protein	25.93	g	Pantothenic Acid	1.10	mg
Fat	6.83	g	Phosphorus	340.00	mg
% of Calories			Potassium	503.70	mg
from Fat:	21		Pyridoxine (B₆)	0.47	mg
Saturated Fat	1.29	g	Riboflavin (B₂)	0.23	mg
Cholesterol	50.70	mg	Selenium	0.01	mg
Dietary Fiber	4.34	g	Thiamin (B₁)	0.23	mg
Sodium	349.60	mg	Vitamin A	14.15	RE
Beta-Carotene	18.10	RE	Vitamin C	1.59	mg
Calcium	129.00	mg	Copper	0.24	mg
Cobalamin (B₁₂)	0.38	µg	Folate	53.32	µg
Iron	3.06	mg	Vitamin E	1.30	mg
Magnesium	68.27	mg	Zinc	2.36	mg

CRUNCHY APPLE SALSA WITH GRILLED CHICKEN

   2 cups Washington Gala apples, halved, cored, and chopped
  ¾ cup (1 large) Anaheim chile pepper, seeded and chopped
  ½ cup chopped onion
  ¼ cup lime juice
     Salt and pepper to taste
     Grilled Chicken (recipe follows)

Combine all ingredients except chicken and mix well; allow flavors to blend about ½ hour. Serve salsa over or alongside Grilled Chicken.

Makes 4 servings (3 cups salsa)

Grilled Chicken: Marinate 2 whole boneless, skinless chicken breasts in a mixture of ¼ cup dry white wine, ¼ cup apple juice, ½ teaspoon grated lime peel, ½ teaspoon salt and dash pepper for 20 to 30 minutes. Drain and grill over medium-hot coals, turning once, until center is no longer pink.

NUTRITIONAL INFORMATION PER SERVING

Calories	272.00	kc	Magnesium	67.11	mg
Protein	26.00	g	Niacin (B_3)	4.95	mg
Fat	5.75	g	Pantothenic Acid	0.79	mg
% of Calories			Phosphorus	315.30	mg
from Fat:	19		Potassium	529.70	mg
Saturated Fat	1.36	g	Pyridoxine (B_6)	0.40	mg
Cholesterol	35.96	mg	Riboflavin (B_2)	0.25	mg
Dietary Fiber	1.88	g	Thiamin (B_1)	0.16	mg
Sodium	199.10	mg	Vitamin A	40.64	RE
Beta-Carotene	64.92	RE	Vitamin C	27.51	mg
Soluble Fiber	0.31	g	Copper	0.19	mg
Calcium	202.10	mg	Folate	80.88	µg
Cobalamin (B_{12})	0.28	µg	Vitamin E	0.47	mg
Iron	2.58	mg	Zinc	2.44	mg

Poultry
Turkey-Potato Casserole

- ½ cup chopped green bell pepper
- ½ cup sliced green onions
- 3 tablespoons margarine
- 1 can (15 ounces) cream-style corn
- 2 cups skim milk
- ½ teaspoon salt
- ⅛ teaspoon ground black pepper
- 2 cups cooked turkey, cut into ½-inch cubes
- 2 cups instant potato flakes
- ¼ cup grated Parmesan cheese
- 2 tablespoons sliced green onion tops

Preheat oven to 375°F. In large saucepan, over medium-high heat, cook and stir bell pepper and sliced onions in margarine until tender. Add corn, milk, salt and pepper. Reduce heat and cook until mixture bubbles; remove from heat. Fold in turkey and potato flakes. Pour turkey mixture into greased 9-inch square casserole. Sprinkle with cheese and onion tops. Bake 25 minutes or until lightly browned.
Makes 6 servings

NUTRITIONAL INFORMATION PER SERVING

Calories	300.70	kc	Niacin (B$_3$)	3.70	mg
Protein	18.83	g	Pantothenic Acid	0.78	mg
Fat	7.67	g	Phosphorus	244.90	mg
% of Calories			Potassium	776.50	mg
from Fat:	23		Pyridoxine (B$_6$)	0.35	mg
Saturated Fat	2.14	g	Riboflavin (B$_2$)	0.24	mg
Cholesterol	36.13	mg	Selenium	0.01	mg
Dietary Fiber	1.48	g	Thiamin (B$_1$)	0.09	mg
Sodium	619.10	mg	Vitamin A	189.00	RE
Beta-Carotene	308.90	RE	Vitamin C	24.72	mg
Soluble Fiber	0.19	g	Copper	0.13	mg
Calcium	175.00	mg	Folate	44.23	µg
Cobalamin (B$_{12}$)	0.52	µg	Vitamin D	1.42	µg
Iron	1.18	mg	Vitamin E	4.44	mg
Magnesium	38.31	mg	Zinc	1.55	mg

TURKEY SPLIT PEA SOUP

- 1 pound dried split peas, washed and drained
- 7 cups Turkey Broth (page 445) *or* low sodium chicken bouillon
- 2 cups chopped onions
- 1 cup chopped carrots
- ½ cup chopped celery
- 1 clove garlic, minced
- 3 tablespoons dried parsley
- 1 bay leaf
- 1 pound turkey ham, cut into ½-inch cubes

In 5-quart saucepan, over high heat, combine peas, Turkey Broth, onions, carrots, celery, garlic, parsley, and bay leaf; bring to a boil. Reduce heat to simmer; cover and cook 1 hour. Remove saucepan from heat; discard bay leaf.

With wire whisk, gently whisk soup to blend peas. If desired, soup may be puréed in blender for smoother texture.

Return soup to medium-high heat, add turkey ham and bring to a boil. Reduce heat to simmer, and cook, uncovered, 10 to 15 minutes.

Makes 8 servings

TURKEY BROTH

- 4 cups water
  Turkey giblets
- 1 stalk celery, sliced
- 1 carrot, sliced
- 1 onion, sliced
- 1 bay leaf
- 3 sprigs parsley
- 4 peppercorns

In large saucepan, over high heat, bring water, giblets, celery, carrot, onion, bay leaf, parsley, and peppercorns to a boil. Reduce heat to low, cover and simmer 1 hour.

Strain broth and refrigerate until needed. Store giblets in refrigerator until ready to make gravy or dressing.

NUTRITIONAL INFORMATION PER SERVING

Calories	242.50	kc	Niacin (B_0)	5.26	mg
Protein	23.42	g	Pantothenic Acid	0.09	mg
Fat	4.15	g	Phosphorus	232.10	mg
% of Calories			Potassium	662.80	mg
from Fat:	15		Pyridoxine (B_6)	0.27	mg
Saturated Fat	1.05	g	Riboflavin (B_2)	0.37	mg
Cholesterol	33.94	mg	Thiamin (B_1)	0.26	mg
Dietary Fiber	7.18	g	Vitamin A	400.60	RE
Sodium	754.10	mg	Vitamin C	5.37	mg
Beta-Carotene	2,331	RE	Copper	0.38	mg
Calcium	51.94	mg	Folate	88.58	µg
Cobalamin (B_{12})	0.14	µg	Vitamin E	3.29	mg
Iron	4.53	mg	Zinc	2.99	mg
Magnesium	57.89	mg			

APRICOT-STUFFED TURKEY THIGHS

- ⅓ cup dried apricots, chopped
- 2 tablespoons raisins, chopped
- 1 small clove garlic, minced
- ¼ cup green onions, finely chopped
- ½ cup celery, finely chopped
- ⅔ cup plain dry bread cubes
- 1½ pounds boneless turkey thighs, skin removed

Creamy Mustard Sauce:

- 1 teaspoon cornstarch
- ⅓ cup reduced-sodium chicken bouillon
- 1½ teaspoons country-style (grainy) mustard
- 1½ teaspoons honey
- 1 teaspoon lemon juice
- 3 tablespoons reduced-calorie mayonnaise

Preheat oven to 325°F.

In medium microwavable bowl, combine apricots and raisins. Cover with hot water. Microwave at HIGH (100% power) 1½ to 2 minutes or until fruit is soft; drain well. Add garlic, onion, celery, and bread cubes. Cover bowl with vented plastic wrap. Microwave at HIGH (100% power) 1½ minutes or until onion and celery are soft. Set aside.

Place turkey thighs between 2 pieces of waxed paper; flatten with meat mallet to ¾-inch thickness. Divide stuffing evenly among thighs. Place stuffing on edge of each flattened thigh. Fold opposite end over stuffing and secure with string or metal skewers.

Arrange thighs, seam side down, on lightly greased rack in shallow roasting pan. Roast 1½ to 1¾ hours or until meat thermometer placed in thigh registers 180° to 185°F.

For Creamy Mustard Sauce, in small saucepan, over medium heat, combine cornstarch, bouillon, mustard, honey, and lemon juice. Cook and stir until sauce thickens. Remove from heat and fold in mayonnaise.

To serve, remove string or skewers from thighs. Slice into rolls and top with Creamy Mustard Sauce.   Makes 4 servings

NUTRITIONAL INFORMATION PER SERVING

Calories	333.30	kc	Pantothenic Acid	1.47	mg
Protein	41.37	g	Phosphorus	321.60	mg
Fat	10.24	g	Potassium	660.60	mg
% of Calories			Pyridoxine (B_6)	0.68	mg
from Fat:	28		Riboflavin (B_2)	0.31	mg
Saturated Fat	2.68	g	Selenium	0.04	mg
Cholesterol	107.80	mg	Thiamin (B_1)	0.13	mg
Dietary Fiber	1.62	g	Vitamin A	106.20	RE
Sodium	179.50	mg	Vitamin C	4.57	mg
Beta-Carotene	637.10	RE	Copper	0.21	mg
Calcium	61.73	mg	Folate	18.14	µg
Cobalamin (B_{12})	0.51	µg	Vitamin D	0.11	µg
Iron	3.43	mg	Vitamin E	7.44	mg
Magnesium	46.93	mg	Zinc	4.42	mg
Niacin (B_3)	8.21	mg			

SHOTGUN BILLY'S TURKEY CHILI WITH BLACK BEANS

- 1 cup coarsely chopped onion
- 1 red bell pepper, cut into ¼-inch cubes
- 2 garlic cloves, minced
- 2 jalapeño peppers, seeded and minced
- 1 can (28 ounces) tomatoes, coarsely chopped, undrained
- 1 tablespoon chili powder
- 1½ teaspoons ground cumin
- 1½ teaspoons ground coriander
- ½ teaspoon dried oregano
- ½ teaspoon dried marjoram
- ¼ teaspoon red pepper flakes
- ¼ teaspoon cinnamon
- 1 can (16 ounces) black beans, drained and rinsed
- 2 cups cooked turkey, cut into ½-inch cubes
- ½ cup fresh cilantro, coarsely chopped
- 4 tablespoons grated reduced-fat Cheddar cheese

In 3-quart microwavable dish combine onion, bell pepper, garlic, jalapeño peppers, and tomatoes. Stir in chili powder, cumin, coriander, oregano, marjoram, red pepper flakes, and cinnamon; cover dish.

Microwave at HIGH (100% power) 10 minutes; stir halfway through. Stir in beans and turkey; cover dish. Microwave at HIGH (100% power) 4 minutes; stir in cilantro.

To serve, ladle into bowls and garnish with cheese.

Makes 4 servings

Note: For full blending of flavors, make one day prior to serving.

Tip: Beans are available in a wide variety—black, pinto, kidney, and navy, to name just a few. They are very high in fiber, and recent studies have shown that eating ½ cup of cooked beans daily may help to reduce cholesterol levels.

NUTRITIONAL INFORMATION PER SERVING

Calories	322.80	kc	Niacin (B_3)	6.76	mg
Protein	32.15	g	Pantothenic Acid	1.10	mg
Fat	3.30	g	Phosphorus	394.60	mg
% of Calories			Potassium	1,231	mg
from Fat:	9		Pyridoxine (B_6)	0.74	mg
Saturated Fat	1.15	g	Riboflavin (B_2)	0.25	mg
Cholesterol	52.24	mg	Selenium	0.01	mg
Dietary Fiber	8.55	g	Thiamin (B_1)	0.44	mg
Sodium	620.90	mg	Vitamin A	264.10	RE
Beta-Carotene	1,549	RE	Vitamin C	61.45	mg
Calcium	180.10	mg	Copper	0.58	mg
Cobalamin (B_{12})	0.28	µg	Folate	218.70	µg
Iron	6.27	mg	Vitamin E	1.22	mg
Magnesium	140.70	mg	Zinc	3.07	mg

435

CHICKEN WITH MANDARIN ORANGE AND WATER CHESTNUT SAUCE

- 2 teaspoons cornstarch
- ¼ cup water
- 1 can (11 ounces) mandarin oranges, drained
- 1 can (8 ounces) sliced water chestnuts, drained
- 4 teaspoons brown sugar
- 2 tablespoons white vinegar
- 1 tablespoon low sodium soy sauce
- 1½ cups chicken broth or stock
- 4 split chicken breast halves, skinned and boned

Dissolve cornstarch in water. In small saucepan, combine mandarin oranges, water chestnuts, brown sugar, vinegar, soy sauce, and cornstarch dissolved in water. Cook over medium-high heat until mixture is clear and thickened, about 4 to 5 minutes, stirring occasionally. Remove from heat.

In large skillet, bring broth to simmer. Pound chicken breasts with meat mallet to ½-inch thickness. Place chicken breasts in skillet; cover and simmer over medium-low heat about 8 to 10 minutes or until chicken is no longer pink in center.

Remove chicken from poaching liquid. Place on serving platter. Heat sauce if needed; spoon sauce over chicken.   Makes 4 servings

Tip: Pounding boned chicken breasts to a uniform thickness allows them to cook faster and more evenly. Place the chicken breast between two pieces of plastic wrap to prevent it from tearing. Using the flat side of a meat mallet, pound the chicken breast with a downward motion until it is evenly flattened.

NUTRITIONAL INFORMATION PER SERVING

Calories	252.60	kc	Niacin (B_3)	13.22	mg
Protein	29.05	g	Pantothenic Acid	0.97	mg
Fat	4.84	g	Phosphorus	252.90	mg
% of Calories			Potassium	447.80	mg
from Fat:	18		Pyridoxine (B_6)	0.67	mg
Saturated Fat	1.03	g	Riboflavin (B_2)	0.20	mg
Cholesterol	73.00	mg	Selenium	0.03	mg
Dietary Fiber	0.48	g	Thiamin (B_1)	0.13	mg
Sodium	754.80	mg	Vitamin A	31.43	RE
Beta-Carotene	157.70	RE	Vitamin C	22.60	mg
Calcium	34.60	mg	Copper	0.19	mg
Cobalamin (B_{12})	0.37	µg	Folate	24.59	µg
Iron	1.84	mg	Vitamin E	0.72	mg
Magnesium	40.09	mg	Zinc	1.38	mg

CHICKEN AND VEGETABLE COUSCOUS

- 1 tablespoon vegetable oil
- 3 (3-ounce) boneless chicken breasts, cut into 3-inch cubes
- 3 garlic cloves, minced
- ½ cup chopped green onions
- 1¼ cups tomato sauce
- 1½ cups water, divided
- 1¼ cups chopped carrots
- 1 large potato, cut into cubes
- 1 yellow squash, chopped
- 1 medium tomato, chopped
- 1 cup canned small white beans, rinsed and drained
- ¼ cup chopped red bell pepper
- ¼ cup raisins
- 2 tablespoons brown sugar
- 2 teaspoons ground cumin
- ¾ teaspoon ground cinnamon
- 3 to 4 drops hot sauce
- 1 cup dry couscous

Place oil in medium skillet. Add chicken breasts and brown over medium heat. Add garlic and green onions; cook and stir for 1 minute. Stir in tomato sauce and ¼ cup water. Add carrots, potato, squash, tomato, beans, red bell pepper, raisins, brown sugar, cumin, cinnamon, and hot sauce. Bring to a simmer and cook 15 minutes.

Meanwhile, bring remaining 1¼ cups water to a boil. Add couscous; cover and remove from heat. Let stand 5 minutes. Serve chicken and vegetables over couscous.   Makes 6 servings

Tip: Couscous is a granular pasta that is a staple in North African cuisine. It is readily available in large supermarkets, usually shelved with rice and other grains.

NUTRITIONAL INFORMATION PER SERVING

Calories	322.40	kc	Niacin (B_3)	6.25	mg
Protein	16.93	g	Pantothenic Acid	1.19	mg
Fat	4.12	g	Phosphorus	229.40	mg
% of Calories			Potassium	833.00	mg
from Fat:	11		Pyridoxine (B_6)	0.50	mg
Saturated Fat	0.71	g	Riboflavin (B_2)	0.17	mg
Cholesterol	21.72	mg	Selenium	0.01	mg
Dietary Fiber	9.25	g	Thiamin (B_1)	0.27	mg
Sodium	347.70	mg	Vitamin A	757.80	RE
Beta-Carotene	4,109	RE	Vitamin C	26.13	mg
Calcium	80.07	mg	Copper	0.39	mg
Soluble Fiber	1.60	g	Folate	70.55	µg
Cobalamin (B_{12})	0.09	µg	Vitamin E	2.51	mg
Iron	3.32	mg	Zinc	1.34	mg
Magnesium	77.37	mg			

LEMON TURKEY STIR-FRY AND PASTA

1   pound linguine or other long pasta
1½ pounds turkey cutlets, cut into ½-inch
     strips
1   tablespoon soy sauce
1   tablespoon white wine vinegar
2   teaspoons cornstarch
1   teaspoon lemon pepper
2   tablespoons olive oil
6   medium green onions, sliced
1   medium fresh lemon, cut into 10 thin slices
     and slivered
1   clove garlic, finely minced
1   (10-ounce) bag fresh spinach, washed,
     drained, and chopped
   Parsley (optional)
   Lemon slices (optional)

In resealable plastic food storage bag, combine turkey cutlets, soy sauce, white wine vinegar, cornstarch, and lemon pepper. Shake bag to coat turkey cutlets thoroughly. Refrigerate 30 minutes to allow flavors to blend. Cook linguine according to package directions; drain.

In large skillet, over medium heat, cook and stir turkey cutlets and marinade in olive oil 2 to 3 minutes or until turkey is no longer pink. Add sliced green onions, lemon slivers, and garlic;

continue to cook until onions are soft. Stir in chopped spinach and cook until spinach is just wilted. Spoon mixture over hot linguine and garnish with parsley and lemon slices, if desired.

Makes 6 servings

NUTRITIONAL INFORMATION PER SERVING

Calories	433.00	kc	Niacin (B$_3$)	7.34	mg
Protein	33.48	g	Pantothenic Acid	0.97	mg
Fat	9.12	g	Phosphorus	314.10	mg
% of Calories			Potassium	579.40	mg
from Fat:	19		Pyridoxine (B$_6$)	0.58	mg
Saturated Fat	1.71	g	Riboflavin (B$_2$)	0.50	mg
Cholesterol	114.80	mg	Thiamin (B$_1$)	0.51	mg
Dietary Fiber	4.57	g	Vitamin A	354.70	RE
Sodium	267.20	mg	Vitamin C	29.97	mg
Beta-Carotene	2,058	RE	Copper	0.34	mg
Calcium	89.48	mg	Folate	112.20	µg
Cobalamin (B$_{12}$)	0.54	µg	Vitamin E	2.43	mg
Iron	4.92	mg	Zinc	2.88	mg
Magnesium	97.85	mg			

TURKEY, CORN, AND SWEET POTATO SOUP

- ½ cup chopped onion
- 1 small jalapeño pepper, minced
- 1 teaspoon margarine
- 5 cups turkey broth *or* reduced-sodium chicken bouillon
- 1½ pounds sweet potatoes, peeled and cut into 1-inch cubes
- 2 cups cooked turkey, cut into ½-inch cubes
- ½ teaspoon salt
- 1½ cups frozen corn
   Cilantro (optional)

In 5-quart saucepan, over medium-high heat, cook and stir onion and pepper in margarine 5 minutes or until onion is soft. Add broth, potatoes, turkey, and salt; bring to a boil. Reduce heat to low; cover and simmer 20 to 25 minutes or until potatoes are tender. Stir in corn. Increase heat to medium and cook 5 to 6 minutes. Spoon 1 cup soup. Garnish with cilantro, if desired.   Makes 8 servings

NUTRITIONAL INFORMATION PER SERVING

Calories	154.70	kc	Niacin (B$_3$)	4.36	mg
Protein	12.14	g	Pantothenic Acid	0.71	mg
Fat	1.27	g	Phosphorus	119.70	mg
% of Calories			Potassium	376.70	mg
from Fat:	7		Pyridoxine (B$_6$)	0.37	mg
Saturated Fat	0.18	g	Riboflavin (B$_2$)	0.20	mg
Cholesterol	23.63	mg	Thiamin (B$_1$)	0.10	mg
Dietary Fiber	3.30	g	Vitamin A	1,462	RE
Sodium	254.20	mg	Vitamin C	18.22	mg
Beta-Carotene	1,863	RE	Copper	0.18	mg
Soluble Fiber	0.43	g	Folate	25.74	µg
Calcium	36.24	mg	Vitamin D	0.05	µg
Cobalamin (B$_{12}$)	0.11	µg	Vitamin E	5.62	mg
Iron	1.32	mg	Zinc	0.82	mg
Magnesium	29.02	mg			

Sweet 'n' Sour with Rice

- 4 (3-ounce) boneless skinless chicken breasts
- 1½ cups water
- ¼ cup vinegar
- 1 cup uncooked converted rice
- 2 tablespoons brown sugar
- 8 ounces canned chunk pineapple, drained, reserving 2 tablespoons juice

Broil chicken for 10 to 15 minutes or until cooked through, turning once. Meanwhile, in medium saucepan, bring water and vinegar to a boil. Add rice and brown sugar. Cover; cook 20 minutes or until water is absorbed and rice is fluffy. Stir in pineapple and reserved juice. Serve chicken over rice.

Makes 4 servings

NUTRITIONAL INFORMATION PER SERVING

Calories	283.80	kc	Niacin (B$_3$)	7.41	mg
Protein	15.94	g	Pantothenic Acid	0.97	mg
Fat	1.75	g	Phosphorus	160.00	mg
% of Calories			Potassium	256.70	mg
from Fat:	6		Pyridoxine (B$_6$)	0.45	mg
Saturated Fat	0.48	g	Riboflavin (B$_2$)	0.10	mg
Cholesterol	34.30	mg	Selenium	0.03	mg
Dietary Fiber	1.29	g	Thiamin (B$_1$)	0.36	mg
Sodium	34.61	mg	Vitamin A	3.39	RE
Beta-Carotene	1.13	RE	Vitamin C	4.36	mg
Calcium	49.36	mg	Copper	0.20	mg
Cobalamin (B$_{12}$)	0.14	µg	Folate	11.88	µg
Iron	2.62	mg	Vitamin E	0.47	mg
Magnesium	37.58	mg	Zinc	0.93	mg

PERUVIAN CHICKEN WITH PLUMS

- 1 chicken (3½ pounds), skinned, cut up
- 1 teaspoon vegetable oil
- 1 cup chopped onion
- 1 cup diced green bell pepper
- 2 teaspoons minced garlic
- 1 tomato, chopped
- 1 fresh jalapeño pepper, seeded, diced
- ¼ teaspoon powdered saffron (optional)
- 3½ cups low-sodium chicken broth
- 1 bay leaf
- 4 fresh California plums, quartered
- 4 cups cooked brown rice

Cook chicken in oil in large nonstick skillet, turning often until golden brown on all sides, about 12 minutes. Add onion, bell pepper, and garlic; cook and stir 2 minutes longer. Add tomato, chili, saffron, broth, and bay leaf. Bring to a boil; cover and simmer 10 minutes. Add plums and rice; heat through. Discard bay leaf.　　　Makes 8 servings

NUTRITIONAL INFORMATION PER SERVING

Calories	344.20	kc	Niacin (B$_3$)	12.04	mg
Protein	33.23	g	Pantothenic Acid	1.50	mg
Fat	9.36	g	Phosphorus	296.80	mg
% of Calories			Potassium	432.10	mg
from Fat:	25		Pyridoxine (B$_6$)	0.75	mg
Saturated Fat	2.32	g	Riboflavin (B$_2$)	0.26	mg
Cholesterol	89.61	mg	Selenium	0.04	mg
Dietary Fiber	3.06	g	Thiamin (B$_1$)	0.22	mg
Sodium	173.90	mg	Vitamin A	50.96	RE
Beta-Carotene	96.78	RE	Vitamin C	30.61	mg
Calcium	42.72	mg	Copper	0.22	mg
Cobalamin (B$_{12}$)	0.33	µg	Folate	23.51	µg
Iron	2.33	mg	Vitamin E	3.62	mg
Magnesium	75.22	mg	Zinc	2.84	mg

PERSIAN CHICKEN

- 2 cups low-sodium chicken broth
- 1 cup cracked wheat
- ½ teaspoon dried basil leaves, crushed
- ½ teaspoon grated lemon peel
- ¼ teaspoon mint flakes
- ¼ cup whole natural California almonds, chopped
- 1 tablespoon almond or olive oil
- ½ cup sliced green onions
- ⅓ cup raisins
- 2 tablespoons chopped parsley
- 1 tablespoon lemon juice
- 1 cup diced cooked chicken or turkey

Combine broth, wheat, basil, lemon peel, and mint flakes in large saucepan; heat to boiling. Cover; reduce heat to low and cook 15 minutes. Meanwhile, lightly brown almonds in oil in small skillet, stirring constantly, over medium heat. When wheat is cooked, add almonds, onions, raisins, parsley, and lemon juice; toss lightly to mix. Add chicken; heat 1 minute before serving.   Makes 3 servings

NUTRITIONAL INFORMATION PER SERVING

Calories	370.30	kc	Magnesium	60.65	mg
Protein	21.70	g	Niacin (B_3)	6.84	mg
Fat	11.29	g	Pantothenic Acid	0.42	mg
% of Calories			Phosphorus	330.10	mg
from Fat:	27		Potassium	410.40	mg
Saturated Fat	0.88	g	Pyridoxine (B_6)	0.28	mg
Cholesterol	31.50	mg	Riboflavin (B_2)	0.31	mg
Dietary Fiber	3.18	g	Thiamin (B_1)	0.25	mg
Sodium	70.45	mg	Vitamin A	84.27	RE
Beta-Carotene	501.20	RE	Vitamin C	12.03	mg
Soluble Fiber	0.32	g	Copper	0.26	mg
Calcium	96.00	mg	Folate	10.32	µg
Cobalamin (B_{12})	0.15	µg	Vitamin E	5.12	mg
Iron	3.93	mg	Zinc	1.27	mg

TURKEY WALDORF SANDWICH

- 6 ounces cooked turkey breast, cubed
- ½ cup diced celery
- 1 small Red Delicious apple, cored and cut into small cubes
- 2 tablespoons walnuts, chopped
- 1 tablespoon reduced-calorie mayonnaise
- 1 tablespoon nonfat yogurt
- ⅛ teaspoon nutmeg
- ⅛ teaspoon cinnamon
- 4 lettuce leaves
- 8 slices reduced-calorie raisin bread

In medium bowl, combine turkey, celery, apple, walnuts, mayonnaise, yogurt, nutmeg, and cinnamon. Cover and refrigerate at least 1 hour to allow flavors to blend. To serve, arrange 1 lettuce leaf on each bread slice. Spoon ¾ cup turkey mixture over lettuce and top with 1 bread slice. Turkey mixture will keep up to four days in refrigerator.   Makes 4 servings

NUTRITIONAL INFORMATION PER SERVING

Calories	187.80	kc	Pantothenic Acid	0.53	mg
Protein	16.37	g	Phosphorus	151.30	mg
Fat	4.72	g	Potassium	335.80	mg
% of Calories			Pyridoxine (B_6)	0.31	mg
from Fat:	22		Riboflavin (B_2)	0.24	mg
Saturated Fat	0.61	g	Selenium	0.01	mg
Cholesterol	36.75	mg	Thiamin (B_1)	0.13	mg
Dietary Fiber	1.95	g	Vitamin A	19.94	RE
Sodium	136.80	mg	Vitamin C	4.38	mg
Beta-Carotene	30.05	RE	Copper	0.13	mg
Calcium	54.39	mg	Folate	30.63	µg
Cobalamin (B_{12})	0.19	µg	Vitamin D	0.04	µg
Iron	1.75	mg	Vitamin E	3.29	mg
Magnesium	32.42	mg	Zinc	1.13	mg
Niacin (B_3)	4.36	mg			

CHICKEN WILD RICE SOUP

- ⅓ cup instant nonfat dry milk
- 2 tablespoons cornstarch
- 2 teaspoons low-sodium instant chicken bouillon
- ¼ teaspoon dried onion flakes
- ¼ teaspoon dried basil
- ¼ teaspoon dried thyme leaves
- ⅛ teaspoon ground black pepper
- 4 cups low sodium chicken broth
- ½ cup sliced celery
- ½ cup sliced carrots
- ½ cup chopped onion
- 2 cups cooked wild rice
- 1 cup cooked cubed chicken breasts

In small bowl, combine dry milk, cornstarch, bouillon, onion flakes, basil, thyme, and pepper. Stir in small amount of chicken broth; set aside. In large saucepan, combine remaining broth, celery, carrots, and onion. Cook until vegetables are crisp-tender. Gradually add dry milk mixture. Stir in wild rice and chicken. Simmer 5 to 10 minutes.

Makes 8 servings

NUTRITIONAL INFORMATION PER SERVING

Calories	102.90	kc	Niacin (B₃)	3.78	mg
Protein	8.48	g	Pantothenic Acid	0.33	mg
Fat	1.11	g	Phosphorus	102.70	mg
% of Calories			Potassium	188.60	mg
from Fat:	10		Pyridoxine (B₆)	0.18	mg
Saturated Fat	0.19	g	Riboflavin (B₂)	0.15	mg
Cholesterol	12.53	mg	Thiamin (B₁)	0.07	mg
Dietary Fiber	1.19	g	Vitamin A	216.00	RE
Sodium	70.21	mg	Vitamin C	2.07	mg
Beta-Carotene	1,169	RE	Copper	0.07	mg
Calcium	54.97	mg	Folate	17.71	µg
Cobalamin (B₁₂)	0.16	µg	Vitamin E	0.30	mg
Iron	0.87	mg	Zinc	0.87	mg
Magnesium	24.00	mg			

STUFFED TURKEY TENDERLOINS

   3   cups cooked wild rice
1¼   pounds boneless turkey tenderloins
   2   cups thawed frozen spinach
¼   cup extra light margarine, softened
¼   cup raisins
¼   cup chopped almonds (optional)
¼   cup chopped onion
   1   teaspoon grated orange peel
   1   teaspoon lemon pepper
¼   teaspoon dried thyme
   1   tablespoon sherry (optional)
   2   tablespoons extra light margarine, melted

Preheat oven to 325°F. Butterfly turkey tenderloin by slicing horizontally, almost cutting all the way through, starting at curved edge. Open each tenderloin. Drain spinach and squeeze out excess liquid. Spoon half the spinach evenly over each butterflied tenderloin.

In large bowl, combine wild rice, ¼ cup margarine, raisins, almonds, onion, orange peel, lemon pepper, thyme, and sherry. Spoon ½ cup wild rice mixture evenly over spinach layers. Roll up each tenderloin, starting at pointed short edge. Secure with string or wooden toothpicks. Set aside.

Grease 2½-quart square baking dish. Spoon remaining wild rice stuffing into dish. Place turkey rolls over stuffing. Cover. Bake 45 minutes. Remove cover; brush with melted margarine and bake 15 minutes more. Slice turkey rolls and serve over stuffing.   Makes 6 servings

Tip: Wild rice is actually *not* a rice, but a cereal grain. It has a nutty flavor and is higher in protein than traditional rice.

NUTRITIONAL INFORMATION PER SERVING

Calories	249.20	kc	Niacin (B₃)	5.44	mg
Protein	23.38	g	Pantothenic Acid	0.60	mg
Fat	8.07	g	Phosphorus	233.50	mg
% of Calories			Potassium	485.40	mg
from Fat:	29		Pyridoxine (B₆)	0.54	mg
Saturated Fat	1.68	g	Riboflavin (B₂)	0.27	mg
Cholesterol	41.29	mg	Thiamin (B₁)	0.12	mg
Dietary Fiber	3.02	g	Vitamin A	662.50	RE
Sodium	229.90	mg	Vitamin C	9.73	mg
Beta-Carotene	3,193	RE	Copper	0.24	mg
Soluble Fiber	0.51	g	Folate	99.66	µg
Calcium	118.10	mg	Vitamin D	1.50	µg
Cobalamin (B₁₂)	0.22	µg	Vitamin E	3.67	mg
Iron	2.53	mg	Zinc	2.83	mg
Magnesium	91.62	mg			

DAD'S TURKEY DAGWOOD

Mock Guacamole (page 451)
16 slices low-calorie whole wheat bread
2 tomatoes, sliced
8 cups shredded iceberg lettuce
2 packages (6 ounces) smoked turkey breast
slices
8 slices (1 ounce *each*) reduced-fat Cheddar
cheese
8 tablespoons sweet hot mustard

Spread 3 tablespoons Mock Guacamole on each
bread slice. Arrange 2 tomato slices, 1 cup lettuce,
2 turkey slices and 1 cheese slice on top of guacamole
on each bread slice.

Spread 1 tablespoon mustard on each remaining
bread slice and place, mustard side down, on top of
each sandwich. To serve, cut each sandwich in half.

Makes 8 servings

MOCK GUACAMOLE

2 large cloves garlic
2 cups frozen peas, cooked and drained
½ cup fresh cilantro
¼ cup chopped onion
1 tablespoon lemon juice
¼ teaspoon ground black pepper
⅛ teaspoon hot pepper sauce

In food processor bowl, process garlic cloves 10 seconds. Add peas, cilantro, onion, lemon juice, black pepper, and hot pepper sauce; process until smooth. Chill at least 1 hour. Makes 8 servings.

NUTRITIONAL INFORMATION PER SERVING

Calories	254.60	kc	Niacin (B_3)	5.50	mg
Protein	23.84	g	Pantothenic Acid	0.37	mg
Fat	8.18	g	Phosphorus	379.10	mg
% of Calories			Potassium	470.40	mg
from Fat:	28		Pyridoxine (B_6)	0.34	mg
Saturated Fat	3.83	g	Riboflavin (B_2)	0.19	mg
Cholesterol	34.94	mg	Selenium	0.01	mg
Dietary Fiber	5.73	g	Thiamin (B_1)	0.28	mg
Sodium	1,044	mg	Vitamin A	102.50	RE
Beta-Carotene	203.40	RE	Vitamin C	17.29	mg
Calcium	269.60	mg	Copper	0.24	mg
Cobalamin (B_{12})	1.10	µg	Folate	88.71	µg
Iron	2.84	mg	Vitamin E	1.93	mg
Magnesium	64.93	mg	Zinc	2.40	mg

WASHINGTON APPLE TURKEY GYROS

- 1 cup onion slices
- 1 cup *each* thinly sliced red and green bell peppers
- 2 tablespoons lemon juice
- 1 tablespoon vegetable oil
- ½ pound cooked turkey breast, cut into thin strips
- 1 medium Washington Golden Delicious or Winesap apple, cored and thinly sliced
- 6 pita rounds, lightly toasted
- ½ cup plain low-fat yogurt

Cook and stir onion, peppers, and lemon juice in oil in nonstick skillet until crisp-tender. Stir in turkey; cook until turkey is thoroughly heated. Remove from heat; stir in apple. Fill each pita with apple mixture; drizzle with yogurt. Serve warm.

Makes 6 servings

NUTRITIONAL INFORMATION PER SERVING

Calories	219.5	kc	Niacin (B₃)	4.45	mg
Protein	16.83	g	Pantothenic Acid	0.45	mg
Fat	3.60	g	Phosphorus	165.33	mg
% of Calories			Potassium	316.67	mg
from Fat:	15		Pyridoxine (B₆)	0.32	mg
Saturated Fat	0.60	g	Riboflavin (B₂)	0.18	mg
Cholesterol	32.50	mg	Thiamin (B₁)	0.23	mg
Dietary Fiber	1.95	g	Vitamin A	20.66	RE
Sodium	250.5	mg	Vitamin C	26.50	mg
Beta-Carotene	48.01	RE	Copper	.072	mg
Calcium	79.67	mg	Folate	16.01	µg
Iron	1.73	mg	Zinc	.91	mg
Magnesium	20.83	mg			

LAMB TORTELLINI MINESTRONE

2 cups cooked cubed lean American lamb (leg or shoulder) *or* 1 pound ground lamb, cooked and drained

2 cans (14 ounces each) reduced-sodium beef broth

1 can (8 ounces) tomato sauce

1 clove garlic, minced *or* ¼ teaspoon garlic powder

1 package (8 ounces) dry cheese tortellini *or* 16 ounces fresh cheese tortellini

1 bag (16 ounces) frozen cauliflower, zucchini, carrot, and red pepper combination

1 can (15 ounces) white northern beans or kidney beans, drained

1½ teaspoon dried Italian seasonings

Bring broth and tomato sauce to a boil in large saucepan over high heat. Add all other ingredients and reduce heat to medium-low. Simmer 10 to 15 minutes until tortellini and vegetables are tender, stirring occasionally.   Makes 8 servings

NUTRITIONAL INFORMATION PER SERVING

Calories	218.70	kc	Magnesium	40.81	mg
Manganesium	0.31	mg	Niacin (B₃)	3.29	mg
Protein	16.74	g	Pantothenic Acid	0.44	mg
Fat	4.27	g	Phosphorus	140.50	mg
% of Calories			Potassium	504.50	mg
from Fat:	18		Pyridoxine (B₆)	0.15	mg
Saturated Fat	1.86	g	Riboflavin (B₂)	0.18	mg
Cholesterol	30.23	mg	Selenium	0.01	mg
Dietary Fiber	1.68	g	Thiamin (B₁)	0.16	mg
Sodium	277.10	mg	Vitamin A	29.72	RE
Beta-Carotene	11.70	RE	Vitamin C	4.50	mg
Soluble Fiber	0.16	g	Copper	0.18	mg
Calcium	62.90	mg	Folate	52.40	µg
Cobalamin (B₁₂)	0.75	µg	Vitamin E	0.02	mg
Iron	1.91	mg	Zinc	1.83	mg

SWEET AND SOUR PORK

   1   **Florida grapefruit**
   1¼ **pounds boneless pork tenderloin, trimmed of
         all fat**
   ⅓   **cup Florida grapefruit juice**
   2   **tablespoons low sodium soy sauce**
   1   **garlic clove, minced**
   2   **teaspoons light brown sugar, divided**
   2   **tablespoons cornstarch**
   1   **tablespoon vegetable oil**
   2   **teaspoons finely minced fresh ginger root**
   8   **medium green onions, cut into 2-inch pieces**
   1   **medium red pepper, cut into 1-inch pieces**
   ⅓   **cup reduced-sodium chicken broth**
   ¼   **cup ketchup**

Peel grapefruit and carefully remove white pith from
fruit. Using a paring knife, carefully section grapefruit, peeling fruit away from the membrane. Set
aside sections. Cut pork into 1-inch cubes.

Combine grapefruit juice, soy sauce, garlic, and
1 teaspoon brown sugar in medium bowl. Add
pork cubes; stir to combine. Cover; set aside for
30 minutes to marinate. Remove pork from
marinade with slotted spoon; reserve marinade. Toss
pork in cornstarch until lightly coated.

Heat oil in large nonstick skillet over medium-high
heat until hot, but not smoking. Add pork pieces
and cook on all sides, about 7 to 10 minutes, until
golden brown. Remove pork and transfer to warm

plate. Add ginger, green onions, and red pepper to skillet. Cook and stir 2 to 3 minutes, until green onions are slightly limp. Add chicken broth, ketchup, remaining 1 teaspoon brown sugar, and reserved marinade. Bring to a boil over medium-high heat. Add browned pork and grapefruit sections; cook 1 to 2 minutes until pork is cooked through and sauce has thickened slightly. Serve immediately.   Makes 6 servings

NUTRITIONAL INFORMATION PER SERVING

Calories	198.2	kc	Niacin (B_3)	4.11	mg
Protein	22.13	g	Pantothenic Acid	0.74	mg
Fat	5.98	g	Phosphorus	232.00	mg
% of Calories			Potassium	589.50	mg
from Fat:	27		Pyridoxine (B_6)	0.40	mg
Saturated Fat	1.52	g	Riboflavin (B_2)	0.33	mg
Cholesterol	67.21	mg	Selenium	0.02	mg
Dietary Fiber	1.03	g	Thiamin (B_1)	0.73	mg
Sodium	388.70	mg	Vitamin A	54.86	RE
Beta-Carotene	221.30	RE	Vitamin C	34.46	mg
Calcium	23.88	mg	Copper	0.19	mg
Soluble Fiber	0.14	g	Folate	15.87	µg
Cobalamin (B_{12})	0.40	µg	Vitamin E	2.95	mg
Iron	1.73	mg	Zinc	2.34	mg
Magnesium	31.64	mg			

Meat
Apple-icious Lamb Kebabs

1½ pounds fresh American lamb (leg or
    shoulder), cut into 1¼-inch cubes
1 cup apple juice or cider
2 tablespoons Worcestershire sauce
½ teaspoon lemon pepper
2 cloves garlic, peeled and sliced
1 large apple, cut into 12 wedges
  Assorted vegetables, such as 1 large green or
    red bell pepper, 1 large onion, 1 small
    summer squash, cut into wedges
  Apple Barbecue Sauce (page 457)

Mix apple juice, Worcestershire sauce, lemon
pepper, and garlic in plastic bag or nonmetal
container. Add lamb cubes and coat well. To
marinate, place in refrigerator for at least 2 hours or
up to 24 hours.

Preheat grill or broiler. Remove meat from marinade
and thread onto skewers, alternating meat, apple,
and vegetables.

To grill, place kebabs 4 inches from medium coals.
Cook about 10 to 12 minutes for medium-rare,
turning occasionally and brushing with Apple
Barbecue Sauce. (To broil, place kebabs on broiler
pan which has been lightly oiled or sprayed with
nonstick cooking spray. Broil lamb 4 inches from
heat source. Cook about 10 to 12 minutes for
medium-rare, turning occasionally and brushing with
Apple Barbecue Sauce.)   Makes 6 servings

APPLE BARBECUE SAUCE

- ½ cup apple juice or cider
- ½ cup finely chopped onion
- 1 cup chili sauce
- ½ cup unsweetened applesauce
- 2 tablespoons packed brown sugar
- 1 tablespoon Worcestershire sauce
- 1 teaspoon dry mustard
- 5 drops hot pepper sauce

Combine apple juice and onion in 1-quart saucepan; bring to a boil. Reduce heat and simmer for 2 minutes. Stir in chili sauce, applesauce, brown sugar, Worcestershire sauce, dry mustard, and hot pepper sauce. Simmer 10 minutes, stirring occasionally. Remove from heat.

NUTRITIONAL INFORMATION PER SERVING
(includes about 1½ tablespoons sauce)

Calories	224.38	kc	Niacin(B_3)	5.81	mg
Protein	25.20	g	Pantothenic Acid	0.56	mg
Fat	6.85	g	Phosphorus	159.30	mg
% of Calories			Potassium	513.97	mg
from Fat:	29		Pyridoxine (B_6)	0.21	mg
Saturated Fat	2.36	g	Riboflavin (B_2)	0.29	mg
Cholesterol	75.65	mg	Selenium	0.01	mg
Dietary Fiber	2.11	g	Thiamin (B_1)	0.15	mg
Sodium	242.60	mg	Vitamin A	14.97	RE
Beta-Carotene	22.77	RE	Vitamin C	12.90	mg
Calcium	25.72	mg	Copper	0.15	mg
Cobalamin (B_{12})	1.70	µg	Folate	29.28	µg
Iron	2.30	mg	Vitamin E	0.44	mg
Magnesium	29.73	mg	Zinc	3.38	mg

Thai Beef with Noodles

- 1 **pound boneless beef top sirloin, 1 inch thick**
- ¼ **cup dry sherry**
- 1½ **tablespoons reduced-sodium soy sauce**
- 1 **teaspoon** *each* **grated fresh ginger, minced garlic and Oriental dark roasted sesame oil**
- ¼ **to ½ teaspoon crushed red pepper**
- 2 **teaspoons cornstarch**
- ¼ **cup water**
- 2 **cups cooked ramen noodles or linguine**
- ¼ **cup chopped green onion tops**

Combine sherry, soy sauce, ginger, garlic, sesame oil, and pepper. Place beef in plastic bag; add marinade. Close bag securely and marinate 15 minutes. Pour off marinade; reserve. Heat nonstick skillet over medium heat 5 minutes. Add steak; cook 12 to 15 minutes for rare (140°F) to medium (160°F), turning once. Remove beef; keep warm. Dissolve cornstarch in reserved marinade and water; add to skillet. Bring to a boil, stirring constantly. Stir in noodles. Cut beef into thin slices and serve over noodles. Sprinkle with onions.   Makes 4 servings

NUTRITIONAL INFORMATION PER SERVING

Calories	310.3	kc	Niacin (B$_3$)	4.86	mg
Protein	31.32	g	Pantothenic Acid	0.40	mg
Fat	10.55	g	Phosphorus	270.40	mg
% of Calories			Potassium	452.30	mg
from Fat:	30		Pyridoxine (B$_6$)	0.46	mg
Saturated Fat	2.33	g	Riboflavin (B$_2$)	0.33	mg
Cholesterol	98.86	mg	Thiamin (B$_1$)	0.21	mg
Dietary Fiber	1.15	g	Vitamin A	135.60	RE
Sodium	673.40	mg	Vitamin C	2.34	mg
Beta-Carotene	248.90	RE	Copper	0.21	mg
Calcium	24.62	mg	Folate	14.34	µg
Cobalamin (B$_{12}$)	2.59	µg	Vitamin E	0.63	mg
Iron	4.30	mg	Zinc	6.31	mg
Magnesium	43.14	mg			

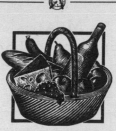

Vitamin and Mineral Counter

The Vitamin and Mineral Counter will give you a good idea of your vitamin intake (pages 460–503) and your mineral intake (pages 504–546), using the following abbreviations.

VIT A = vitamin A
BETA-C = beta-carotene
VIT E = vitamin E
VIT D = vitamin D
VIT C = vitamin C
FOL = folate
VIT B$_6$ = vitamin B$_6$
VIT B$_{12}$ = vitamin B$_{12}$
PANT = pantothenic acid
CALC = calcium
IRON = iron
MAG = magnesium
PHOS = phosphorus
SOD = sodium
POTA = potassium
COP = copper
ZINC = zinc
SELE = selenium

BOX = box
CAK = cake
CI = cubic inch
CP = cup
EA = each
FO = fluid ounce
LG = large
LK = link
MD = medium
MDE = medium egg used
OZ = ounce
PC = piece
PKG = package
PKT = packet
POD = pod
PTY = patty
REB = regular bar
REG = regular
RG = ring

SET = set
SI = square inch
SL = slice
SM = small
STK = stick
STR = strip
SUG = sugar cone
SV = serving
SW = sandwich
TB = tablespoon
TS = teaspoon

mg = milligram
μg = microgram
IU = international unit
g = gram

NA = value not available

FOOD	WEIGHT (g)	VIT A (IU)	BETA-C (µg)	VIT E (mg)	VIT D (µg)	VIT C (mg)	FOL (µg)	VIT B₆ (mg)	PANT (mg)	VIT B₁₂ (mg)
BEVERAGES										
Club soda (CP)	236.80	0	0	0	0	0	0	0	0	0
Coffee, brewed, hot or iced, without sugar (CP)	237	0	0	0	0	0	0.24	0	0	0
Coffee, decaffeinated, instant, dry powder (TS)	1	0	0	0	0	0	0	0	0	0
Coffee, instant, dry powder (TS)	0.9	0	0	0	0	0	0	0	0	0
Cola (CP)	246.40	0	0	0	0	0	0	0	0	0
Cola, diet, with aspartame (CP)	236.80	0	0	0	0	0	0	0	0	0
Cola, diet, with saccharin (CP)	240	0	0	0	0	0	0	0	0	0
Noncola (CP)	245.60	0	0	0	0	0	0	0	0	0
Noncola, diet, with aspartame (CP)	240	0	0	0	0	0	0	0	0	0
Noncola, diet, with saccharin (CP)	236.80	0	0	0	0	0	0	0	0	0
Noncola, diet, with saccharin, sodium free (CP)	236.80	0	0	0	0	0	0	0	0	0
Postum, dry powder (TS)	3.06	0	0	0.02	0	0	4.80	0.03	0.03	0
Root beer, cream soda, birch beer, near beer (CP)	246.40	0	0	0	0	0	0	0	0	0
Root beer, diet, with aspartame (CP)	240	0	0	0	0	0	0	0	0	0

											(g)
Root beer, diet, with saccharin (CP)	0	0	0	0	0	0	0	0	0	0	240
Tea, herbal (CP)	0	0.02	0	1.42	0	0	0	0	0	0	237
Tea, hot or iced, with aspartame, reconstituted (CP)	0	0.02	0	4.50	0	0	0	0	0	0	238
Tea, hot or iced, with saccharin, reconstituted (CP)	0	0.02	0	6.90	0	0	0	0	0	0	238
Tea, hot or iced, without sugar, brewed (CP)	0	0.02	0	12.32	0	0	0	0	0	0	237
Tea, hot or iced, with sugar, reconstituted, presweetened, instant (CP)	0	0.02	0	8.88	0	0	0	0	0	0	240
Tea, instant, decaffeinated, dry powder (TS)	0	0.03	0.01	0.72	0	0	0	0	0	0	0.70
Tea, instant, decaffeinated, dry powder, with aspartame (TS)	0	0	0	0	4.68	0	0	0	0	0	0.80
Tea, instant, decaffeinated, dry powder, with sugar (TS)	0	0.02	0	0.47	0	0	0	0	0	0	3.80
Tea, instant, decaffeinated, with saccharin, dry powder (TS)	0	0.01	0	0.38	0	0	0	0	0	0	1.20
Tea, instant, dry powder (TS)	0	0.03	0.01	0.72	0	0	0	0	0	0	0.70
Tea, instant, dry powder, with aspartame (TS)	0	0.01	0	2.25	0	0	0	0	0	0	0.78
Tea, instant, dry powder, with saccharin (TS)	0	0.01	0	3.46	0	0	0	0	0	0	1.20

FOOD	WEIGHT (g)	VIT A (IU)	BETA-C (µg)	VIT E (mg)	VIT D (µg)	VIT C (mg)	FOL (µg)	VIT B$_6$ (mg)	PANT (mg)	VIT B$_{12}$ (mg)
EGGS AND EGG PRODUCTS										
Egg, scrambled with whole milk (LG)	122.20	983.9	170.8	1.27	2.34	0.30	48.61	0.15	1.35	1.12
Egg, whole (LG)	50	317.5	57.03	0.37	0.63	0	23.50	0.07	0.63	0.50
Egg, yolk (LG)	16.60	322.8	57.93	0.36	0.67	0	24.24	0.06	0.63	0.52
Egg Beaters egg substitute, prepared as directed (CP)	210.14	2295.36	1004.27	1.39	4.28	0.03	147.6	0.27	3.70	3.32
Eggnog, commercial (CP)	254	894.0	223.5	0.38	3.07	3.81	2.29	0.13	1.07	1.14
Egg white (LG)	33.40	0	0	0	0	0	1	0	0.04	0.07
Scramblers egg substitute, prepared as directed (CP)	217.18	4827.95	2519.46	3.39	5.96	0.03	7.69	0.76	4.58	4.84
Second Nature egg substitute, prepared as directed (CP)	217.20	2428.53	986.1	3.05	4.47	0.41	127.9	0.33	3.19	1.91
FATS AND OILS										
Butter, salted (TS)	4.73	144.6	38.03	0.08	0.02	0	0.13	0	0.01	0.01
Butter, unsalted (TS)	4.73	144.6	38.03	0.08	0.02	0	0.14	0	0.01	0.01
Butter, whipped (TS)	3.15	96.33	25.51	0.05	0.02	0	0.09	0	0	0
Butter, whipped, unsalted (TS)	3.15	96.33	25.55	0.05	0.02	0	0.09	0	0	0

Lard, rendered (TS)	4.27	0	0	0.05	0	0	0	0
Margarine, corn, diet (40% fat) (TS)	4.80	246.6	52.85	0.44	0.53	0	0.03	0
Margarine, corn, liquid (80% fat) (TS)	4.70	207.3	31.07	0.81	0.52	0.01	0.06	0
Margarine, corn, spread (52% fat) (TS)	4.80	235.3	46.03	0.59	0.53	0	0.05	0
Margarine, corn, stick/tub (80% fat) (TS)	4.70	206.9	31.07	0.89	0.52	0.01	0.05	0
Margarine, corn, stick/tub (80% fat), unsalted (TS)	4.70	206.9	31.07	0.89	0.52	0.01	0.05	0
Margarine, corn, whipped (80% fat) (TS)	3.16	162.3	34.79	0.56	0.35	0	0.03	0
Margarine, safflower, stick/tub (80% fat) (TS)	4.70	206.9	31.07	0.43	0.52	0.01	0.05	0
Margarine, safflower, stick/tub (80% fat), unsalted (TS)	4.70	207.2	31.07	1.01	0.52	0.01	0.06	0
Margarine, soybean, diet (40% fat) (TS)	4.80	246.6	52.85	0.17	0.53	0	0.03	0
Margarine, soybean, spread (52% fat) (TS)	4.80	171.4	46.03	0.37	0.53	0	0.05	0
Margarine, soybean, stick/tub (80% fat) (TS)	4.70	206.9	31.07	0.40	0.52	0.01	0.05	0
Margarine, sunflower, diet (40% fat) (TS)	4.80	246.9	52.85	0.60	0.53	0	0.03	0
Margarine, sunflower, spread (52% fat) (TS)	4.80	179.9	12.86	0.82	0.53	0.01	0.04	0
Margarine, sunflower, stick/tub (80% fat) (TS)	4.70	207.3	31.07	1.21	0.78	0.01	0.05	0

FOOD	WEIGHT (g)	VIT A (IU)	BETA-C (µg)	VIT E (mg)	VIT D (µg)	VIT C (mg)	FOL (µg)	VIT B6 (mg)	PANT (mg)	VIT B12 (mg)
Oil, canbra or canola (rapeseed) (TS)	4.54	0	0	0.92	0	0	0	0	0	0
Oil, coconut (TS)	4.54	0	0	0.02	0	0	0	0	0	0
Oil, cod liver (TS)	4.54	4540	271.8	1	11.35	0	0	0	0	0
Oil, corn (TS)	4.54	0	0	0.95	0	0	0	0	0	0
Oil, cottonseed (TS)	4.54	0	0	1.74	0	0	0	0	0	0
Oil, olive (TS)	4.50	0	0	0.54	0	0	0	0	0	0
Oil, palm (TS)	4.54	0	0	0.67	0	0	0	0	0	0
Oil, palm kernel (TS)	4.54	0	0	0.17	0	0	0	0	0	0
Oil, peanut (TS)	4.50	0	0	0.58	0	0	0	0	0	0
Oil, safflower (TS)	4.54	0	0	1.56	0	0	0	0	0	0
Oil, sesame (TS)	4.54	0	0	0.18	0	0	0	0	0	0
Oil, soybean, partially hydrogenated (TS)	4.54	0	0	0.68	0	0	0	0	0	0
Oil, sunflower seed (TS)	4.54	0	0	2.72	0	0	0	0	0	0
Olives, black (ripe) (MD)	4	16.12	9.65	0.05	0	0.04	0	0	0	0
Olives, green, plain or stuffed (MD)	4	12	7.20	0.06	0	0	0.04	0	0	0
Salad dressing, blue cheese, commercial (TB)	15.30	32.13	7.65	1.08	0.06	0.31	1.24	0.01	0.06	0.04

Food										
Salad dressing, blue cheese, low calorie, commercial (TB)	15.30	12.24	2.91	0	0.02	0.31	0.02	0	0.02	0
Salad dressing, French, commercial (TB)	15.60	10.45	6.24	0.97	0	0	0.65	0	0.02	0.02
Salad dressing, French, low calorie, commercial (TB)	16.30	264.3	158.2	0.02	0	0	0.25	0	0	0
Salad dressing, French, no salt added, commercial (TB)	16.30	0	0	0.15	0	0	0	0	0	0
Salad dressing, Italian, commercial (TB)	14.70	11.47	6.91	1.05	0.03	0	0.72	0	0.03	0.02
Salad dressing, Italian, low calorie, commercial (TB)	15	0	0	0.22	0	0	0	0	0	0
Salad dressing, mayonnaise type, commercial (33% fat) (TB)	14.70	32.34	5.88	0.72	0.04	0	0.92	0	0.04	0.03
Salad dressing, mayonnaise, commercial (79% fat) (TB)	13.80	38.64	6.90	1.62	0.04	0	1.06	0.08	0.03	0.03
Salad dressing, mayonnaise, imitation (19% fat) (TB)	15	18.15	3.30	0.43	0.04	0	0	0	0.03	0
Salad dressing, Thousand Island, commercial (TB)	15.60	49.92	22.93	0.82	0.04	0	0.98	0	0.04	0.03
Salad dressing, Thousand Island, low calorie, commercial (TB)	15.30	48.96	22.49	0.23	0.04	0	0.85	0	0.03	0.03
Salad dressing, yogurt based, commercial (TB)	15	18.67	11.13	0.31	0	0.34	0.44	0	0.02	0.01
Sandwich spread (TB)	15.30	15.30	2.75	0.91	0.05	0.11	0.15	0	0.02	0.01

FOOD	WEIGHT (g)	VIT A (IU)	BETA-C (µg)	VIT E (mg)	VIT D (µg)	VIT C (mg)	FOL (µg)	VIT B$_6$ (mg)	PANT (mg)	VIT B$_{12}$ (mg)
Shortening, household (TS)	4.27	0	0	1.14	0	0	0	0	0	0
Tartar sauce (TB)	14.38	31.64	5.61	1.36	0.02	0.14	1.11	0.04	0.03	0.03
FRUITS AND FRUIT PRODUCTS										
Apple, fresh, with skin (MD)	138	73.14	44.16	0.54	0	7.87	3.86	0.07	0.08	0
Apple juice, sweetened (CP)	248	0	0	0.02	0	2.18	0	0.07	0.07	0
Apple juice, unsweetened, bottled or canned (CP)	248	2.48	1.49	0.02	0	2.23	0.25	0.07	0.15	0
Apples, dried, uncooked (CP)	86	0	0	0.38	0	3.35	0	0.11	0.21	0
Applesauce, sweetened, canned (CP)	255	28.05	17.85	0.48	0	4.33	1.53	0.08	0.13	0
Applesauce, unsweetened (CP)	244	70.76	41.48	0.46	0	2.93	1.46	0.07	0.22	0
Apricots, dried, uncooked (CP)	130	9412	5647.20	1.20	0	3.12	13.39	0.21	0.97	0
Apricots, dried, unsweetened, cooked (CP)	250	5907.50	3545	0.82	0	4	0	0.27	0.52	0
Apricots, fresh (MD)	35.33	369.55	221.17	0.33	0	3.53	3.04	0.02	0.08	0
Apricots, sweetened, canned (CP)	258	3173.40	1904.04	2.37	0	8	4.39	0.13	0.23	0
Avocado (SM)	173	1058.76	634.91	2.16	NA	13.67	107.09	0.48	1.68	0
Banana, fresh (MD)	114	92.34	55.86	0.31	0	10.37	21.77	0.66	0.30	0

Food									
Blackberries, fresh (CP)	144	237.60	142.56	1.04	0	30.24	48.96	0.09	0.35	0
Blueberries, fresh (CP)	145	145	87	1.04	0	18.85	9.28	0.06	0.13	0
Cantaloupe, fresh (MD)	922.75	23375.62	15197.69	1.29	0	389.4*	156.87	1.02	1.20	0
Cherries, fresh, sweet (CP)	145	310.30	185.60	0.19	0	10.15	6.09	0.06	0.19	0
Cherries, sweetened, canned (CP)	200	308	184	0.26	0	7.20	8.40	0.06	0.26	0
Cranberries, fresh (CP)	95	43.70	26.60	0	0	12.82	1.61	0.06	0.21	0
Cranberry-apple juice, sweetened (CP)	245	7.35	4.90	0.02	0	78.40	0.49	0.05	0.15	0
Cranberry juice, sweetened (CP)	253	10.12	6.07	0	0	89.56	0.51	0.05	0.15	0
Dates, dried (CP)	178	89	53.40	0	0	0	22.43	0.34	1.39	0
Figs, canned in heavy syrup (CP)	259	95.83	56.98	0	0	2.59	5.18	0.18	0.18	0
Figs, dried (CP)	199	264.67	159.20	0	0	1.59	14.92	0.44	0.86	0
Figs, fresh (MD)	50	71	42.50	0	0	1	3.50	0.05	0.15	0
Fruit-flavored drink or juice, low calorie (CP)	237	9.48	5.69	0	NA	76.31	0.47	0.05	0.14	0
Grapefruit juice, sweetened, frozen or canned (CP)	250	0	0	0.52	0	67.25	26	0.05	0.32	0
Grapefruit juice, unsweetened, fresh, frozen, or canned (CP)	247	17.29	9.88	0.52	0	72.12	25.69	0.05	0.32	0
Grapefruit sections, sweetened, canned (CP)	254	0	0	1.02	0	54.10	21.59	0.05	0.30	0
Grapefruit, fresh (MD)	291.20	361.09	215.49	0.70	0	100.17	29.70	0.12	0.82	0

FOOD	WEIGHT (g)	VIT A (IU)	BETA-C (µg)	VIT E (mg)	VIT D (µg)	VIT C (mg)	FOL (µg)	VIT B_6 (mg)	PANT (mg)	VIT B_{12} (mg)
Grape juice, sweetened, frozen (CP)	250	20	12.50	0	0	59.75	3.25	0.10	0.05	0
Grape juice, unsweetened (CP)	253	20.24	12.65	0	0	0.25	6.58	0.15	0.10	0
Grapes, fresh (CP)	160	116.80	70.40	0.54	0	17.28	6.24	0.18	0.03	0
Guava, fresh (MD)	90	712.80	426.82	1.01	0	165.15	12.60	0.13	0.13	0
Honeydew melon, fresh (MD)	1290	516	309.60	0	0	319.92	387	0.77	2.71	0
Kiwifruit, fresh (MD)	76	133	79.80	1.15	0	74.48	28.88	0.07	0.13	0
Kumquats, fresh (MD)	19	57.38	34.39	0	0	7.11	3.04	0.01	NA	0
Lemon, fresh (MD)	58	16.82	9.86	0	0	30.74	6.15	0.05	0.11	0
Lemonade or limeade, sweetened, other than fruit-flavored beverage mix (CP)	248	52.08	31.17	0	0	9.67	5.46	0.02	0.02	0
Lemon juice, unsweetened, fresh, frozen, bottled, or canned (1 whole or 4 wedges = 1.50 oz) (CP)	244	36.60	21.96	0.54	0	60.51	24.64	0.10	0.22	0
Mandarin orange, fresh (MD)	84	772.80	463.68	0	0	25.87	17.14	0.06	0.17	0
Mango, fresh (MD)	207	8060.58	4835.52	2.32	0	57.34	74.52	0.27	0.33	0
Nectarine, fresh (MD)	136	150.96	89.76	1.21	0	7.34	5.03	0.03	0.22	0
Nectars, apricot, sweetened (CP)	251	3303.16	1982.90	2.33	0	1.51	3.26	0.05	0.25	0
Nectars, peach, sweetened, canned (CP)	249	642.42	385.95	0.25	0	13.20	3.49	0.02	0.17	0

Food									
Orange, fresh (MD)	131	268.55	161.13	0.24	0	69.69	39.69	0.08	0.33	0
Orange juice, sweetened, canned or frozen (CP)	250	424.38	254.12	0.22	0	83.42	43.90	0.20	0.40	0
Orange juice, unsweetened, fortified with calcium (CP)	249	194.22	117.03	0.47	0	96.86	109.06	0.10	0.40	0
Orange juice, unsweetened; fresh, frozen, or canned (CP)	249	194.22	117.03	0.47	0	96.86	109.06	0.10	0.40	0
Papaya, fresh (CP)	140	397.60	238	0	0	86.52	53.20	0.03	0.31	0
Papaya juice, canned (CP)	250	277.50	167.50	0	0	7.50	5.25	0.02	0.12	0
Peach, fresh (MD)	87	465.45	279.27	1.17	0	5.74	2.96	0.02	0.15	0
Peaches, dried, unsweetened, cooked (CP)	258	508.26	304.44	0	0	9.55	0.26	0.10	0.46	0
Peaches, sweetened, canned or frozen (CP)	256	849.92	509.44	3.43	0	7.17	8.19	0.05	0.13	0
Pear, fresh (MD)	166	33.20	19.92	0.86	0	6.64	12.12	0.03	0.12	0
Pears, dried, unsweetened, cooked (CP)	255	107.10	63.75	0	0	10.20	0	0.08	0.18	0
Pears, sweetened, canned (CP)	255	0	0	1.43	0	2.80	3.06	0.03	0.05	0
Persimmons, Japanese, raw (MD)	168	3640.56	2184	0	0	12.60	12.60	0.17	NA	0
Pineapple, canned, unsweetened or juice pack (CP)	250	95	57.50	0.25	0	23.75	12	0.17	0.25	0
Pineapple, fresh (SL)	84	19.32	11.76	0.08	0	12.94	8.90	0.08	0.13	0

FOOD	WEIGHT (g)	VIT A (IU)	BETA-C (µg)	VIT E (mg)	VIT D (µg)	VIT C (mg)	FOL (µg)	VIT B$_6$ (mg)	PANT (mg)	VIT B$_{12}$ (mg)
Pineapple, sweetened, canned (SL)	58	8.70	5.22	0.06	0	4.35	2.73	0.04	0.06	0
Pineapple juice, frozen or canned (CP)	250	12.50	7.50	0.05	0	26.75	57.75	0.25	0.25	0
Plum, fresh (MD)	66	213.18	128.04	0.47	0	6.27	1.45	0.05	0.12	0
Plums, sweetened, canned (CP)	258	668.22	399.90	1.81	0	1.03	6.45	0.08	0.18	0
Pomegranate, fresh (MD)	154	0	0	0	0	9.39	9.24	0.15	0.92	0
Prunes, dried, cooked (CP)	212	648.72	390.08	0.83	0	6.15	0.21	0.47	0.23	0
Prunes, dried, uncooked (CP)	161	3199.07	1919.12	2.33	0	5.31	5.96	0.42	0.74	0
Prune juice, bottled (CP)	256	7.68	5.12	0.84	0	10.50	1.02	0.56	0.28	0
Raisins (TB)	9.69	0.78	0.46	0.03	0	0.32	0.32	0.02	0	0
Raspberries, fresh (CP)	123	159.90	95.94	0.59	0	30.75	31.98	0.07	0.30	0
Raspberries, sweetened, canned or frozen (CP)	250	150	90	1.20	0	41.25	65	0.07	0.37	0
Rhubarb, stewed, unsweetened (CP)	240	256.80	153.77	0.43	0	12	19.68	0.05	0.19	0
Rhubarb, sweetened, cooked (CP)	240	165.60	98.40	0.48	0	7.92	12.72	0.05	0.12	0
Strawberries, fresh or frozen, unsweetened (CP)	149	40.23	23.84	0.36	0	84.48	26.37	0.09	0.51	0
Strawberries, sweetened, canned or frozen (CP)	255	61.20	35.70	0.59	0	105.57	37.99	0.08	0.28	0
Watermelon, fresh (SL)	482	1764.12	1060.40	0	0	46.27	10.60	0.67	1.01	0

Bagel, egg (MD)	55	17.60	3.30	0.33	0.05	0	13.20	0.02	0.20	0.05
Bagel, plain (MD)	55	0	0	0.19	0	0	13.20	0.02	0.20	0
Bagel, rye (MD)	55	0	0	0.13	0	0	31.27	0.05	0.24	0
Bagel, whole wheat (MD)	55	0	0	0.16	0	0	35.13	0.07	0.32	0
Barley, pearled, cooked with salt (CP)	157	12.03	7.21	0.02	0	0	12.58	0.14	0.16	0
Barley, pearled, dry (CP)	200	44	26.34	0.04	0	0	46	0.52	0.56	0
Biscuit, baking powder (MD)	45	33.51	3.10	1.56	0.17	0.15	7.33	0.02	0.16	0.06
Bran, unprocessed (TB)	3.75	0	0	0.07	0	0	2.96	0.05	0.08	0
Bread, Boston brown (SL)	48	33.60	20.16	0.29	NA	0	14.40	0.07	0.20	0
Bread, diet, with fiber added (SL)	23	0	0	0.50	0	0	9.66	0.01	0.04	0
Bread, egg (SL)	32.70	98.82	14.22	0.13	0.29	0.10	15.83	0.02	0.18	0.07
Bread, Italian (SL)	30	0	0	0.07	0	0	9.90	0.02	0.15	0
Bread, nut (SL)	48.90	57.47	9.15	0.51	0.22	0.31	9.14	0.04	0.19	0.09
Bread, oatmeal (SL)	35.50	5.11	3.06	0.41	0	0	14.96	0.02	0.17	0
Bread, pumpkin, without nuts (SL)	56.20	3268.81	1940.17	1.12	0.08	0.69	8.32	0.02	0.20	0.06
Bread, raisin (SL)	22.50	0.41	0.25	0.04	NA	0.17	7.87	0.01	0.10	0
Bread, rye (SL)	28.69	0	0	0.06	0	0	11.19	0.03	0.13	0
Bread, white (SL)	25	0	0	0.04	0	0	8.75	0.01	0.07	0

FOOD	WEIGHT (g)	VIT A (IU)	BETA-C (µg)	VIT E (mg)	VIT D (µg)	VIT C (mg)	FOL (µg)	VIT B$_6$ (mg)	PANT (mg)	VIT B$_{12}$ (mg)
Bread, white, low sodium (SL)	25	0	0	0.04	0	0	8.75	0.08	0.11	0
Bread, whole wheat, low sodium (SL)	25	0	0	0.04	0	0	13.75	0.03	0.15	0
Bread, zucchini, without nuts (SL)	37.10	47.22	16.18	0.57	0.06	0.40	5.85	0.01	0.11	0.04
Buckwheat groats, cooked with salt (CP)	198	0	0	0.53	0	0	21.60	0.18	0.63	0
Buckwheat groats, dry (CP)	164	0	0	1.69	NA	0	68.88	0.57	2.02	0
Bulgur, cooked with salt (CP)	182	0	0	0.05	0	0	11.68	0.15	0.45	0
Bulgur, dry (CP)	140	0	0	0.15	0	0	37.80	0.48	1.46	0
Cereal, cream of rice, cooked with salt (CP)	244	0	0	0.02	0	0	10.96	0.07	0.22	0
Cereal, cream of wheat, instant, cooked with salt (CP)	241	0	0	0.34	0	0	14.22	0.02	0.19	0
Cereal, cream of wheat, regular, cooked with salt (CP)	251	0	0	0.33	0	0	12.35	0.05	0.20	0
Cereal, dry, All-Bran (CP)	85	2242.77	0	1.31	3.73	44.84	297.63	1.49	1.47	0
Cereal, dry, Apple Jacks (CP)	28.35	749.57	29.42	0.02	1.25	14.99	99.92	0.50	0.04	0
Cereal, dry, Cap'n Crunch (CP)	37	0	0	0.73	0	0	227.18	0.73	3.58	1.99
Cereal, dry, Cheerios (CP)	22.68	995.51	13.03	0.33	0.82	12.02	79.45	0.41	0.27	0
Cereal, dry, Cinnamon Toast Crunch (CP)	42.50	1873.82	0	0.86	1.50	22.49	150.02	0.75	0.16	0

Food										
Cereal, dry, Common Sense Oat Bran (CP)	37.80	1015.33	9.97	0.23	1.60	0	202.06	1	0.74	0
Cereal, dry, Cracklin' Oat Bran (CP)	56.70	1448.14	29.94	0.88	2.40	30	132.75	0.67	0.41	2.64
Cereal, dry, Frosted Flakes (CP)	37.80	1000.19	39.26	0.03	1.67	20	133.33	0.67	0.05	0
Cereal, dry, Frosted Mini-Wheats (CP)	56.70	0	0	0.28	0	0	201.56	1	0.47	3.99
Cereal, dry, Fruitful Bran (CP)	59.10	1131.56	0	1.02	2.09	0	149.71	0.75	0.44	2.25
Cereal, dry, Grape-Nuts (CP)	113.40	4999.81	0	1.47	5	0	400.30	2	1.08	6
Cereal, dry, Honeycomb (CP)	21.26	938.08	0	0.01	0.94	0	75.11	0.37	0.06	1.12
Cereal, dry, Just Right, with raisins, dates, and nuts (CP)	50.30	6631.27	24	26.84	1.60	0.16	534.52	2.67	13.33	8
Cereal, dry, Kellogg's Corn Flakes (CP)	28.35	749.57	0	0.04	1.25	14.99	100	0.50	0.16	0
Cereal, dry, Kix (CP)	18.90	830.56	0	0.02	0.83	10	66.73	0.33	0.11	0
Cereal, dry, Life (CP)	44	0	0	0.15	0	0	32.56	0.07	0.37	0
Cereal, dry, Oatmeal Raisin Crisp (CP)	68	2525.90	17.50	0.08	2.02	2.04	189.80	1.06	0.36	0
Cereal, dry, Product 19 (CP)	28.35	750.14	0	20.13	1.25	60.10	400.02	2.01	10	6.01
Cereal, dry, Raisin Bran (Ralston) (CP)	50.40	1664.65	0.12	5.09	1.32	0.08	130.10	0.86	0.49	2
Cereal, dry, Rice Chex (CP)	25.20	0	0	0.02	0	13.33	88.60	0.44	0.19	1.33
Cereal, dry, Rice Krispies (CP)	28.35	749.57	0	0.04	1.25	14.99	100	0.50	0.16	0
Cereal, dry, Special K (CP)	28.35	750.14	0	0.15	1.25	15.03	100.08	0.70	0.15	0.01
Cereal, dry, Total (CP)	33	5820.21	0	23.43	1.16	69.96	465.63	2.34	11.55	7

FOOD	WEIGHT (g)	VIT A (IU)	BETA-C (µg)	VIT E (mg)	VIT D (µg)	VIT C (mg)	FOL (µg)	VIT B₆ (mg)	PANT (mg)	VIT B₁₂ (mg)
Cereal, dry, Wheat Chex (CP)	42.50	0	0	0.41	0	22.52	149.62	0.75	0.39	2.25
Cereal, dry, puffed rice (CP)	14	0	0	0.01	NA	0	2.66	0.01	0.04	0
Cereal, dry, puffed wheat (CP)	12	0	0	0.08	0	0	3.84	0.02	0.06	0
Coffeecake, yeast, without nuts, without topping (PC)	39.60	28.19	5.66	0.27	0.04	0.11	24.72	0.03	0.26	0.11
Cornbread (PC)	67.40	189.46	55.75	1.30	0.42	0.26	17.58	0.07	0.34	0.21
Corn grits, cooked with salt, regular or instant (CP)	242	0	0	0.05	0	0	1.91	0.05	0.17	0
Corn grits, dry (CP)	156	0	0	0.25	0	0	7.80	0.23	0.75	0
Cornmeal, cooked with salt (CP)	240	135.70	81.26	0.07	0	0	15.77	0.10	0.10	0
Cornmeal, dry (CP)	138	569.94	341.29	0.28	NA	0	66.24	0.36	0.43	0
Cornstarch (TB)	8	0	0	0	NA	0	0.16	0	0	0
Couscous, cooked with salt (CP)	179	0	0	0.09	0	0	10.72	0.05	0.66	0
Couscous, dry (CP)	184	0	0	0.33	0	0	36.80	0.20	2.28	0
Cracker, graham (PC)	3.50	0.07	0.04	0.03	0	0	0.74	0	0.02	0
Cracker, saltine (PC)	3.50	0	0	0.04	0	0	0.63	0	0.01	0
Cracker, saltine, unsalted top (PC)	3.50	0	0	0.05	0	0	0.77	0	0.01	0
Cracker, zwieback (PC)	3.50	2.03	0.36	0.03	0	0	0.70	0	0.02	0
Donut, cake (MD)	42	144.03	21.66	0.45	0.38	0.08	6.73	0.02	0.15	0.07

Donut, yeast (MD)	60	59.42	8.75	1.08	0.19	0.10	42.47	0.04	0.31	0.10
Flour, all-purpose (CP)	125	0	0	0.06	0	0	32.50	0.05	0.55	0
Flour, amaranth (whole grain) (CP)	195	0	0	NA	0	8.19	95.55	0.43	2.05	0
Flour, buckwheat (whole groat) (CP)	120	0	0	1.42	0	0	64.80	0.70	0.53	0
Flour, cake or pastry (CP)	109	0	0	0.05	0	0	20.71	0.03	0.50	0
Flour, corn, masa, enriched (CP)	114	0	0	0.17	0	0	27.36	0.42	0.75	0
Flour, rice (CP)	158	0	0	0.11	0	0	6.32	0.70	1.30	0
Flour, rice, brown (CP)	158	0	0	2.01	0	0	25.28	1.17	2.51	0
Flour, rye, medium (CP)	102	0	0	1.03	0	0	19.38	0.28	0.50	0
Flour, triticale (whole grain) (CP)	130	0	0	0.26	0	0	96.20	0.52	2.82	0
Flour, whole wheat (CP)	120	0	0	1.30	0	0	52.80	0.41	1.21	0
Hominy, canned (CP)	160	0	0	0.06	NA	0	1.60	0	0.24	0
Macaroni, whole wheat, cooked without salt (CP)	140	0	0	0.15	0	0	7	0.11	0.59	0
Matzos (PC)	3.50	0	0	0	0	0	0.50	0	0.02	0
Melba toast, unsalted (PC)	3.50	0	0	0	0	0	0.91	0	0.02	0
Millet, cooked with salt (CP)	240	0	0	0.14	0	0	64.75	0.29	0.65	0
Millet, dry (CP)	200	0	0	0.36	0	0	170	0.76	1.70	0
Muffin, bran, homemade (MD)	50	250.87	5.29	0.86	0.41	4.64	34.85	0.16	0.28	0.07
Muffin, corn, commercial mix or homemade (MD)	52	112.01	34.78	1.12	0.25	0.17	11.50	0.05	0.21	0.11

FOOD	WEIGHT (g)	VIT A (IU)	BETA-C (µg)	VIT E (mg)	VIT D (µg)	VIT C (mg)	FOL (µg)	VIT B6 (mg)	PANT (mg)	VIT B12 (mg)
Muffin, English, whole wheat (MD)	58	55.58	5.15	0.59	0.28	0.26	45.25	0.08	0.41	0.10
Noodles, chow mein (CP)	45	38.25	6.87	2.07	0	0	9.90	0.05	0.24	0
Noodles, egg, cooked without salt (CP)	160	32	5.74	0.13	0.05	0	11.20	0.06	0.22	0.14
Noodles, macaroni, white, cooked without salt (CP)	140	0	0	0.04	0	0	9.80	0.04	0.15	0
Noodles, macaroni, whole wheat, cooked with salt (CP)	140	0	0	0.15	0	0	7	0.11	0.59	0
Noodles, manicotti, cooked without salt (CP)	140	0	0	0.04	0	0	9.80	0.06	0.15	0
Noodles, ramen, cooked, all varieties (CP)	227	17.02	10.21	1.66	0	0	7.99	0.07	0.16	0
Noodles, rice, cooked without salt (CP)	160	0	0	0.03	0	0	3.46	0.10	0.45	0
Noodles, rice, fried (CP)	9.45	0	0	0.62	0	0	0.11	0	0.02	0
Oat bran, cooked with salt (CP)	219	36.79	22.03	0.15	0	0	19.14	0.07	0.55	0
Oat bran, dry (CP)	94	94	56.29	0.40	0	0	48.88	0.15	1.40	0
Oatmeal, cooked with salt (CP)	234	38.05	22.79	0.58	0	0	12.05	0.05	0.47	0
Oatmeal, dry (CP)	81	81.81	48.99	1.25	0	0	25.92	0.10	1	0
Pancake, homemade, all varieties except whole wheat and buckwheat (MD)	40	76.96	10.20	0.48	0.28	0.19	7.26	0.02	0.20	0.13
Pancake, homemade, whole wheat (MD)	40	76.96	10.20	0.62	0.28	0.19	9.53	0.06	0.27	0.13

Quinoa (CP)	170	0	0	8.28	0	0	83.30	0.37	1.78	0
Rice, brown, cooked without salt (CP)	195	0	0	0.80	0	0	7.80	0.27	0.55	0
Rice, white, cooked without salt (CP)	158	0	0	0.05	0	0	4.74	0.14	0.62	0
Rice, wild, cooked without salt (CP)	164	0	0	0	0	0	42.64	0.21	0.25	0
Rice bran, dry (CP)	83	0	0	5.69	0	0	52.29	3.38	6.13	0
Rice cakes, plain, no salt added (PC)	9	0	0	0.13	0	0	1.89	0.01	0.09	0
Rice cakes, plain, salted (PC)	9	0	0	0.13	0	0	1.91	0.01	0.09	0
Roll, croissant (MD)	69.70	731.46	182.03	0.43	0.39	0.19	32	0.04	0.38	0.16
Roll, hamburger (MD)	43	0	0	0.03	0	0	16.77	0.03	0.13	0
Roll, hamburger, whole wheat (MD)	43	0	0	0.07	0	0	23.65	0.06	0.26	0
Roll, hard (MD)	37	0	0	0.15	0	0	9.25	0.02	0.11	0
Roll, hot dog (MD)	43	0	0	0.03	0	0	16.77	0.03	0.13	0
Roll, hot dog, whole wheat (MD)	43	0	0	0.07	0	0	23.65	0.06	0.26	0
Roll, kaiser (MD)	50	0	0	0.08	0	0	29.89	0.02	0.15	0
Roll, rye (MD)	36	0	0	0.07	0	0	14.04	0.03	0.16	0
Roll, sourdough (MD)	45	0	0	0.10	0	0	14.85	0.03	0.22	0
Roll, submarine (MD)	94	0	0	0.14	0.46	0	34.78	0.04	0.50	0
Roll, white, dinner (MD)	36	0	0	0.03	0.14	0.11	13.68	0.02	0.11	0.04
Roll, whole wheat (MD)	36	0	0	0.06	0	0	19.25	0.05	0.21	0
Rye (whole grain) (CP)	169	0	0	2.60	0	0	101.40	0.49	2.47	0

FOOD	WEIGHT (g)	VIT A (IU)	BETA-C (µg)	VIT E (mg)	VIT D (µg)	VIT C (mg)	FOL (µg)	VIT B$_6$ (mg)	PANT (mg)	VIT B$_{12}$ (mg)
Stuffing, bread, all types except cornbread (CP)	114.20	50.54	30.27	4.84	0	3.11	29.27	0.08	0.25	0
Stuffing, cornbread (CP)	213.60	551.86	177.78	7.34	1.09	3.78	56.86	0.26	0.96	0.56
Tortilla, corn, fried (MD)	25.57	36.21	21.73	0.22	0	0	4.05	0.06	0.04	0
Tortilla, corn, plain (MD)	21.30	36.21	21.73	0.17	NA	0	4.05	0.06	0.04	0
Tortilla, flour, plain, commercial (PC)	42.50	0	0	0.05	NA	0	5.95	0.02	0.09	0
Tortilla, flour, whole wheat, commercial (PC)	36.90	0	0	0.44	0	0	8.61	0.07	0.20	0
Tortilla, taco shell (MD)	13	55.12	32.76	0.25	NA	0	3.77	0.04	0.04	0
Waffle, frozen, all varieties including bran (LG)	34	38.39	2.92	0.20	0.14	0.05	5.03	0.01	0.12	0.06
Waffle, homemade with whole milk, bran (PC)	75	135.85	30.11	1.14	0.67	0.49	20.80	0.17	0.60	0.30
Wheat, rolled, dry (CP)	94	0	0	1.20	0	0	73.32	0.37	0.86	0
Wheat germ (CP)	113	0	0	19.58	0.79	6.78	397.76	1.11	1.57	0
MEAT AND MEAT PRODUCTS (BEEF, FISH, AND POULTRY)										
Abalone, cooked, canned (OZ)	28.35	1.42	0.09	0.01	0.03	0.57	1.42	0.03	0.09	27.57
Anchovies, smoked, canned in oil (PC)	4	2.80	0.17	0.29	NA	0	0.50	0.01	0.04	0.04

Bacon, beef, kosher, cooked (SL)	6.50	0	0	0.03	0.08	2.01	0.52	0.02	0.03	0.25
Bacon, Canadian, cooked, drained (SL)	21	0	0	0.02	0	4.54	0.84	0.09	0.11	0.16
Bacon, low salt, cooked, drained (SL)	6.33	0	0	0.03	NA	2.12	0.32	0.02	0.07	0.11
Bacon, regular, cooked, drained (SL)	6.33	0	0	0.04	0	2.12	0.32	0.02	0.07	0.11
Bacon, turkey, cooked, drained (SL)	8	2.11	0.12	0.09	0	0	0.56	0.04	0.09	0.03
Beef, arm roast (9% fat), no visible fat, cooked (OZ)	28.35	0	0	0.07	0	0	2.27	0.12	0.10	0.57
Beef, chipped (OZ)	28.35	0	0	0.31	0	4.20	3.12	0.10	0.17	0.75
Beef, ground, regular (22.56% fat), cooked (OZ)	28.35	0	0	0.17	0.09	0	2.55	0.07	0.10	0.77
Beef, hamburger, ground chuck (20% fat), cooked (OZ)	28.35	0	0	0.11	0	0	3.12	0.10	0.09	0.73
Beef, pot roast (26% fat), cooked (moist heat) (OZ)	28.35	0	0	0.20	0	0	1.98	0.09	0.08	0.82
Beef, prime rib (30% fat), cooked (OZ)	28.35	0	0	0.22	0	0	1.98	0.07	0.10	0.66
Beef, rib eye steak (20% fat), cooked (OZ)	28.35	0	0	0.15	0	0	1.98	0.10	0.09	0.55
Beef, short ribs (42% fat), cooked (OZ)	28.35	0	0	0.31	0	0	1.42	0.06	0.07	0.74
Beef, top round roast/steak (5% fat), no visible fat, cooked (OZ)	28.35	0	0	0.04	0	0	3.40	0.16	0.14	0.70
Breakfast strips, beef, cooked (SL)	11.33	0	0	0.10	0.07	4.08	0.91	0.04	0.04	0.39

FOOD	WEIGHT (g)	VIT A (IU)	BETA-C (µg)	VIT E (mg)	VIT D (µg)	VIT C (mg)	FOL (µg)	VIT B_6 (mg)	PANT (mg)	VIT B_{12} (mg)
Breakfast strips, pork, cooked (SL)	11.33	0	0	0.05	0	4.92	0.45	0.04	0.10	0.20
Chicken, canned (OZ)	28.35	33.17	1.98	0.08	0	0.57	1.13	0.10	0.24	0.08
Chicken, dark meat, without skin, cooked (OZ)	28.35	10.21	0.57	0.18	0	0	2.41	0.10	0.35	0.10
Chicken, dark meat, with skin, cooked (OZ)	28.35	28.49	1.71	0.18	0	0	2.27	0.09	0.32	0.09
Chicken, light meat, without skin, cooked (OZ)	28.35	4.11	0.25	0.10	0	0	1.42	0.16	0.23	0.10
Chicken, light meat, without skin, without visible fat, cooked (OZ)	28.35	3.83	0.23	0.05	0	0	1.42	0.16	0.23	0.10
Chicken, light meat, with skin, cooked (OZ)	28.35	15.59	0.85	0.10	0	0	1.28	0.14	0.22	0.10
Chicken-fried steak (untrimmed beef round) (PC)	102.50	58.29	10.09	1.71	0.13	0.02	12.28	0.31	0.42	1.50
Chitterlings, cooked (CP)	161	0	0	0.61	NA	0	4.83	0.02	0.35	1.66
Clams, cooked or canned (MD)	12.50	71.25	4.27	0.20	0.01	2.76	3.60	0.01	0.08	12.36
Corned beef, canned (OZ)	28.35	0	0	0.10	0	0.43	2.55	0.04	0.18	0.46
Crab, all types, cooked, fresh or frozen (OZ)	28.35	1.70	0.10	0.35	NA	0.94	14.40	0.05	0.12	2.07
Crabmeat, canned (OZ)	28.35	1.42	0.09	0.35	NA	0.77	12.05	0.04	0.10	0.13

Duck, domestic, with skin, cooked (OZ)	28.35	59.53	3.69	0.23	0	0	1.70	0.05	0.31	0.09
Duck, domestic, without skin, cooked (OZ)	28.35	21.83	0	0.07	0	0	1.70	0.10	0.43	0.11
Fish, carp, cooked (OZ)	28.35	17.86	1.07	0.43	2.30	0.14	4.25	0.11	0.64	2.12
Fish, chinook salmon, smoked (OZ)	28.35	24.95	1.49	0.24	0.85	0	0.54	0.08	0.25	0.92
Fish, cisco, smoked (OZ)	28.35	267.34	16.01	0.43	0.85	0	0.60	0.08	0.09	1.21
Fish, cod, dried, salted, soaked in water, cooked (OZ)	28.35	15.03	0.90	0.08	0.41	0	0.58	0.04	0.16	0.08
Fish, flounder, cooked (OZ)	28.35	10.77	0.65	0.10	0.43	0	2.61	0.07	0.16	0.71
Fish, gefilte (PC)	102.70	78.32	8.69	0.46	1.85	0.66	8.97	0.21	0.45	0.77
Fish, haddock, smoked (OZ)	28.35	20.70	1.24	0.11	0.85	0	4.34	0.11	0.05	0.45
Fish, mackerel, Atlantic, cooked (OZ)	28.35	51.03	0	0.43	2.55	0.11	0.43	0.13	0.28	5.39
Fish, salmon, chinook (king) and sockeye (red), cooked (OZ)	28.35	34.02	2.04	0.38	3.54	0	4.90	0.07	0.25	0.34
Fish, salmon, pink, canned (CP)	177	97.35	5.82	2.05	22.12	0	27.26	0.53	0.97	7.79
Fish, salmon, pink, canned without salt (CP)	177	97.35	5.82	2.05	22.12	0	27.26	0.53	0.97	7.79
Fish, sardines, canned, drained (MD)	12	26.88	1.61	0.13	0.90	0	1.42	0.02	0.08	1.07
Fish, whitefish, cooked (OZ)	28.35	39.97	2.39	0.36	1.59	0.34	2.78	0.14	0.25	0.07
Fish fillet, breaded, commercial (approx. 18% fat) (OZ)	28.35	4.49	0.27	0.76	0.18	0	2.70	0.03	0.10	0.30

FOOD	WEIGHT (g)	VIT A (IU)	BETA-C (µg)	VIT E (mg)	VIT D (µg)	VIT C (mg)	FOL (µg)	VIT B$_6$ (mg)	PANT (mg)	VIT B$_{12}$ (mg)
Fish stick, breaded, commercial (approx. 10% fat) (OZ)	28.35	3.75	0.22	0.43	0.15	0	3.13	0.03	0.09	0.25
Fowl, wild, cooked, with or without skin (OZ)	28.35	53.54	3.21	0.10	0	0.65	1.70	0.21	0.34	0.20
Frankfurter, beef, low salt (REG)	45	0	0	0.31	0	0	1.54	0.08	0.07	0.52
Frankfurter, beef, regular (REG)	45	0	0	0.34	0.27	10.84	1.80	0.05	0.13	0.69
Frankfurter, beef and pork, low salt, regular (REG)	45	2.05	0.12	0.19	0	0	1.04	0.06	0.12	0.30
Frankfurter, beef and pork, reduced fat (LK)	57	1.92	0.11	0.20	0	0	2.10	0.13	0.20	0.76
Frankfurter, beef and pork, regular (REG)	45	0	0	0.22	0.40	11.70	1.80	0.06	0.16	0.58
Frankfurter, chicken, regular (REG)	45	0	0	0.24	0	0	3.60	0.10	0.32	0.13
Game, wild, cooked (OZ)	28.35	0	0	0.15	0	0	1.13	0.14	0.23	3.40
Goose, domestic, with skin, cooked (OZ)	28.35	19.84	1.13	0.31	0	0	0.57	0.10	0.43	0.12
Herring, canned or smoked (MD)	40	51.20	3.06	0.92	10	0.40	5.48	0.16	0.35	7.48
Herring, pickled (PC)	15	129.15	7.73	0.34	3.75	0	0.36	0.03	0.01	0.64
Lamb, chop, arm (9% fat), no visible fat, cooked (OZ)	28.35	0	0	0.05	0	0	5.95	0.05	0.20	0.73
Lamb, chop, breast (36% fat), cooked (OZ)	28.35	0	0	0.04	0	0	0.85	0.04	0.11	0.28

Food										
Lamb, chop, loin (24% fat), cooked (OZ)	28.35	0	0	0.03	0	0	5.39	0.03	0.18	0.63
Lamb, crown roast (30% fat), cooked (OZ)	28.35	0	0	0.03	0	0	4.25	0.03	0.18	0.63
Lamb, leg (20% fat), cooked (OZ)	28.35	0	0	0.04	0	0	5.95	0.04	0.20	0.75
Lamb, shank roast (13% fat), cooked (OZ)	28.35	0	0	0.04	0	0	6.24	0.04	0.19	0.61
Liver, beef, cooked (OZ)	28.35	10115	605.69	0.18	6.52	0.32	61.52	0.26	1.30	20.13
Liver, calves or veal, cooked (OZ)	28.35	7621.33	456.37	0.10	8.79	0.07	215.18	0.14	0.65	10.35
Liver, chicken, cooked (OZ)	28.35	4642.31	281.23	0.41	4.48	0.06	218.29	0.16	1.53	5.50
Liver, lamb, cooked (OZ)	28.35	7071.91	423.47	0.22	1.13	0.14	20.70	0.14	1.12	21.69
Liver, pork, cooked (OZ)	28.35	5102.15	305.52	0.13	6.69	0.32	46.21	0.16	1.35	5.29
Liverwurst (SL)	18	4980.06	298.21	0.08	0	0.11	5.40	0.03	0.53	2.42
Lobster, cooked (MD)	104	90.48	5.42	1.53	0	NA	11.54	0.08	0.29	3.23
Luncheon meat, bologna, beef (SL)	28.35	0	0	0.22	6.04	0.28	1.42	0.04	0.08	0.40
Luncheon meat, bologna, beef and pork (SL)	28.35	0	0	0.02	5.95	0.28	1.42	0.05	0.08	0.38
Luncheon meat, bologna, pork (SL)	23	0	0	0.05	8.12	0.05	1.15	0.06	0.17	0.21
Luncheon meat, bologna, turkey or chicken (SL)	28.35	0	0	0.14	0	0	1.56	0.07	0.17	0.07
Luncheon meat, chicken breast (SL)	28.35	3.67	0.21	0.06	0	0	0.97	0.08	0.12	0.06
Luncheon meat, corned beef (SL)	17	0	0	0.01	0	0	1.22	0.06	0.05	0.25

FOOD	WEIGHT (g)	VIT A (IU)	BETA-C (µg)	VIT E (mg)	VIT D (µg)	VIT C (mg)	FOL (µg)	VIT B$_6$ (mg)	PANT (mg)	VIT B$_{12}$ (mg)
Luncheon meat, pastrami, beef (OZ)	28.35	0	0	0.22	0	0.85	1.98	0.05	0.09	0.50
Luncheon meat, pastrami, turkey (SL)	28.35	0	0	0.10	NA	0	1.42	0.08	0.16	0.07
Luncheon meat, salami, beef (SL)	23	0	0	0.01	0.26	3.98	0.46	0.04	0.22	0.70
Luncheon meat, salami, beef and pork (SL)	23	0	0	0.09	0.21	2.76	0.46	0.05	0.20	0.84
Luncheon meat, salami, beef and pork, low salt (SL)	28.35	76.74	0.29	0.14	0.35	0.21	1.98	0.03	0.17	0.31
Luncheon meat, salami, dry or hard, pork (SL)	10	0	0	0.01	0.15	0	0.20	0.05	0.11	0.28
Luncheon meat, salami, dry or hard, pork and beef (SL)	10	0	0	0.06	0.19	2.60	0.20	0.05	0.11	0.19
Luncheon meat, turkey breast (SL)	21	1.95	0.12	0.05	0	0	0.67	0.08	0.11	0.05
Oyster, raw (MD)	14	14	0.84	0.12	1.12	0.52	1.40	0.01	0.03	2.72
Oysters, cooked (MD)	7	12.60	0.75	0.06	0.56	0.42	0.98	0.01	0.02	2.45
Pepperoni, pork and beef (SL)	5.50	0	0	0.04	0	0	0.22	0.01	0.10	0.14
Pork, arm picnic (14% fat), fresh, no visible fat, cooked (OZ)	28.35	2.55	0.15	0.05	0	0.11	2.27	0.10	0.15	0.16
Pork, chop, center loin (21% fat), fresh, cooked (OZ)	28.35	2.55	0.15	0.07	0	0.09	1.42	0.11	0.18	0.19
Pork, chop, loin (23% fat), smoked, cooked (OZ)	28.35	0	0	0.07	0	6.24	0.85	0.06	0.22	0.30

Food										
Pork, chop, rib (25% fat), fresh, cooked (OZ)	28.35	2.55	0.15	0.09	0	0.06	1.13	0.11	0.14	0.21
Pork, ham, Polish (15% fat), smoked, cooked (OZ)	28.35	0	0	0.08	0	3.97	1.42	0.09	0.21	0.30
Pork, ham, extra lean (6% fat), smoked, cooked (OZ)	28.35	0	0	0.02	0	5.95	0.85	0.11	0.11	0.18
Pork, ham, rump (11% fat), fresh, no visible fat, cooked (OZ)	28.35	2.27	0.14	0.03	0	0.11	2.55	0.11	0.16	0.16
Pork, ham, shank (21% fat), smoked, cooked (OZ)	28.35	0	0	0.08	0	6.24	0.85	0.08	0.16	0.26
Pork, loin ribs (30% fat), fresh, cooked (OZ)	28.35	2.83	0.17	0.10	0	0	1.13	0.10	0.21	0.31
Pork, salt, cooked (SL)	17	0	0	0.11	0	0	0.14	0.01	0.02	0.04
Pork, smoked (5% fat), low salt (OZ)	28.35	0	0	0.01	0	5.95	0.85	0.11	0.11	0.18
Pork, tenderloin roast (5% fat), fresh, cooked (OZ)	28.35	1.98	0.12	0.02	0	0.11	1.70	0.12	0.20	0.16
Sausage, braunschweiger (SL)	18	2529.18	151.74	0.06	0.11	1.80	7.92	0.06	0.61	3.62
Sausage, chorizo (LK)	60	0	0	0.27	0	0	1.20	0.32	0.67	1.20
Sausage, Italian (LK)	68	0	0	0.21	0	1.36	3.40	0.22	0.31	0.88
Sausage, knackwurst or bratwurst (LK)	68	0	0	0.38	0	18.36	1.36	0.12	0.22	0.80
Sausage, Polish (LK)	75.60	0	0	0.29	0	0.76	1.51	0.14	0.34	0.74
Sausage, pork, fresh, cooked (LK)	13	0	0	0.02	0.26	0.26	0.26	0.04	0.09	0.22

FOOD	WEIGHT (g)	VIT A (IU)	BETA-C (µg)	VIT E (mg)	VIT D (µg)	VIT C (mg)	FOL (µg)	VIT B₆ (mg)	PANT (mg)	VIT B₁₂ (mg)
Sausage, pork and beef, fresh, cooked (LK)	13	0	0	0.06	0.26	0	0.26	0.01	0.06	0.06
Sausage, turkey, fresh, cooked (LK)	24	19.52	1.17	0.12	0	0	1.55	0.06	0.22	0.06
Sausage, turkey, smoked (OZ)	28.35	18.22	1.09	0.12	0	0	1.45	0.06	0.21	0.06
Sausage, Vienna, cooked (LK)	16	0	0	0.09	NA	0	0.64	0.02	0.06	0.16
Scallops, cooked (LG)	15	25.50	1.53	0.09	NA	0	2.55	0.02	0.02	0.20
Shrimp, cooked, canned without salt (OZ)	28.35	62.09	3.72	0.81	0.74	0.62	0.99	0.04	0.10	0.42
Shrimp, cooked, canned with salt (OZ)	28.35	17.01	0	0.71	0.74	0.65	0.51	0.03	0.06	0.32
Squid, cooked (OZ)	28.35	34.30	1.98	0.34	NA	1.75	1.20	0.02	0.15	0.48
Surimi (OZ)	28.35	18.71	1.32	0.10	NA	0	0.45	0.01	0.02	0.45
Sushi or sashimi (raw tuna) (OZ)	28.35	619.16	37.08	0.42	1.53	0	0.54	0.13	0.30	2.67
Tuna, canned, oil pack, drained (CP)	160	124.80	7.47	1.84	9.28	0	8.48	0.18	0.59	3.52
Tuna, canned, oil pack, drained, no salt added (CP)	160	124.80	7.47	1.84	9.28	0	8.48	0.18	0.59	3.52
Tuna, canned, water pack, drained (CP)	160	124.80	7.47	0.85	9.28	0	7.52	0.61	0.59	3.52
Tuna, canned, water pack, drained, low sodium (CP)	160	124.80	7.47	0.85	9.28	0	7.52	0.61	0.59	3.52
Tuna, canned, water pack, drained, no salt (CP)	160	124.80	7.47	0.85	9.28	0	7.52	0.61	0.59	3.52

Food										
Turkey breast, processed (OZ)	28.35	0	0	0.03	0.14	0	1.42	0.09	0.14	0.09
Turkey ham (OZ)	28.35	0	0	0.12	0	0	1.70	0.07	0.24	0.07
Veal, breast (25% fat), cooked (OZ)	28.35	0	0	0.01	0	0	3.69	0.09	0.36	0.41
Veal, cutlet (10% fat), cooked (OZ)	28.35	0	0	0.12	0	0	4.25	0.09	0.36	0.40
Veal, rib roast (14% fat), cooked (OZ)	28.35	0	0	0.10	0	0	3.69	0.07	0.36	0.41
Veal, rump roast (6% fat), cooked (OZ)	28.35	0	0	0.14	0	0	4.82	0.09	0.34	0.45

MILK, DAIRY, AND RELATED PRODUCTS

Food										
Buttermilk, 1% fat (CP)	245	80.85	22.05	0.05	0.07	2.40	12.25	0.07	0.66	0.54
Buttermilk, whole (CP)	240	336	84	0.17	0.05	2.35	12	0.12	0.67	1.32
Cheese foods and spreads, pasteurized processed, 20–26% fat (TB)	16	136	36.64	0.07	0.05	0	1.12	0.02	0.09	0.18
Cheese, 17–26% fat (feta) (OZ)	28.35	126.72	5.10	0.01	NA	0	9.07	0.12	0.27	0.48
Cheese, 22–28% fat (Camembert, Brie, Jarlsberg) (OZ)	28.35	261.67	20.41	0.14	NA	0	17.63	0.07	0.39	0.37
Cheese, 25–30% fat (Edam, Gouda, Romano, provolone, Tilsit) (OZ)	28.35	259.69	18.14	0.16	NA	0	4.59	0.02	0.08	0.43
Cheese, 26–31% fat (blue, Roquefort, Limburger, Liederkranz) (OZ)	28.35	204.40	13.61	0.17	NA	0	10.32	0.05	0.49	0.35
Cheese, 28–32% fat (Muenster, brick, Monterey Jack, fontina, Cheshire) (OZ)	28.35	317.52	22.11	0.18	NA	0	3.43	0.02	0.05	0.42

FOOD	WEIGHT (g)	VIT A (IU)	BETA-C (µg)	VIT E (mg)	VIT D (µg)	VIT C (mg)	FOL (µg)	VIT B$_6$ (mg)	PANT (mg)	VIT B$_{12}$ (mg)
Cheese, 29–33% fat (process American) (OZ)	28.35	342.92	88.74	0.19	0.05	0	2.21	0.02	0.14	0.20
Cheese, 31–37% fat (cheddar, colby, Havarti) (OZ)	28.35	300.23	93.84	0.20	0.05	0	5.16	0.02	0.12	0.24
Cheese, Parmesan, fresh or dry (TB)	5	35.05	15	0.03	0.01	0	0.40	0	0.03	0.07
Cheese, imitation, low cholesterol, 19–26% fat (OZ)	28.35	257.98	68.04	2.57	0	0	5.10	0.02	0.11	0.24
Cheese, mozzarella, part skim milk, low moisture (OZ)	28.35	178.04	48.48	0.10	0.03	0	2.81	0.02	0.03	0.26
Cheese, ricotta, part skim milk (CP)	246	1062.72	194.34	0.42	0.10	0	32.23	0.05	0.59	0.71
Cheese, ricotta, whole milk (CP)	246	1205.40	317.34	0.66	0.20	0	30.01	0.10	0.52	0.84
Cottage cheese, 1% fat (CP)	226	83.62	22.60	0.05	0.05	0	28.02	0.16	0.47	1.42
Cottage cheese, 2% fat (CP)	226	158.20	42.94	0.09	NA	0	29.61	0.18	0.54	1.60
Cottage cheese, 2% fat, no salt added (CP)	226.80	158.76	43.09	0.09	0.05	0	29.71	0.18	0.54	1.61
Cottage cheese, 4% fat (CP)	210	342.30	94.50	0.19	0.04	0	25.62	0.15	0.44	1.30
Cottage cheese, 4% fat, no salt added (CP)	210	342.30	94.50	0.19	0.04	0	25.62	0.15	0.44	1.30
Cottage cheese, low fat (CP)	226	158.20	42.94	0.09	0.05	0	29.61	0.18	0.54	1.60

Food										
Cottage cheese, uncreamed (CP)	145	43.50	5.80	0.01	0	0	21.46	0.12	0.23	1.19
Cream, half and half (CP)	242	1050.28	278.30	0.27	0.19	2.08	6.05	0.10	0.70	0.80
Cream, heavy whipping (CP)	238	3498.60	880.60	1.50	3.09	1.38	8.81	0.07	0.59	0.43
Cream, light (CP)	240	1728	463.20	0.36	0.26	1.82	5.52	0.07	0.67	0.53
Cream, whipping (CP)	239	2693.53	738.51	1.58	2.99	1.46	8.84	0.07	0.62	0.45
Cream, whipping, unsweetened (TB)	7.50	84.52	23.17	0.05	0.09	0.05	0.28	0	0.02	0.01
Cream cheese, 35% fat (TB)	14	199.78	48.86	0.10	0.03	0	1.85	0.01	0.04	0.06
Cream cheese, Neufchâtel (TB)	14	158.76	32.80	0.07	0	0	1.58	0.01	0.08	0.04
Cream cheese, light, 18% fat (TB)	14.69	109.99	27.04	0.06	0.02	0	1.93	0.01	0.04	0.08
Ice cream, 7% fat (light), all flavors except chocolate or coffee (CP)	121.50	350.01	93.29	0.16	0.05	0.85	6.71	0.06	0.66	0.63
Ice cream, 7% fat (light), chocolate or coffee (CP)	121.50	354.27	93.29	0.16	0.05	0.91	13.41	0.07	0.63	0.57
Ice cream, 11% fat (average), all flavors except chocolate and coffee (CP)	132	539.88	145.20	0.26	0.08	0.79	6.60	0.07	0.77	0.51
Ice cream, 11% fat (average), chocolate or coffee (CP)	132	549.12	145.20	0.26	0.08	0.92	21.12	0.08	0.73	0.38
Ice cream, 16% fat (rich), all flavors except chocolate or coffee (CP)	148	951.64	239.76	0.41	0.13	1.04	7.40	0.06	0.53	0.53
Ice cream, 16% fat (rich), chocolate or coffee (CP)	148	951.64	239.76	0.41	0.13	1.04	7.40	0.06	0.53	0.53

FOOD	WEIGHT (g)	VIT A (IU)	BETA-C (µg)	VIT E (mg)	VIT D (µg)	VIT C (mg)	FOL (µg)	VIT B6 (mg)	PANT (mg)	VIT B12 (mg)
Ice milk, hardened, 4% fat, all flavors except chocolate (CP)	132	217.80	56.76	0.09	0.04	1.06	7.92	0.08	0.66	0.88
Milk, 1% fat (CP)	244	500.20	26.84	0.05	2.49	2.37	12.44	0.10	0.78	0.90
Milk, 2% fat (CP)	244	500.20	46.36	0.07	2.49	2.32	12.44	0.10	0.78	0.88
Milk, canned, condensed, sweetened (CP)	306	1003.68	266.22	0.55	0.15	7.96	34.27	0.15	2.29	1.35
Milk, canned, evaporated skim, undiluted (CP)	256	1003.52	5.12	0	5.32	3.17	22.02	0.13	1.89	0.61
Milk, canned, evaporated whole, undiluted (CP)	252	612.36	191.52	0.40	5.24	4.74	19.91	0.13	1.61	0.40
Milk, low fat (CP)	244	500.20	46.36	0.07	2.49	2.32	12.44	0.10	0.78	0.88
Milk, powdered, nonfat, instant (TS)	1.42	33.65	0.10	0	0.16	0.08	0.71	0	0.05	0.06
Milk, powdered, nonfat, regular (TS)	2.50	59.22	0.17	0	0.27	0.14	1.24	0.01	0.08	0.10
Milk, skim (CP)	245	499.80	4.90	0	2.50	2.40	12.74	0.10	0.81	0.93
Milk, whole (CP)	244	307.44	81.50	0.10	2.49	2.29	12.20	0.10	0.76	0.88
Sherbet (CP)	192	145.92	38.40	0.08	0.02	8.26	7.68	0.06	0.29	0.25
Sour cream, low fat (CP)	248	1599.60	159.96	0.35	0.47	1.54	15.77	0.27	2.43	1.12
Whipped topping, aerosol, saturated vegetable fat (TB)	4.38	20.72	12.48	0	NA	0	0	0	0	0

Food										
Whipped topping, frozen, saturated vegetable fat (TB)	4.69	40.38	24.18	0	0	0	0	0	0	0
Whipped topping, powdered, reduced calorie, with aspartame (TB)	4.94	8.45	4.94	0.04	0	0	0.04	0	0.02	0.01
Yogurt, 1% fat, all flavors (CP)	245	862.40	154.35	0.10	0	1.71	22.05	0.05	0.64	0.98
Yogurt, 1% fat, sweetened with aspartame, all flavors (CP)	245	409.25	10.53	0.10	2.01	1.84	0.10	0.78	0.73	248.48
Yogurt, 2–4% fat, all flavors (CP)	245	311.15	78.40	0.17	0.05	1.57	0.22	22.29	0.10	0.96
Yogurt, 2–4% fat, unflavored or plain (CP)	245	301.35	79.62	0.17	0.05	1.30	18.13	0.07	0.96	0.91
Yogurt, frozen, 1–2% fat, all flavors except chocolate (CP)	193	88.78	21.23	0.04	0.04	1.27	17.95	0.08	0.95	0.91
Yogurt, frozen, 1–2% fat, chocolate (CP)	193	86.27	21	0.02	0.02	1.22	18.91	0.08	0.89	0.87
Yogurt, low fat, all flavors except coffee (CP)	245	112.70	26.95	0.05	0.05	1.62	22.78	0.10	1.20	1.15
Yogurt, low fat, coffee flavor (CP)	245	111.99	26.78	0.05	0.05	1.59	22.64	0.10	1.20	1.15
Yogurt, low fat, unflavored or plain (CP)	245	161.70	39.20	0.07	0	1.96	27.44	0.12	1.45	1.37
NUTS AND SEEDS										
Almonds, unsalted (CP)	142	0	0	22.83	0	0.85	83.35	0.16	0.67	0
Brazil nuts, unsalted (CP)	140	0	0	10.64	0	0.98	5.60	0.35	0.34	0
Cashews, salted (CP)	130	0	0	1.96	0	0	88.01	0.32	1.55	0

FOOD	WEIGHT (g)	VIT A (IU)	BETA-C (µg)	VIT E (mg)	VIT D (µg)	VIT C (mg)	FOL (µg)	VIT B$_6$ (mg)	PANT (mg)	VIT B$_{12}$ (mg)
Cashews, unsalted (CP)	130	0	0	1.96	0	0	88.01	0.32	1.55	0
Chestnuts, unsalted (CP)	143	0	0	1.72	0	21.45	156.30	0.94	1.29	0
Coconut, fresh (PC)	45	0	0	0.04	0	1.48	11.88	0.02	0.13	0
Coconut, shredded, sweetened (TS)	1.94	0	0	0	0	0.01	0.16	0.01	0.01	0
Coconut, shredded, unsweetened (TS)	1.67	0	0	0	0	0.03	0.15	0.01	0.01	0
Filberts, hazelnuts, unsalted (CP)	135	90.45	54.16	32.29	0	1.35	96.93	0.82	1.55	0
Hickory nuts, unsalted (CP)	100	131	78.44	3.84	0	2	40	0.19	1.75	0
Macadamia nuts, salted (CP)	134	12.06	7.22	0	0	0	21.04	0.27	0.59	0
Peanut butter, no salt added, creamy or chunky (TS)	5.33	0	0	0.44	0	0	4.17	0.02	0.05	0
Peanut butter, with salt, creamy or chunky (TS)	5.33	0	0	0.44	0	0	4.17	0.02	0.05	0
Peanuts, salted (CP)	144	0	0	13.15	0	0	181.01	0.36	2	0
Peanuts, unsalted (CP)	144	0	0	13.15	0	0	181.01	0.36	2	0
Pecans, salted (CP)	110	141.90	84.97	2.91	0	2.20	43.34	0.21	1.89	0
Pecans, unsalted (CP)	108	138.24	82.78	2.86	0	2.16	42.34	0.21	1.85	0
Pine nuts, unsalted (CP)	120	34.80	20.84	4.25	0	2.40	69.36	0.13	0.25	0
Pistachio nuts, salted (CP)	128	304.64	182.41	6.67	0	9.34	75.65	0.32	1.55	0

Pumpkin seeds, salted (CP)	138	524.40	314.01	2.26	0	2.48	79.21	0.12	0.47	0
Pumpkin seeds, unsalted (CP)	138	524.40	314.01	2.26	0	2.48	79.21	0.12	0.47	0
Sesame seeds (TB)	8	5.28	3.16	0.18	0	0	7.68	0.01	0.05	0
Sunflower seeds, hulled, salted (CP)	144	72	43.11	72.19	0	2.02	327.46	1.11	9.71	0
Sunflower seeds, hulled, unsalted (CP)	144	72	43.11	72.19	0	2.02	327.46	1.11	9.71	0
Tahini (sesame butter) (TS)	5	3.35	2.01	0.90	0	0	4.88	0.01	0.03	0
Walnuts, unsalted (CP)	100	124	74.25	2.63	0	3.20	66	0.56	0.63	0

VEGETABLES AND LEGUMES

Artichokes, cooked, without salt (CP)	168	297.36	178.06	0.32	0	16.80	85.68	0.18	0.57	0
Arugula, raw (CP)	20	474.60	284.19	0.50	0	18.20	19.40	0.01	0.09	0
Asparagus, canned, drained solids, with salt (CP)	242	1285.02	769.46	2.20	0	44.53	231.35	0.27	0.34	0
Asparagus, fresh or frozen, cooked without salt (CP)	180	1472.40	881.68	2.59	0	43.92	242.46	0.04	0.29	0
Baked beans with franks, canned (CP)	257	248.47	148.78	1.16	0.33	16.55	83.06	0.23	0.33	0.49
Bamboo shoots, canned, cooked, with salt (CP)	131	10.48	6.27	0	0	1.44	4.19	0.18	0.12	0
Beans, kidney, dry, cooked or canned, without fat, without salt (CP)	177	0	0	0.14	0	2.12	229.39	0.21	0.39	●

FOOD	WEIGHT (g)	VIT A (IU)	BETA-C (µg)	VIT E (mg)	VIT D (µg)	VIT C (mg)	FOL (µg)	VIT B$_6$ (mg)	PANT (mg)	VIT B$_{12}$ (mg)
Beans, kidney, dry, cooked or canned, without fat, with salt (CP)	177	0	0	0.14	0	2.14	231.43	0.21	0.39	0
Beans, lima, cooked, fresh or frozen, without salt (CP)	170	323	193.41	0.49	0	21.76	36.04	0.20	0.27	0
Beans, lima, dry, cooked or canned, without fat, without salt (CP)	188	0	0	0.45	0	0	156.23	0.30	0.79	0
Beans, lima, dry, cooked or canned, without fat, with salt (CP)	188	0	0	0.45	0	0	156.79	0.30	0.79	0
Beans, navy, dry, cooked or canned, without fat, without salt (CP)	182	3.64	2.18	0.33	0	1.64	254.62	0.29	0.45	0
Beans, navy, dry, cooked or canned, without fat, with salt (CP)	182	3.64	2.18	0.33	0	1.64	254.36	0.29	0.45	0
Beans, northern dry, cooked or canned, without fat, without salt (CP)	179	0	0	0.23	0	0	144.45	0.16	0.41	0
Beans, northern dry, cooked or canned, without fat, with salt (CP)	179	0	0	0.23	0	0	144.45	0.16	0.41	0
Beans, pinto, dry, cooked or canned, without fat, without salt (CP)	171	3.42	2.05	0.02	0	3.59	294.12	0.26	0.48	0
Beans, pinto, dry, cooked or canned, without fat, with salt (CP)	171	3.45	2.07	0.02	0	3.63	296.55	0.26	0.48	0

Beans, yellow, canned, drained solids, with salt (CP)	136	142.80	85.50	0.39	0	6.53	43.25	0.05	0.18	0
Beans, yellow, cooked, fresh or frozen, without salt (CP)	135	151.20	90.54	0.39	0	11.07	11.07	0.08	0.07	0
Beets, Harvard (CP)	246	374.07	64.72	0.87	0.89	7.12	52.60	0.10	0.28	0.01
Beets, pickled (CP)	169	62.38	37.37	0.30	0	6.49	135.99	0.12	0.24	0
Beets, red, canned, drained solids, with salt (CP)	170	18.70	11.20	0.27	0	6.97	51.34	0.10	0.27	0
Beets, red, cooked, fresh or frozen, without salt (CP)	170	59.50	35.63	0.29	0	6.12	136	0.12	0.24	0
Broccoli, cooked, fresh or frozen, without salt (CP)	184	3481.28	2084.72	1.90	0	73.78	103.78	0.24	0.50	0
Broccoli, raw (CP)	88	1121.12	671.44	0.42	0	82.02	62.48	0.14	0.47	0
Brussels sprouts, cooked, fresh or frozen, without salt (CP)	155	912.95	546.67	1.32	0	70.83	156.86	0.45	0.53	0
Cabbage, Chinese (pak-choi), cooked, drained (CP)	170	4365.60	2614.60	0.20	0	44.20	69.02	0.29	0.14	0
Cabbage, Chinese (pak-choi), raw, shredded (CP)	70	2100	1257.20	0.09	0	31.50	45.99	0.13	0.06	0
Cabbage, Chinese (pe-tsai), cooked, drained (CP)	119	1150.73	689.01	0.14	0	18.80	63.55	0.21	0.10	0
Cabbage, Chinese (pe-tsai), raw, shredded (CP)	76	912	546.44	0.09	0	20.52	59.81	0.17	0.08	0

FOOD	WEIGHT (g)	VIT A (IU)	BETA-C (µg)	VIT E (mg)	VIT D (µg)	VIT C (mg)	FOL (µg)	VIT B$_6$ (mg)	PANT (mg)	VIT B$_{12}$ (mg)
Cabbage, cooked, without salt (CP)	150	198	118.56	2.50	0	30.15	30	0.16	0.21	0
Cabbage, raw (CP)	70	93.10	55.75	1.17	0	22.54	30.10	0.07	0.10	0
Carrot, raw (CP)	110	17022.50	10192.60	0.49	0	10.23	15.40	0.16	0.22	0
Carrot juice (CP)	246	63347.46	37933.20	0.84	0	20.91	9.35	0.54	0.57	0
Carrots, canned, drained solids, with salt (CP)	146	20110.04	12041.93	0.61	0	3.94	13.43	0.16	0.19	0
Carrots, fresh or frozen, cooked, without salt (CP)	156	38304.24	22936.66	1.34	0	3.59	21.68	0.39	0.47	0
Cauliflower, fresh or frozen, cooked, without salt (CP)	180	39.60	23.71	0.07	0	56.34	73.80	0.16	0.18	0
Cauliflower, raw (CP)	100	19	11.38	0.04	0	46.40	57	0.22	0.65	0
Celery, raw (CP)	120	160.80	96.29	0.43	0	8.40	33.60	0.11	0.23	0
Chard, Swiss, fresh or frozen, cooked, without salt (CP)	175	5493.25	3289.37	0	0	31.50	15.05	0.14	0.28	0
Chickpeas, dry, cooked or canned, without fat, with salt (CP)	164	44.28	26.52	0.51	0	2.13	282.08	0.23	0.48	0
Chickpeas, dry, cooked or canned, without fat, without salt (CP)	164	44.28	26.52	0.51	0	2.13	282.08	0.23	0.48	0
Corn, ear, cooked (MD)	77	167.09	100.05	0.08	0	4.77	35.73	0.05	0.68	0

Food									
Corn, whole kernel, drained solids, canned, with salt (CP)	164	255.84	153.19	0.10	0	13.94	79.70	0.08	1.10	0
Corn, whole kernel, fresh or frozen, without salt (CP)	164	406.72	243.54	0.23	0	4.26	37.39	0.16	0.36	0
Cucumber, raw (CP)	104	223.60	133.89	0.14	0	5.51	13.52	0.04	0.19	0
Eggplant, cooked, boiled, without salt, diced (CP)	96	61.44	36.79	0.03	0	1.25	13.82	0.09	0.07	0
Endive, raw (CP)	29	594.50	355.99	0.13	0	1.88	41.18	0.01	0.26	0
Fennel, bulb, raw (CP)	87	203.41	121.80	NA	0	10.44	23.49	0.04	0.20	0
Garlic, fresh (TS)	3.12	0	0	0	0	0.97	0.10	0.04	0.02	0
Ginger root, raw (CP)	96	0	0	NA	0	4.80	10.75	0.15	0.19	0
Green beans, canned, drained solids, with salt (CP)	136	474.64	284.21	0.04	0	6.53	43.25	0.05	0.18	0
Green beans, fresh or frozen, cooked, without salt (CP)	135	712.80	426.83	0.11	0	11.07	11.07	0.08	0.07	0
Greens, collard, fresh or frozen, cooked, without salt (CP)	128	3490.56	2090.15	2.87	0	15.49	7.68	0.06	0.06	0
Greens, turnip, fresh or frozen, cooked, without salt (CP)	144	7917.12	4740.80	3.23	0	39.46	170.50	0.26	0.39	0
Jicama, cooked, without salt (CP)	135.20	25.69	15.39	0.07	0	19.06	10.82	0.05	0.16	0
Jicama, raw (CP)	130	0	0	0.16	0	26	71.50	0.03	0.06	0

FOOD	WEIGHT (g)	VIT A (IU)	BETA-C (µg)	VIT E (mg)	VIT D (µg)	VIT C (mg)	FOL (µg)	VIT B$_6$ (mg)	PANT (mg)	VIT B$_{12}$ (mg)
Kohlrabi, fresh or frozen, cooked, without salt (CP)	165	57.75	34.58	0	0	89.10	19.96	0.25	0.26	0
Lentils, dry, cooked or canned, without fat, without salt (CP)	198	15.84	9.48	0.08	0	2.97	357.98	0.36	1.27	0
Lentils, dry, cooked or canned, without fat, with salt (CP)	198	15.68	9.39	0.08	0	2.95	354.52	0.36	1.25	0
Lettuce (CP)	55	181.50	108.68	0.24	0	2.14	30.80	0.02	0.03	0
Mushrooms, canned, drained solids, with salt (CP)	156	0	0	0.16	0	0	19.19	0.09	1.26	0
Mushrooms, fresh or frozen, cooked, without salt (CP)	156	0	0	0	0	6.24	28.39	0.14	3.37	0
Mushrooms, raw, whole or sliced (CP)	70	0	0	0.07	0	2.45	14.77	0.07	1.54	0
Okra, fresh or frozen, cooked, without salt (CP)	184	945.76	566.32	0	0	22.45	267.90	0.09	0.44	0
Onions, fresh or frozen, cooked, without salt (CP)	210	0	0	0.25	0	10.92	31.50	0.27	0.23	0
Onions, raw (CP)	160	0	0	0.19	0	10.24	30.40	0.19	0.18	0
Parsley, fresh (TB)	3.75	195	116.77	0.07	0	4.99	5.70	0	0.01	0
Parsnips, fresh or frozen, cooked, without salt (CP)	156	0	0	1.56	0	20.28	90.79	0.14	0.92	0

Food									
Peas and carrots, fresh or frozen, cooked, without salt (CP)	160	12417.60	7435.70	0.82	0	12.96	41.60	0.14	0.26	0
Peas, blackeye, dry, cooked or canned, without fat, without salt (CP)	171	25.65	15.36	0	0	0.68	355.51	0.17	0.70	0
Peas, blackeye, dry, cooked or canned, without fat, with salt (CP)	171	25.65	15.36	0	0	0.68	355.51	0.17	0.70	0
Peas, blackeye, fresh, cooked (CP)	165	1305.15	781.52	0	0	3.63	209.55	0.10	0.25	0
Peas, edible podded, fresh or frozen, cooked without salt (CP)	160	209.60	125.50	0.50	0	76.64	46.56	0.22	1.07	0
Peas, green, canned, drained solids, with salt (CP)	170	1305.60	781.80	0.03	0	16.32	75.31	0.10	0.22	0
Peas, green, fresh or frozen, cooked, without salt (CP)	160	1068.80	640	0.26	0	15.84	93.76	0.18	0.22	0
Peas, split, dry, cooked or canned, without fat, without salt (CP)	196	13.72	8.21	0.59	0	0.78	127.20	0.10	1.16	0
Peas, split, dry, cooked or canned, without fat, with salt (CP)	196	13.72	8.21	0.59	0	0.78	127.20	0.10	1.16	0
Pepper, chili, Mexican, canned (CP)	136	829.60	497.76	4.03	0	92.48	13.60	0.20	0.04	0
Pepper, chili, fresh, cooked, without salt (CP)	136	13158	7878.48	.94	0	263.84	22.28	0.34	0.07	0
Pepper, green, fresh or frozen, cooked, without salt (CP)	136	805.12	482.11	0.79	0	101.18	21.76	0.31	0.11	0
Pepper, green, raw (CP)	100	632	378.44	0.58	0	89.30	22	0.25	0.08	0

FOOD	WEIGHT (g)	VIT A (IU)	BETA-C (µg)	VIT E (mg)	VIT D (µg)	VIT C (mg)	FOL. (µg)	VIT B$_6$ (mg)	PANT (mg)	VIT B$_{12}$ (mg)
Pepper, red, fresh or frozen, cooked, without salt (CP)	136	5113.60	3061.36	0.79	0	232.56	21.76	0.31	0.11	0
Pepper, red, raw (CP)	100	5700	3420	0.58	0	190	22	0.25	0.08	0
Plantains, fresh, cooked, without salt (CP)	154	1399.86	838.24	7.70	0	16.79	40.04	0.37	0.35	0
Potatoes, French fried (REG)	4.20	0	0	0.12	0	0.49	0.59	0.02	0.03	0
Potatoes, French fried, without salt (REG)	4.20	0	0	0.12	0	0.49	0.59	0.02	0.03	0
Potatoes, baked, without skin, without salt (MD)	93	0	0	0.03	0	11.90	8.46	0.28	0.52	0
Potatoes, baked, with skin, without salt (CP)	122	0	0	0.05	0	15.74	13.42	0.43	0.67	0
Potatoes, boiled, without skin, without salt (CP)	156	0	0	0.06	0	11.54	13.88	0.42	0.80	0
Potatoes, boiled, with skin, without salt (MD)	142	0	0	0.04	0	14.74	12.57	0.40	0.62	0
Pumpkin, canned, cooked (CP)	245	54037.20	32357.15	2.60	0	10.29	30.13	0.15	0.98	0
Radicchio, raw (CP)	40	10.80	6.47	0.18	0	3.20	24	0.02	0.11	0
Radish, raw (CP)	116	9.28	5.56	0	0	26.45	31.32	0.08	0.10	0
Refried beans, canned (CP)	253	0	0	0.03	0	15.18	211.25	0.25	0.33	0
Romaine, raw (CP)	30	780	467.07	0.13	0	7.20	40.71	0.01	0.05	0

Food									
Rutabaga, fresh or frozen, cooked, without salt (CP)	170	953.70	571.08	0.25	0	31.96	25.50	0.17	0.27	0
Sauerkraut, cooked, canned, solids and liquid (CP)	236	42.48	25.44	3.94	0	34.69	55.93	0.31	0.21	0
Scallion, cooked (CP)	219	10312.71	6175.80	1.07	0	72.18	21.90	0.13	0.31	0
Scallion, raw (CP)	100	385	230.54	0.46	0	18.80	64	0.06	0.07	0
Seaweed, kelp, raw (CP)	80	92.80	55.57	0.72	0	9	144	0	0.51	●
Soybean curd (tofu) (OZ)	28.35	24.10	14.46	0.18	0	0.03	4.25	0.01	0.02	0
Soybeans, dry, cooked or canned, without salt (CP)	172	15.48	9.27	3.51	0	2.92	92.54	0.40	0.31	0
Soybeans, roasted (CP)	172	344	206.40	9.91	0	3.78	362.92	0.36	0.77	0
Soy flour (CP)	85	102	61.08	3.01	0	0	293.25	0.39	1.35	0
Spinach, canned, drained solids, with salt (CP)	214	18780.64	11245.89	0.04	0	30.60	209.29	0.21	0.11	0
Spinach, fresh or frozen, cooked, without salt (CP)	190	14789.60	8856.05	3.50	0	23.37	204.25	0.28	0.15	0
Spinach, raw (CP)	56	4705.12	2817.36	1.06	0	15.74	108.86	0.11	0.03	0
Sprouts, alfalfa, raw (CP)	33	51.15	30.63	0	0	2.71	11.88	0.01	0.18	0
Sprouts, soybean, raw (CP)	70	7.70	4.61	0.18	0	10.71	120.26	0.13	0.65	0
Squash, summer, all varieties, fresh or frozen, cooked, without salt (CP)	180	516.60	309.35	0.22	0	9.90	36.18	0.11	0.25	0

FOOD	WEIGHT (g)	VIT A (IU)	BETA-C (µg)	VIT E (mg)	VIT D (µg)	VIT C (mg)	FOL (µg)	VIT B$_6$ (mg)	PANT (mg)	VIT B$_{12}$ (mg)
Squash, winter, all varieties, fresh or frozen, cooked, without salt (CP)	245	8714.65	5218.35	0.29	0	23.52	68.60	0.17	0.86	0
Sweet potato, canned, syrup pack, drained solids, with salt (CP)	196	14027.72	8400.56	0.86	0	21.17	15.48	0.12	0.78	0
Sweet potatoes, candied (MD)	132.50	25187.55	14942.98	1.02	0.78	28.05	26.02	0.28	0.77	0.01
Sweet potatoes, canned, vacuum pack, drained solids, with salt (CP)	200	15966	9560.48	0.88	0	52.80	33.20	0.38	1.04	0
Sweet potatoes, fresh or frozen, cooked, without salt (CP)	255	55646.10	33320.85	1.12	0	62.73	57.63	0.61	1.66	0
Tempeh, fresh or frozen (PTY)	226.80	1555.85	931.65	3.95	0	0	117.94	0.68	0.82	2.27
Tomatillos, raw (CP)	132	150.48	90.10	NA	0	15.44	9.24	0.08	0.20	0
Tomatoes, canned, no salt added (CP)	240	1449.60	868.03	3.05	0	36.24	18.72	0.22	0.41	0
Tomatoes, canned, with salt (CP)	240	1449.60	868.03	3.05	0	36.24	18.72	0.22	0.41	0
Tomatoes, fresh, cooked, without salt (CP)	240	1783.20	1067.78	3.05	0	54.72	31.20	0.22	0.70	0
Tomatoes, raw (CP)	180	1121.40	671.49	0.85	0	34.38	27	0.14	0.45	0
Tomatoes, sun dried (CP)	54	471.96	282.61	2.28	0	21.17	36.72	0.18	1.13	0
Tomatoes, sun dried, oil pack, drained (CP)	110	1414.60	847.07	3.64	0	111.98	25.30	0.35	0.53	0
Tomato juice, no salt added (CP)	242.64	1349.08	807.82	0	0	44.40	48.29	0.27	0.61	0
Tomato juice, salt added (CP)	242.64	1349.08	807.82	0.53	0	44.40	48.29	0.27	0.61	0

Tomato paste, canned, no salt added (CP)	262	6466.16	3871.94	4.93	0	110.83	58.69	1	1.96	0
Tomato paste, canned, with salt (CP)	262	6466.16	3871.94	4.93	0	110.83	58.69	1	1.96	0
Tomato sauce, canned, without fat, no salt added (CP)	245	2398.55	1436.26	3.45	0	32.09	23.03	0.37	0.76	0
Tomato sauce, canned, without fat, with salt (CP)	245	2398.55	1436.26	3.45	0	32.09	23.03	0.37	0.76	0
Turnips, fresh or frozen, cooked, without salt (CP)	156	0	0	0.05	0	18.10	14.35	0.11	0.22	0
Vegetable juice, cocktail, no salt added (CP)	242	2831.40	1695.45	0	0	67.03	51.06	0.34	0.65	0
Vegetable juice, cocktail, salt added (CP)	242	2831.40	1695.45	0	0	67.03	51.06	0.34	0.65	0
Water chestnuts, cooked, canned (CP)	140	0	0	0	0	8.40	8.12	0.22	0.31	0
Watercress, raw (CP)	34	1598	956.89	0.34	0	14.62	3.13	0.04	0.11	0
Zucchini, fresh or frozen, cooked, without salt (CP)	180	432	258.68	0.70	0	8.28	30.24	0.14	0.20	0
Zucchini, raw (CP)	130	442	264.67	0.51	0	11.70	28.73	0.12	0.10	0

FOOD	CALC (mg)	IRON (mg)	MAG (mg)	PHOS (mg)	SOD (mg)	POTA (mg)	COP (mg)	ZINC (mg)	SELE (µg)
BEVERAGES									
Club soda (CP)	11.84	0.02	2.37	0	49.73	4.74	0.02	0.24	0.24
Coffee, brewed, hot or iced, without sugar (CP)	4.74	0.12	11.85	2.37	4.74	127.98	0.02	0.05	0.12
Coffee, decaffeinated, instant, dry powder (TS)	1.40	0.04	3.11	2.86	0.23	35.01	0	0	0.05
Coffee, instant, dry powder (TS)	1.27	0.04	2.94	2.73	0.33	31.81	0	0	0.12
Cola (CP)	7.39	0.07	2.46	29.57	9.86	2.46	0.02	0.02	0.49
Cola, diet, with aspartame (CP)	9.47	0.07	2.37	21.31	14.21	0	0.02	0.19	0
Cola, diet, with aspartame and saccharin blend (CP)	0	0.31	2.40	39	24	1.99	0.05	0	0
Cola, diet, with saccharin (CP)	9.60	0.10	2.40	26.40	38.40	4.80	0.05	0	0
Noncola (CP)	4.91	0.17	2.46	0	27.02	2.46	0.02	0.12	0.25
Noncola, diet, with aspartame (CP)	9.60	0.31	2.40	9.60	22.10	4.80	0.05	0.53	0.24
Noncola, diet, with aspartame and saccharin blend (CP)	9.60	0.31	2.40	9.60	52.80	4.80	0.05	0.53	0.24
Noncola, diet, with saccharin (CP)	9.47	0.09	2.37	26.05	37.89	4.74	0.05	0.12	0.24
Noncola, diet, with saccharin, sodium free (CP)	9.47	0.09	2.37	26.05	37.89	4.74	0.05	0.12	0.24

Food									
Postum, dry powder (TS)	8.26	0.21	10.23	21.11	3.03	97.61	0.06	0.25	1.7
Root beer, cream soda, birch beer, near beer (CP)	12.32	0.12	2.46	0	32.03	2.46	0.02	0.17	0.25
Root beer, diet, with aspartame (CP)	5.90	0.96	2.40	5.93	45.60	69.60	0.05	0.53	0.24
Root beer, diet, with aspartame and saccharin blend (CP)	5.90	0.96	2.40	5.93	14.40	69.60	0.05	0.53	0.24
Root beer, diet, with saccharin (CP)	9.60	0.10	2.40	26.40	38.40	4.80	0.05	0.12	0.24
Tea, herbal (CP)	4.74	0.19	2.37	0	2.37	21.33	0.02	0.09	0.05
Tea, hot or iced, with aspartame, reconstituted (CP)	0.33	0.14	1.95	2.19	0	25.01	0	0	0.07
Tea, hot or iced, without sugar, brewed (CP)	0	0.05	7.11	2.37	7.11	87.69	0.02	0.05	0.05
Tea, hot or iced, with saccharin, reconstituted (CP)	0.50	0.21	3	3.36	25.13	61.19	0	0.02	0.12
Tea, hot or iced, with sugar, reconstituted, presweetened, instant (CP)	4.80	0.05	4.80	2.40	7.20	45.60	0.02	0.07	0.05
Tea, instant, decaffeinated, dry powder (TS)	0.38	0.03	2.54	3.09	0.91	46.17	0.01	0.02	0.03
Tea, instant, decaffeinated, dry powder, with aspartame (TS)	0.03	0	6.22	0	0.31	11.77	0	0	0.01
Tea, instant, decaffeinated, dry powder, with saccharin, (TS)	0.28	0.01	1.27	1.55	4.94	23.09	0	0.01	0.02
Tea, instant, decaffeinated, dry powder, with sugar (TS)	0.28	0.02	1.65	2.08	0.63	30.14	0.01	0.02	0.06

FOOD	CALC (mg)	IRON (mg)	MAG (mg)	PHOS (mg)	SOD (mg)	POTA (mg)	COP (mg)	ZINC (mg)	SELE (µg)
Tea, instant, dry powder (TS)	0.38	0.03	2.54	3.09	0.91	46.17	0.01	0.02	0.03
Tea, instant, dry powder, with aspartame (TS)	0.16	0.07	0.97	1.09	0	12.50	0	0.01	0.04
Tea, instant, dry powder, with saccharin (TS)	0.25	0.11	1.50	1.68	12.56	30.60	0	0.01	0.06
Tea, instant, dry powder, with sugar (TS)	0.11	0.01	0.42	0.53	0.19	8.22	0	0	0.05
EGGS AND EGG PRODUCTS									
Egg, scrambled with whole milk (LG)	88.14	1.45	14.73	208.09	740.37	170.29	0.01	1.23	24.53
Egg, whole (LG)	24.50	0.72	5	89	63	60.50	0	0.55	12
Egg, yolk (LG)	22.74	0.59	1.49	81.01	7.14	15.60	0	0.52	6.81
Egg Beaters egg substitute, prepared as directed (CP)	153.01	3.96	20.29	162.71	650.36	293.97	0.12	2.25	29.57
Eggnog, commercial (CP)	330.20	0.51	46.99	277.88	138.18	419.61	0.03	1.17	5.13
Egg white (LG)	2	0.01	3.67	4.34	54.78	47.76	0	0	4.68
Scramblers egg substitute, prepared as directed (CP)	165.23	2.90	21.01	174.17	633.35	368.21	0.18	3.23	21.26
Second Nature egg substitute, prepared as directed (CP)	165.24	4.30	64.32	100.08	537.61	418.36	0.02	2.43	30.4

FATS AND OILS

Butter, salted (TS)	1.11	0.01	0.10	1.08	25.49	1.23	0	0	0.08
Butter, unsalted (TS)	1.11	0.01	0.10	1.08	0.52	1.23	0	0	0.08
Butter, whipped (TS)	0.74	0.01	0.07	0.72	16.98	0.82	0	0	0.05
Butter, whipped, unsalted (TS)	0.74	0.01	0.07	0.72	0.35	0.82	0	0	0.05
Lard, rendered (TS)	0	0	0	0	0	0	0	0	NA
Margarine, corn, diet (40% fat) (TS)	0.85	0	0.07	0.66	46.06	1.21	0	0	0.04
Margarine, corn, liquid (80% fat) (TS)	1.41	0	0.12	1.08	31.91	1.99	0	0.01	0.08
Margarine, corn, spread (52% fat) (TS)	0.96	0	0.08	0.72	46.90	1.34	0	0.01	0.05
Margarine, corn, stick/tub (80% fat) (TS)	1.25	0	0.11	1.08	44.34	1.99	0	0.01	0.08
Margarine, corn, stick/tub (80% fat), unsalted (TS)	1.25	0	0.11	0.95	1.32	1.77	0	0.01	0.08
Margarine, corn, whipped (80% fat) (TS)	0.84	0	0.07	0.64	34.09	1.19	0	0.01	0.05
Margarine, safflower, stick/tub (80% fat) (TS)	1.25	0	0.11	0.95	50.70	1.77	0	0.01	0.08
Margarine, safflower, stick/tub (80% fat), unsalted (TS)	1.41	0	0.12	1.08	0.66	1.99	0	0.01	0.08
Margarine, soybean, diet (40% fat) (TS)	0.85	0	0.07	0.66	46.06	1.21	0	0	0.04
Margarine, soybean, spread (52% fat) (TS)	0.29	0	0.08	0.38	37.25	1.10	0	0.01	0.05
Margarine, soybean, stick/tub (80% fat) (TS)	1.25	0	0.11	0.95	50.71	1.77	0	0.01	0.08

FOOD	CALC (mg)	IRON (mg)	MAG (mg)	PHOS (mg)	SOD (mg)	POTA (mg)	COP (mg)	ZINC (mg)	SELE (µg)
Margarine, sunflower, diet (40% fat) (TS)	0.86	0	0.07	0.67	28.80	1.34	0	0	0.04
Margarine, sunflower, spread (52% fat) (TS)	0.95	0	0.08	0.48	24.29	1.44	0	0.01	0.05
Margarine, sunflower, stick/tub (80% fat) (TS)	1.25	0	0.11	0.95	33.37	0.47	0	0.01	0.08
Oil, canbra or canola (rapeseed) (TS)	0	0	0	0	0	0	0	0	0
Oil, cocoanut (TS)	0	0	0.01	0	0	0	0	0.01	0
Oil, cod liver (TS)	0	0	NA	0	0	0	NA	NA	0.23
Oil, corn (TS)	0	0	0.02	0	0	0	0	0.01	0
Oil, cottonseed (TS)	0	0	0	0	0	0	0	0	0
Oil, olive (TS)	0.01	0.02	0	0.05	0	0	0	0	0.95
Oil, palm (TS)	0	0	0	0.01	0	0	0	0	0
Oil, palm kernel (TS)	0	0	0	0	0	0	0	0	0
Oil, peanut (TS)	0	0	0	0	0	0	0	0	0.41
Oil, safflower (TS)	0	0	0	0	0	0	0.01	0.01	0
Oil, sesame (TS)	0	0	0	0	0	0	0	0.01	0
Oil, soybean, partially hydrogenated (TS)	0	0	0	0	0	0	0.02	0.01	0
Oil, sunflower seed (TS)	0	0	0.03	0	0	0	0	0	0.48
Olives, black (ripe) (MD)	3.52	0.13	0.16	0.12	34.88	0.32	0.01	0.01	0

Olives, green, plain or stuffed (MD)	2.44	0.06	0.88	0.68	96	2.20	0.02	0	0
Salad dressing, blue cheese, commercial (TB)	12.39	0.03	0	11.32	167.38	5.66	0	0	3.22
Salad dressing, blue cheese, low calorie, commercial (TB)	5.35	0.02	1.63	3.67	173.50	4.44	0	0	0.83
Salad dressing, French, commercial (TB)	1.72	0.06	1.06	2.18	213.72	12.32	0	0.01	0
Salad dressing, French, low calorie, commercial (TB)	1.79	0.07	0.16	2.28	128.28	12.88	0	0.03	0.82
Salad dressing, French, no salt added, commercial (TB)	1.79	0.07	0	2.28	4.89	12.88	0	0.03	2.68
Salad dressing, Italian, commercial (TB)	1.47	0.03	0.09	0.73	115.69	2.20	0.01	0.02	2.28
Salad dressing, Italian, low calorie, commercial (TB)	0.30	0.03	0.27	0.75	118.05	2.25	0	0.02	2.63
Salad dressing, mayonnaise, commercial (79% fat) (TB)	2.48	0.07	0.14	3.86	78.44	4.69	0.03	0.02	0.86
Salad dressing, mayonnaise, imitation (19% fat) (TB)	0	0.03	0	0.01	74.55	1.50	0	0.02	2.56
Salad dressing, mayonnaise type, commercial (33% fat) (TB)	2.06	0.03	0.29	3.82	104.48	1.32	0	0.03	1.59
Salad dressing, Thousand Island, commercial (TB)	1.72	0.09	0.31	2.65	109.20	17.63	0	0.02	2.38
Salad dressing, Thousand Island, low calorie, commercial (TB)	1.68	0.09	0.11	2.60	153	17.29	0	0.02	0.95

FOOD	CALC (mg)	IRON (mg)	MAG (mg)	PHOS (mg)	SOD (mg)	POTA (mg)	COP (mg)	ZINC (mg)	SELE (µg)
Salad dressing, yogurt based, commercial (TB)	5.17	0.04	1.50	4.42	135	15.18	0.01	0.04	2.09
Sandwich spread (TB)	1.38	0.04	0.31	2.29	153	5.35	0	0	0.53
Shortening, household (TS)	0	0	0	0	0	0	0	0	0
Tartar sauce (TB)	2.59	0.13	0.46	4.60	101.67	11.22	0	0.03	1.89

FRUITS AND FRUIT PRODUCTS

FOOD	CALC (mg)	IRON (mg)	MAG (mg)	PHOS (mg)	SOD (mg)	POTA (mg)	COP (mg)	ZINC (mg)	SELE (µg)
Apple, fresh, with skin (MD)	9.66	0.25	6.90	9.66	0	158.70	0.06	0.06	0.83
Apple juice, sweetened (CP)	16.96	0.89	7.24	17.04	7.29	287.85	0.50	0.27	0.52
Apple juice, unsweetened, bottled or canned (CP)	17.36	0.92	7.44	17.36	7.44	295.12	0.05	0.07	0.5
Apples, dried, uncooked (CP)	12.04	1.20	13.76	32.68	74.82	387	0.16	0.17	1.03
Applesauce, sweetened, canned (CP)	10.20	0.89	7.65	17.85	7.65	155.55	0.10	0.10	0.51
Applesauce, unsweetened (CP)	7.32	0.29	7.32	17.08	4.88	183	0.07	0.07	0.49
Apricots, dried, uncooked (CP)	58.50	6.11	61.10	152.10	13	1791.40	0.56	0.96	1.56
Apricots, dried, unsweetened, cooked (CP)	40	4.17	42.50	102.50	7.50	1222.50	0.37	0.65	1.07
Apricots, fresh (MD)	4.95	0.19	2.83	6.71	0.35	104.58	0.03	0.09	0
Apricots, sweetened, canned (CP)	23.22	0.77	18.06	30.96	10.32	361.20	0.21	0.28	0.52

Avocado (SM)	19.03	1.76	67.47	70.93	17.30	1036.27	0.45	0.73	1.73
Banana, fresh (MD)	6.84	0.35	33.06	22.80	1.14	451.44	0.11	0.18	1.25
Blackberries, fresh (CP)	46.08	0.82	28.80	30.24	0	282.24	0.20	0.39	0
Blueberries, fresh (CP)	8.70	0.25	7.25	14.50	8.70	129.05	0.09	0.16	0
Cantaloupe, fresh (MD)	101.50	1.94	101.50	156.87	83.05	2851.30	0.37	1.48	3.69
Cherries, fresh, sweet (CP)	21.75	0.57	15.95	27.55	0	324.80	0.13	0.09	0.58
Cherries, sweetened, canned (CP)	18	0.70	18	36	6	290	0.28	0.20	0.8
Cranberries, fresh (CP)	6.65	0.19	4.75	8.55	0.95	67.45	0.06	0.12	0.19
Cranberry-apple juice, sweetened (CP)	17.15	0.15	4.90	7.35	4.90	66.15	0.02	0.10	0.49
Cranberry juice, sweetened (CP)	7.59	0.38	5.06	5.06	5.06	45.54	0.05	0.18	0.15
Dates, dried (CP)	56.96	2.05	62.30	71.20	5.34	1160.56	0.52	0.52	3.38
Figs, canned in heavy syrup (CP)	69.93	0.73	25.90	25.90	2.59	256.41	0.28	0.28	0.85
Figs, dried (CP)	286.56	4.44	117.41	135.32	21.89	1416.88	0.62	1.01	4.52
Figs, fresh (MD)	17.50	0.18	8.50	7	0.50	116	0.03	0.07	0.2
Fruit-flavored drink or juice, low calorie (CP)	21.33	0.09	4.74	2.37	7.11	52.14	0.02	0.05	0.14
Grapefruit juice, sweetened, frozen or canned (CP)	20	0.90	25	27.50	5	405	0.12	0.15	0.05
Grapefruit juice, unsweetened; fresh, frozen, or canned (CP)	17.29	0.49	24.70	27.17	2.47	377.91	0.10	0.22	0
Grapefruit sections, sweetened, canned (CP)	35.56	1.02	25.40	25.40	5.08	327.66	0.18	0.20	2.24
Grapefruit, fresh (MD)	34.94	0.26	23.30	23.30	0	404.77	0.15	0.20	2.53

FOOD	CALC (mg)	IRON (mg)	MAG (mg)	PHOS (mg)	SOD (mg)	POTA (mg)	COP (mg)	ZINC (mg)	SELE (µg)
Grape juice, sweetened, frozen (CP)	10	0.25	10	10	5	52.50	0.02	0.10	0.25
Grape juice, unsweetened (CP)	22.77	0.61	25.30	27.83	7.59	333.96	0.08	0.13	0
Grapes, fresh (CP)	17.60	0.42	9.60	20.80	3.20	296	0.14	0.08	0.32
Guava, fresh (MD)	18	0.28	9	22.50	2.70	255.60	0.09	0.21	0.54
Honeydew melon, fresh (MD)	77.40	0.90	90.30	129	129	3495.90	0.52	1.29	0
Kiwifruit, fresh (MD)	19.76	0.31	22.80	30.40	3.80	252.32	0.12	0.15	0.3
Kumquats, fresh (MD)	8.36	0.07	2.47	3.61	1.14	37.05	0.02	0.02	0.08
Lemon, fresh (MD)	15.08	0.35	4.64	9.28	1.16	80.04	0.02	0.03	0.23
Lemonade or limeade, sweetened, other than fruit-flavored beverage mix (CP)	7.44	0.40	4.96	4.96	7.44	37.20	0.05	0.10	0.25
Lemon juice, unsweetened, fresh, frozen, bottled, or canned (1 whole or 4 wedges = 1.50 oz) (CP)	26.84	0.32	19.52	21.96	51.24	248.88	0.10	0.15	0
Mandarin orange, fresh (MD)	11.76	0.08	10.08	8.40	0.84	131.88	0.03	0.20	0.17
Mango, fresh (MD)	20.70	0.27	18.63	22.77	4.14	322.92	0.23	0.08	0
Nectarine, fresh (MD)	6.80	0.20	10.88	21.76	0	288.32	0.10	0.12	0.54
Nectars, apricot, sweetened (CP)	17.57	0.95	12.55	22.59	7.53	286.14	0.18	0.23	0.28
Nectars, peach, sweetened, canned (CP)	12.45	0.47	9.96	14.94	17.43	99.60	0.17	0.20	0.65

Orange, fresh (MD)	52.40	0.13	13.10	18.34	0	237.11	0.05	0.09	1.93
Orange juice, sweetened, canned or frozen (CP)	19.40	1.07	26.67	33.95	4.92	424.60	0.15	0.17	14
Orange juice, unsweetened, fortified with calcium (CP)	289.41	0.25	24.90	39.84	2.49	423.10	0.10	0.12	14.94
Orange juice, unsweetened; fresh, frozen, or canned (CP)	22.41	0.25	24.90	39.84	2.49	423.10	0.10	0.12	14.94
Papaya juice, canned (CP)	25	0.85	7.50	0	12.50	77.50	0.02	0.37	NA
Papaya, fresh (CP)	33.60	0.14	14	7	4.20	359.80	0.03	0.10	NA
Peach, fresh (MD)	4.35	0.10	6.09	10.44	0	171.39	0.06	0.12	0.35
Peaches, dried, unsweetened, cooked (CP)	23.22	3.38	33.54	98.04	5.16	825.60	0.31	0.46	1.01
Peaches, sweetened, canned or frozen (CP)	7.68	0.69	12.80	28.16	15.36	255.52	0.13	0.23	0.77
Pear, fresh (MD)	18.26	0.41	9.96	18.26	0	207.50	0.18	0.20	1
Pears, dried, unsweetened, cooked (CP)	40.80	2.60	40.80	71.40	7.65	657.90	0.46	0.48	1.48
Pears, sweetened, canned (CP)	12.75	0.56	10.20	17.85	12.75	166.75	0.13	0.20	0.51
Persimmons, Japanese, raw (MD)	13.44	0.25	15.12	28.56	1.68	270.48	0.18	0.18	0.67
Pineapple juice, frozen or canned (CP)	42.50	0.65	32.50	20	2.50	335	0.22	0.27	0
Pineapple, canned, unsweetened or juice pack (CP)	35	0.70	35	15	2.50	305	0.22	0.25	0.25
Pineapple, fresh (SL)	5.88	0.31	11.76	5.88	0.84	9?-92	0.09	0.07	0.46
Pineapple, sweetened, canned (SL)	8.12	0.23	9.28	4.06	0.58	60.90	0.06	0.07	0.58

FOOD	CALC (mg)	IRON (mg)	MAG (mg)	PHOS (mg)	SOD (mg)	POTA (mg)	COP (mg)	ZINC (mg)	SELE (µg)
Plum, fresh (MD)	2.64	0.07	4.62	6.60	0	113.52	0.03	0.07	0.13
Plums, sweetened, canned (CP)	23.22	2.17	12.90	33.54	49.02	234.78	0.10	0.18	0.7
Pomegranate, fresh (MD)	4.62	0.46	4.62	12.32	4.62	398.86	0.11	0.62	0.62
Prune juice, bottled (CP)	30.72	3.02	35.84	64	10.24	706.56	0.18	0.54	0
Prunes, dried, cooked (CP)	48.76	2.35	42.40	74.20	4.24	708.08	0.40	0.51	0.49
Prunes, dried, uncooked (CP)	82.11	3.99	72.45	127.19	6.44	1199.45	0.69	0.85	0.8
Raisins (TB)	4.75	0.20	3.20	9.40	1.16	72.77	0.03	0.03	0.05
Raspberries, fresh (CP)	27.06	0.70	22.14	14.76	0	186.96	0.09	0.57	0
Raspberries, sweetened, canned or frozen (CP)	37.50	1.62	32.50	42.50	2.50	285	0.25	0.45	0.5
Rhubarb, stewed, unsweetened (CP)	465.60	0.70	43.20	45.60	2.40	552	0.05	0.26	0.96
Rhubarb, sweetened, cooked (CP)	348	0.50	28.80	19.20	2.40	230.40	0.07	0.19	1.37
Strawberries, fresh or frozen, unsweetened (CP)	20.86	0.57	14.90	28.31	1.49	247.34	0.07	0.19	0.3
Strawberries, sweetened, canned or frozen (CP)	28.05	1.50	17.85	33.15	7.65	249.90	0.05	0.15	0.82
Watermelon, fresh (SL)	38.56	0.82	53.02	43.38	9.64	559.12	0.14	0.34	1.93
GRAIN PRODUCTS									
Bagel, egg (MD)	8.80	1.21	11	36.85	226.02	105.10	0.04	0.29	17.6
Bagel, plain (MD)	23.10	2.14	11	36.85	227.49	149.07	0.04	0.29	17.6

Bagel, rye (MD)	8.15	1.68	16.68	62.55	165.39	81.75	0.10	0.48	15.56
Bagel, whole wheat (MD)	10.04	1.96	26.96	86.09	165.73	97.81	0.12	0.65	19.88
Barley, pearled, cooked with salt (CP)	17.93	1.37	43.74	120.86	72.14	153.14	0.24	1.18	17.51
Barley, pearled, dry (CP)	58	5	158	442	18	560	0.84	4.26	64
Biscuit, baking powder (MD)	95.72	1.17	7.91	60.34	186.14	59.05	0.04	0.24	10.25
Bran, unprocessed (TB)	2.74	0.40	22.91	37.99	0.07	44.32	0.04	0.27	3.27
Bread, Boston brown (SL)	43.20	1.01	36	76.80	120.48	140.16	0.13	0.19	8.3
Bread, diet, with fiber added (SL)	17.94	0.61	9.66	29.90	101.66	21.62	0.08	0.25	3.71
Bread, egg (SL)	17.33	0.99	6.56	39.45	55.29	45.30	0.04	0.23	8.73
Bread, Italian (SL)	25.20	0.87	6.90	23.10	175.50	22.20	0.03	0.18	16.7
Bread, nut (SL)	62.92	0.94	13.52	61.30	122.52	71.09	0.10	0.33	8.14
Bread, oatmeal (SL)	7.63	1.11	12.64	46.30	68.25	48.76	0.06	0.30	8.33
Bread, pumpkin, without nuts (SL)	14.60	0.97	7.30	32.52	171.76	53.89	0.04	0.20	6.97
Bread, raisin (SL)	15.97	0.65	5.62	19.57	82.12	52.42	0.03	0.14	6.75
Bread, rye (SL)	22.95	0.78	6.89	41.60	199.97	58.53	0.03	0.36	9.47
Bread, white (SL)	21	0.70	6.50	24.25	126.75	26.25	0.04	0.20	7.5
Bread, white, low sodium (SL)	18.75	0.63	5.25	26	2.50	29	0.03	0.15	7.5
Bread, whole wheat, low sodium (SL)	24.75	0.75	23.25	57	2.50	68.25	0.07	0.50	10.48
Bread, zucchini, without nuts (SL)	8.57	0.56	4.42	22.30	120.72	35.84	0.04	0.13	4.99
Buckwheat groats, cooked with salt (CP)	12.93	1.27	115.37	164.14	1176.87	164.87	0.32	1.25	2.69

FOOD	CALC (mg)	IRON (mg)	MAG (mg)	PHOS (mg)	SOD (mg)	POTA (mg)	COP (mg)	ZINC (mg)	SELE (µg)
Buckwheat groats, dry (CP)	27.88	4.05	362.44	523.16	18.04	524.80	1.02	3.97	8.2
Bulgur, cooked with salt (CP)	19.11	1.07	72.53	129.82	1093.42	177.63	0.15	0.84	27.35
Bulgur, dry (CP)	49	3.44	229.60	420	23.80	574	0.46	2.70	88.2
Cereal, cream of rice, cooked with salt (CP)	14.27	0.49	10.20	46.87	486.88	54.14	0.10	0.41	7.2
Cereal, cream of wheat, instant, cooked with salt (CP)	63.24	11.95	15.42	43.04	368.75	48.13	0.10	0.41	8.39
Cereal, cream of wheat, regular, cooked with salt (CP)	55.80	10.39	11.07	41.79	331.77	43.67	0.08	0.33	7.3
Cereal, dry, All-Bran (CP)	50.61	13.44	414.95	687.11	776.45	801.91	0.69	11.22	59.45
Cereal, dry, Apple Jacks (CP)	0.91	4.50	1.93	9	125.19	24.97	0.02	3.61	1.15
Cereal, dry, Cap'n Crunch (CP)	7.40	6.28	12.95	38.48	262.33	46.99	0.05	3.09	2.96
Cereal, dry, Cheerios (CP)	31.88	6.69	32.08	102.12	232.01	75.46	0.07	0.73	6.06
Cereal, dry, Cinnamon Toast Crunch (CP)	59.92	6.74	16.57	90.10	329.80	59.92	0.05	0.38	7.66
Cereal, dry, Common Sense Oat Bran (CP)	35.32	2.84	119.78	368.58	277.54	307.34	0.22	3	14.14
Cereal, dry, Cracklin' Oat Bran (CP)	15.36	10.80	60.67	175.55	342.20	156.73	0.12	5	14.21
Cereal, dry, Frosted Flakes (CP)	1.33	2.40	2.66	12	266.67	33.33	0.03	0	1.54
Cereal, dry, Frosted Mini-Wheats (CP)	21.64	3.61	75.16	200.99	5.69	205.54	0.37	2.99	2.9
Cereal, dry, Fruitful Bran (CP)	27.81	6.76	100.59	247.93	385.80	364.50	0.33	1.80	6.51

516

Cereal, dry, Grape-Nuts (CP)	41.96	32.43	107.73	283.50	661.12	352.67	0.50	4.81	10.09
Cereal, dry, Honeycomb (CP)	4.36	2.04	5.87	15.96	120	32.83	0.04	1.12	2.22
Cereal, dry, Just Right, with raisins, dates, and nuts (CP)	18.91	24	37.72	95.19	270.03	168.52	0.14	20	10.61
Cereal, dry, Kellogg's Corn Flakes (CP)	3.20	1.80	7.14	26.06	291.20	30.04	0.05	0.19	4.01
Cereal, dry, Kix (CP)	2.11	5.39	4.75	17.39	173.07	20.04	0.03	0	2.67
Cereal, dry, Life (CP)	144.76	12.57	72.16	251.68	241.12	266.20	0.26	1.30	NA
Cereal, dry, Oatmeal Raisin Crisp (CP)	33.74	8.88	61.54	229.30	342.44	231.42	0.26	1.28	23.86
Cereal, dry, Product 19 (CP)	3.40	18	10.49	39.97	324.89	44.23	0.08	15	3.4
Cereal, dry, Raisin Bran (Ralston) (CP)	18.14	5.90	75.97	176.93	374.59	223.22	0.21	1.45	28.72
Cereal, dry, Rice Chex (CP)	2.61	7.19	8.38	22.99	213.82	17.88	0.03	0.19	5.13
Cereal, dry, Rice Krispies (CP)	3.20	1.80	7.14	26.06	291.20	30.04	0.05	0.38	4.01
Cereal, dry, Special K (CP)	8.22	4.51	15.59	55	229.92	49.05	0.13	3.74	16.16
Cereal, dry, Total (CP)	281.82	20.95	36.96	136.95	163.02	123.09	0.14	17.49	3.85
Cereal, dry, Wheat Chex (CP)	13.46	12.16	53.15	132.60	345.01	155.27	0.14	1.12	23.63
Cereal, dry, puffed rice (CP)	0.84	0.15	3.50	13.72	0.42	15.82	0.02	0.14	1.68
Cereal, dry, puffed wheat (CP)	3.36	0.57	17.40	42.60	0.48	41.76	0.05	0.28	14.4
Coffeecake, yeast, without nuts, without topping (PC)	31.20	1.06	8.33	53.10	139.87	67.17	0.05	0.34	8.88
Cornbread (PC)	121.47	1.46	14.25	93.27	273.35	97.02	0.03	0.44	10.02

FOOD	CALC (mg)	IRON (mg)	MAG (mg)	PHOS (mg)	SOD (mg)	POTA (mg)	COP (mg)	ZINC (mg)	SELE (μg)
Corn grits, cooked with salt, regular or instant (CP)	5.35	1.48	11.64	27.78	521.53	52.22	0.02	0.15	2.71
Corn grits, dry (CP)	3.12	6.10	42.12	113.88	1.56	213.72	0.11	0.64	10.92
Cornmeal, cooked with salt (CP)	5.90	1.37	14.28	27.60	255.96	53.28	0.02	0.24	2.33
Cornmeal, dry (CP)	6.90	5.70	55.20	115.92	4.14	223.56	0.11	0.99	9.66
Cornstarch (TB)	0.16	0.04	0.24	1.04	0.72	0.24	0	0	0.25
Couscous, cooked with salt (CP)	15.77	0.57	24.49	91.08	407.53	89.02	0.13	0.45	5.92
Couscous, dry (CP)	44.16	1.99	80.96	312.80	18.40	305.44	0.46	1.53	20.24
Cracker, graham (PC)	1.27	0.10	1.26	4.14	22.22	6.50	0.01	0.03	1.04
Cracker, saltine (PC)	0.73	0.17	0.63	3.15	40.84	4.20	0	0.02	0.43
Cracker, saltine, unsalted top (PC)	5.93	0.21	0.99	3.79	26.33	4.46	0.01	0.03	1.16
Cracker, zwieback (PC)	0.70	0.02	0.49	1.92	8.12	10.67	0	0.02	1.23
Donut, cake (MD)	34.29	0.87	5.25	37.84	85.09	35.73	0.03	0.20	7.9
Donut, yeast (MD)	20.03	1.33	9.26	57.23	76.42	65.85	0.08	0.34	11.18
Flour, all-purpose (CP)	18.75	5.80	27.50	135	2.50	133.75	0.17	0.87	48.75
Flour, amaranth (whole grain) (CP)	298.35	14.80	518.70	887.25	40.95	713.70	1.52	6.20	21.45
Flour, buckwheat (whole groat) (CP)	49.20	4.87	301.20	404.40	13.20	692.40	0.62	3.74	6.84
Flour, cake or pastry (CP)	15.26	7.98	17.44	92.65	2.18	114.45	0.15	0.68	5.45

Flour, corn, masa, enriched (CP)	160.74	3.22	125.40	254.22	5.70	339.72	0.19	2.03	17.1
Flour, rice (CP)	15.80	0.55	55.30	154.84	0	120.08	0.21	1.26	34.33
Flour, rice, brown (CP)	17.38	3.13	176.96	532.46	12.64	456.62	0.36	3.87	12.8
Flour, rye, medium (CP)	24.48	2.16	76.50	211.14	3.06	346.80	0.30	2.03	36.41
Flour, triticale (whole grain) (CP)	45.50	3.37	198.90	417.30	2.60	605.80	0.73	3.46	76.6
Flour, whole wheat (CP)	40.80	4.66	165.60	415.20	6	486	0.46	3.52	73.8
Hominy, canned (CP)	16	0.99	25.60	56	336	14.40	0.05	1.68	NA
Macaroni, whole wheat, cooked without salt (CP)	21	1.48	42	124.60	4.20	61.60	0.24	1.13	32.02
Matzos (PC)	0.46	0.10	0.88	3.10	0.06	3.91	0	0.02	1.55
Melba toast, unsalted (PC)	0.53	0.16	0.77	3.78	4.95	3.75	0	0.02	1.37
Millet, cooked with salt (CP)	10.90	2.28	88.78	217.15	1416.70	148.85	0.58	1.30	1.66
Millet, dry (CP)	16	6.02	228	570	10	390	1.50	3.36	4
Muffin, bran, homemade (MD)	27.62	1.89	46.04	100.72	203.27	120.39	0.09	1.30	11.07
Muffin, corn, commercial mix or homemade (MD)	75.25	1.09	10.02	60.49	145.35	65.73	0.03	0.29	7.42
Muffin, English, whole wheat (MD)	41.55	1.75	27.93	106.60	133.41	134.11	0.13	0.70	18.18
Noodles, chow mein (CP)	9	2.13	23.40	72.45	197.55	54	0.08	0.63	19.35
Noodles, egg, cooked without salt (CP)	19.20	2.54	30.40	110.40	11.20	44.80	0.14	0.99	28.66
Noodles, macaroni, white, cooked without salt (CP)	9.80	1.96	25.20	75.60	1.40	43.40	0.14	0.74	26.6

FOOD	CALC (mg)	IRON (mg)	MAG (mg)	PHOS (mg)	SOD (mg)	POTA (mg)	COP (mg)	ZINC (mg)	SELE (µg)
Noodles, macaroni, whole wheat, cooked with salt (CP)	21	1.48	42	124.60	179.20	61.60	0.24	1.13	32.02
Noodles, manicotti, cooked without salt (CP)	9.80	1.96	25.20	75.60	1.40	43.40	0.14	0.74	26.6
Noodles, ramen, cooked, all varieties (CP)	8.06	1.07	51.76	70.05	978.37	40	0.11	1.25	15.14
Noodles, rice, cooked without salt (CP)	11.20	0.96	14.05	11.20	1.42	40.35	0.08	0.56	7.26
Noodles, rice, fried (CP)	0.37	0.03	0.46	0.37	5.68	1.33	0.02	0.02	0.24
Oat bran, cooked with salt (CP)	25.14	1.99	87.45	269.98	234.26	208.25	0.15	1.16	10.34
Oat bran, dry (CP)	54.52	5.09	220.90	689.96	3.76	532.04	0.38	2.92	26.32
Oatmeal, cooked with salt (CP)	23.77	1.59	56.96	178.59	349.69	131.93	0.14	1.17	10.6
Oatmeal, dry (CP)	42.12	3.40	119.88	383.94	3.24	283.50	0.28	2.49	22.68
Pancake, homemade, all varieties except whole wheat and buckwheat (MD)	109.74	0.74	6.64	64.01	262.53	54.93	0.02	0.24	7.38
Pancake, homemade, whole wheat (MD)	113.47	0.64	22.42	95.46	263.50	99.33	0.06	0.54	10.17
Quinoa (CP)	102	15.72	357	697	35.70	1258	1.39	5.61	18.7
Rice, brown, cooked without salt (CP)	19.50	0.82	83.85	161.85	9.75	83.85	0.19	1.23	25.56
Rice, white, cooked without salt (CP)	15.80	1.90	18.96	67.94	1.58	55.30	0.11	0.77	9.95
Rice, wild, cooked without salt (CP)	4.92	0.98	52.48	134.48	4.92	165.64	0.20	2.20	1.62
Rice bran, dry (CP)	47.31	15.39	648.23	1391.91	4.15	1232.55	0.61	5.01	9.13

Rice cakes, plain, no salt added (PC)	0.99	0.13	11.79	32.40	2.34	26.10	0.04	0.27	4.19
Rice cakes, plain, salted (PC)	1.03	0.14	11.94	32.76	29.87	26.39	0.04	0.27	4.24
Roll, croissant (MD)	38.41	1.97	13.26	81.85	87.84	93.57	0.08	0.46	17.37
Roll, hamburger (MD)	59.34	0.90	12.04	35.26	217.58	40.85	0.07	0.39	12.47
Roll, hamburger, whole wheat (MD)	42.57	1.29	39.99	98.04	226.61	117.39	0.12	0.86	18.02
Roll, hard (MD)	17.39	1.04	11.10	34.04	231.25	35.89	0.06	0.33	10.73
Roll, hot dog (MD)	59.34	0.90	12.04	35.26	217.58	40.85	0.07	0.39	12.47
Roll, hot dog, whole wheat (MD)	42.57	1.29	39.99	98.04	226.61	117.39	0.12	0.86	18.02
Roll, kaiser (MD)	23.50	1.40	17	46	312.50	48.50	0.09	0.45	15.43
Roll, rye (MD)	28.80	0.98	8.64	52.20	250.92	73.44	0.04	0.46	11.88
Roll, sourdough (MD)	37.80	1.30	10.35	34.65	263.25	33.30	0.04	0.27	25.05
Roll, submarine (MD)	84.60	2.63	17.85	79.90	545.20	84.60	0.16	0.58	26.55
Roll, white, dinner (MD)	26.64	1.01	10.08	30.60	182.16	34.20	0.06	0.32	10.44
Roll, whole wheat (MD)	34.65	1.03	32.55	79.80	184.45	95.55	0.09	0.70	14.67
Rye (whole grain) (CP)	55.77	4.51	204.49	632.06	10.14	446.16	0.76	6.30	1.69
Stuffing, bread, all types except cornbread (CP)	67.23	1.84	21.30	68.27	731.13	187.37	0.11	0.54	17.27
Stuffing, cornbread (CP)	343.21	4.17	44.94	262.64	1178.25	387.30	0.13	1.26	27.55
Tortilla, corn, fried (MD)	43.66	0.40	13.84	57.30	37.91	37.06	0.06	0.30	1.45
Tortilla, corn, plain (MD)	43.66	0.40	13.84	57.30	37.91	37.06	0.06	0.30	1.45

FOOD	CALC (mg)	IRON (mg)	MAG (mg)	PHOS (mg)	SOD (mg)	POTA (mg)	COP (mg)	ZINC (mg)	SELE (µg)
Tortilla, flour, plain, commercial (PC)	25.78	1.59	12.62	57.37	159.80	42.07	0.13	0.60	7.65
Tortilla, flour, whole wheat, commercial (PC)	7.14	0.76	27.19	67.67	151.25	79.24	0.07	0.57	12.04
Tortilla, taco shell (MD)	18.46	0.34	13.52	30.03	63.05	31.59	0.04	0.17	0.88
Waffle, frozen, all varieties including bran (LG)	31.16	0.64	4.46	31.75	218.02	33.55	0.02	0.16	5.85
Waffle, homemade with whole milk, bran (PC)	183.90	2.17	73.11	216.04	669	233.80	0.13	1.18	19.88
Wheat, rolled, dry (CP)	37.60	3.19	114.68	356.26	1.88	365.66	0.43	2.50	59.22
Wheat germ (CP)	50.85	10.27	361.60	1294.98	4.52	1070.11	0.70	18.84	89.5
MEAT AND MEAT PRODUCTS (BEEF, FISH, AND POULTRY)									
Abalone, cooked, canned (OZ)	2.83	0.51	13.61	32.89	85.33	31.18	0.06	0.60	3.55
Anchovies, smoked, canned in oil (PC)	9.28	0.19	2.76	10.08	146.72	21.76	0.01	0.10	0.8
Bacon, beef, kosher, cooked (SL)	0.91	0.21	1.69	23.79	66.36	15.34	0.01	0.40	2.62
Bacon, Canadian, cooked, drained (SL)	2.10	0.17	4.41	62.16	324.66	81.90	0.01	0.36	5.25
Bacon, low salt, cooked, drained (SL)	0.76	0.10	1.52	21.27	65.20	30.76	0.01	0.21	1.08
Bacon, regular, cooked, drained (SL)	0.76	0.10	1.52	21.27	101.03	30.76	0.01	0.21	1.08
Bacon, turkey, cooked, drained (SL)	0.72	0.17	2.32	32.32	207.84	33.12	0.01	0.24	1.3

								7
Beef, arm roast (9% fat), no visible fat, cooked (OZ)	2.27	0.70	7.65	61.80	19.28	112.27	0.03	1.48	7
Beef, chipped (OZ)	1.70	1.28	9.07	49.33	984.03	125.87	0.05	1.49	15.03
Beef, ground, regular (22.56% fat), cooked (OZ)	3.12	0.69	5.67	48.48	23.81	85.05	0.02	1.44	7.37
Beef, hamburger, ground chuck (20% fat), cooked (OZ)	1.70	0.82	7.09	62.37	17.86	101.49	0.03	1.20	7.64
Beef, pot roast (26% fat), cooked (moist heat) (OZ)	3.69	0.62	6.24	49.61	17.58	92.14	0.03	1.58	8.54
Beef, prime rib (30% fat), cooked (OZ)	2.83	0.65	5.39	48.19	18.14	81.65	0.03	1.62	9.46
Beef, rib eye steak (20% fat), cooked (OZ)	2.55	0.63	6.52	55	17.86	98.94	0.03	1.30	5.1
Beef, short ribs (42% fat), cooked (OZ)	3.40	0.65	4.25	45.93	14.17	63.50	0.03	1.38	7.37
Beef, top round roast/steak (5% fat), no visible fat, cooked (OZ)	1.70	0.82	8.79	69.74	17.29	125.31	0.03	1.58	6.55
Breakfast strips, beef, cooked (SL)	1.02	0.36	3.06	26.74	255.26	46.68	0.01	0.72	3.83
Breakfast strips, pork, cooked (SL)	1.59	0.22	2.95	30.02	237.82	52.80	0.02	0.42	3.97
Chicken, canned (OZ)	3.97	0.45	3.40	31.47	142.60	39.12	0.01	0.40	4.35
Chicken, dark meat, with skin, cooked (OZ)	6.80	0.52	6.38	51.60	23.11	70.02	0.03	0.94	3.86
Chicken, dark meat, without skin, cooked (OZ)	6.66	0.52	6.66	54.29	24.38	75.13	0.03	1.03	3.86
Chicken, light meat, with skin, cooked (OZ)	5.10	0.36	7.23	57.83	19.56	72.58	0.01	0.46	5.32
Chicken, light meat, without skin, cooked (OZ)	4.82	0.34	7.80	61.66	19.99	78.25	0.01	0.46	4.79

FOOD	CALC (mg)	IRON (mg)	MAG (mg)	PHOS (mg)	SOD (mg)	POTA (mg)	COP (mg)	ZINC (mg)	SELE (μg)
Chicken, light meat, without skin, without visible fat, cooked (OZ)	4.82	0.34	7.80	61.52	19.99	78.25	0.01	0.46	3.71
Chicken-fried steak (untrimmed beef round) (PC)	15.07	2.35	22.82	181.52	385.82	304.33	0.13	3.84	23.39
Chitterlings, cooked (CP)	43.47	5.96	16.10	75.67	62.79	12.88	0.37	8.15	3.22
Clams, cooked or canned (MD)	11.50	3.49	2.25	42.25	14	78.50	0.09	0.34	1.57
Corned beef, canned (OZ)	3.40	0.59	3.97	31.47	285.20	38.56	0.02	1.01	5.39
Crab, all types, cooked, fresh or frozen (OZ)	29.48	0.26	9.36	58.40	79.10	91.85	0.18	1.20	14.46
Crabmeat, canned (OZ)	28.63	0.24	11.06	73.71	94.41	106.03	0.22	1.14	6.24
Duck, domestic, with skin, cooked (OZ)	3.12	0.77	4.54	44.23	16.73	57.83	0.07	0.53	3.86
Duck, domestic, without skin, cooked (OZ)	3.69	0.79	6.38	72.58	20.13	90.72	0.07	0.74	3.86
Fish, carp, cooked (OZ)	15.59	0.54	7.94	89.02	18.99	131.26	0.07	0.24	16.73
Fish, chinook salmon, smoked (OZ)	3.12	0.24	5.10	46.49	222.26	49.61	0.07	0.09	6.8
Fish, cisco, smoked (OZ)	7.37	0.14	4.82	42.52	136.36	83.07	0.06	0.09	9.36
Fish, cod, dried, salted, soaked in water, cooked (OZ)	7.99	0.29	7.47	64.92	146	11.06	0.01	0.16	12.32
Fish, flounder, cooked (OZ)	5.10	0.10	16.44	81.93	29.77	97.52	0.01	0.18	12.76
Fish, gefilte (PC)	17.86	0.62	24.33	154.95	159.48	247.55	0.06	0.48	24.74

Fish, haddock, smoked (OZ)	13.89	0.40	15.31	71.16	216.31	117.65	0.01	0.14	13.61
Fish, mackerel, Atlantic, cooked (OZ)	4.25	0.45	27.50	78.81	23.53	113.68	0.03	0.27	7.37
Fish, salmon, chinook (king) and sockeye (red), cooked (OZ)	12.19	0.19	8.79	96.67	21.55	180.31	0.02	0.20	7.37
Fish, salmon, pink, canned (CP)	377.01	1.49	60.18	582.33	980.58	577.02	0.18	1.63	132.75
Fish, salmon, pink, canned without salt (CP)	377.01	1.49	60.18	582.33	132.75	577.02	0.18	1.63	132.75
Fish, sardines, canned, drained (MD)	45.84	0.35	4.68	58.80	60.60	47.64	0.02	0.16	4.2
Fish, whitefish, cooked (OZ)	8.79	0.40	9.36	69.17	20.13	129.84	0.04	0.25	13.32
Fish fillet, breaded, commercial (approx. 18% fat) (OZ)	3.26	0.33	8.32	40.86	94.90	47.31	0.03	0.12	7.75
Fish stick, breaded, commercial (approx. 10% fat) (OZ)	3.36	0.43	7.75	37.71	158.79	43.08	0.03	0.13	7.78
Fowl, wild, cooked, with or without skin (OZ)	13.89	2.38	9.92	87.88	28.35	116.23	0.02	0.39	14.46
Frankfurter, beef, low salt (REG)	3.87	0.49	4.95	41.28	307.80	315.90	0.02	0.93	3.43
Frankfurter, beef, regular (REG)	9	0.64	1.35	39.15	461.70	74.70	0.03	0.93	4.05
Frankfurter, beef and pork, low salt, regular (REG)	10.61	0.36	4.68	51.55	300.15	307.80	0.02	0.84	5.87
Frankfurter, beef and pork, reduced fat (LK)	12.51	0.77	9.40	83.47	628.21	123.61	0.05	1.95	8.12
Frankfurter, beef and pork, regular (REG)	4.95	0.52	4.50	38.70	504	75.15	0.04	0.83	4.05
Frankfurter, chicken, regular (REG)	47.70	0.83	6.30	85.05	505.35	80.55	0.04	1.40	4.05

FOOD	CALC (mg)	IRON (mg)	MAG (mg)	PHOS (mg)	SOD (mg)	POTA (mg)	COP (mg)	ZINC (mg)	SELE (µg)
Game, wild, cooked (OZ)	1.98	1.27	6.80	64.07	15.31	94.97	0.09	0.78	13.89
Goose, domestic, with skin, cooked (OZ)	3.69	0.80	6.24	76.54	19.84	93.27	0.07	0.74	3.86
Herring, canned or smoked (MD)	33.60	0.60	18.40	130	367.20	178.80	0.05	0.54	10.8
Herring, pickled (PC)	11.55	0.18	1.20	13.35	130.50	10.35	0.01	0.08	4.05
Lamb, chop, arm (9% fat), no visible fat, cooked (OZ)	2.27	0.62	7.09	57.55	20.13	94.41	0.03	1.37	3.38
Lamb, chop, breast (36% fat), cooked (OZ)	2.55	0.31	5.10	44.23	13.95	63.82	0.05	1.02	5.42
Lamb, chop, loin (24% fat), cooked (OZ)	5.10	0.60	6.52	51.03	18.14	69.74	0.03	0.97	4.82
Lamb, crown roast (30% fat), cooked (OZ)	6.24	0.45	5.67	47.06	20.70	76.83	0.03	0.99	4.82
Lamb, leg (20% fat), cooked (OZ)	5.67	0.56	6.52	52.16	18.71	71.16	0.03	1.48	4.82
Lamb, shank roast (13% fat), cooked (OZ)	5.95	0.50	6.52	55.28	22.96	89.30	0.04	1.27	3.76
Liver, beef, cooked (OZ)	1.98	1.92	5.67	114.53	19.84	66.62	1.28	1.72	15.88
Liver, calves or veal, cooked (OZ)	1.98	0.74	5.39	90.44	15.03	58.12	2.25	2.70	17.86
Liver, chicken, cooked (OZ)	3.97	2.40	5.95	88.45	14.46	39.69	0.10	1.23	10.21
Liver, lamb, cooked (OZ)	2.27	2.35	6.24	119.07	15.88	62.65	2	2.24	25.51
Liver, pork, cooked (OZ)	2.83	5.08	3.97	68.32	13.89	42.52	0.18	1.91	18.14
Liverwurst (SL)	4.68	1.15	2.16	41.40	154.80	30.60	0.04	0.41	10.44
Lobster, cooked (MD)	63.44	0.41	36.40	192.40	395.20	366.08	2.02	3.04	82.16

Luncheon meat, bologna, beef (SL)	3.40	0.47	3.40	24.95	278.11	44.51	0.01	0.61	4.82
Luncheon meat, bologna, beef and pork (SL)	3.40	0.43	3.12	25.80	288.89	51.03	0.02	0.55	4.82
Luncheon meat, bologna, pork (SL)	2.53	0.18	3.22	31.97	272.32	64.63	0.02	0.47	6.9
Luncheon meat, bologna, turkey or chicken (SL)	14.74	0.45	4.11	33.59	266.77	62.80	0.01	0.50	9.36
Luncheon meat, chicken breast (SL)	3.40	0.21	4.42	35.74	334.02	51.04	0.01	0.26	2.69
Luncheon meat, corned beef (SL)	0.97	0.29	3.36	25.10	204.01	45.14	0.01	0.57	2.38
Luncheon meat, pastrami, beef (OZ)	2.55	0.54	5.10	42.52	347.85	64.64	0.02	1.21	5.39
Luncheon meat, pastrami, turkey (SL)	2.55	0.47	3.97	56.70	296.26	73.71	0.01	0.61	9.36
Luncheon meat, salami, beef (SL)	2.07	0.50	3.22	25.99	270.48	51.52	0.03	0.50	4.6
Luncheon meat, salami, beef and pork (SL)	2.99	0.61	3.45	26.45	244.95	45.54	0.05	0.49	4.6
Luncheon meat, salami, beef and pork, low salt (SL)	43.54	0.20	5.29	49.11	199.87	199.87	0.01	0.40	3.45
Luncheon meat, salami, dry or hard, pork (SL)	1.30	0.13	2.20	22.90	226	37.80	0.02	0.42	3.3
Luncheon meat, salami, dry or hard, pork and beef (SL)	0.80	0.15	1.70	14.20	186	37.80	0.01	0.32	3.3
Luncheon meat, turkey breast (SL)	2.74	0.16	3.97	29.24	290.43	37.17	0.01	0.22	2.3
Oyster, raw (MD)	6.30	0.93	6.58	18.90	29.54	21.84	0.62	12.71	7.98
Oysters, cooked (MD)	6.30	0.84	6.65	14.21	29.54	19.67	0.53	12.71	3.43
Pepperoni, pork and beef (SL)	0.55	0.08	0.88	6.54	112.20	19.08	0	0.14	1.81

FOOD	CALC (mg)	IRON (mg)	MAG (mg)	PHOS (mg)	SOD (mg)	POTA (mg)	COP (mg)	ZINC (mg)	SELE (µg)
Pork, arm picnic (14% fat), fresh, no visible fat, cooked (OZ)	1.70	0.26	6.24	60.67	13.61	98.09	0.01	0.75	2.42
Pork, chop, center loin (21% fat), fresh, cooked (OZ)	4.25	0.28	6.24	72.86	16.73	95.82	0.03	0.87	2.62
Pork, chop, loin (23% fat), smoked, cooked (OZ)	1.98	0.25	3.69	44.23	275.85	55	0.02	0.69	13.16
Pork, chop, rib (25% fat), fresh, cooked (OZ)	9.64	0.31	5.67	59.53	8.50	92.42	0.02	0.94	2.77
Pork, ham, Polish (15% fat), smoked, cooked (OZ)	2.27	0.39	4.82	68.89	266.77	101.21	0.04	0.71	11.73
Pork, ham, extra lean (6% fat), smoked, cooked (OZ)	2.27	0.42	3.97	55.57	341.05	81.36	0.02	0.82	9.7
Pork, ham, rump (11% fat), fresh, no visible fat, cooked (OZ)	1.70	0.28	6.80	62.94	14.17	102.91	0	0.80	2.23
Pork, ham, shank (21% fat), smoked, cooked (OZ)	2.83	0.27	3.97	62.65	303.91	73.14	0.03	0.71	6.8
Pork, loin ribs (30% fat), fresh, cooked (OZ)	13.32	0.52	6.80	73.99	26.37	90.72	0.04	1.30	3.38
Pork, salt, cooked (SL)	1.36	0.27	1.70	20.40	206.04	7.14	0.01	0.14	7.14
Pork, smoked (5% fat), low salt (OZ)	1.13	0.31	5.10	73.14	234.74	248.35	0.02	0.53	9.7
Pork, tenderloin roast (5% fat), fresh, cooked (OZ)	1.70	0.42	7.94	73.43	15.88	123.89	0.01	0.75	1.91

Sausage, braunschweiger (SL)	1.62	1.68	1.95	30.24	205.74	35.82	0.04	0.51	3.96
Sausage, chorizo (LK)	4.80	0.95	10.80	90	741	238.80	0.05	2.05	15
Sausage, Italian (LK)	16.32	1.02	12.24	115.60	626.96	206.72	0.05	1.63	17
Sausage, knackwurst or bratwurst (LK)	7.48	0.62	7.48	66.64	686.80	135.32	0.04	1.13	17
Sausage, Polish (LK)	9.07	1.09	10.58	102.82	562.26	179.17	0.07	1.46	18.9
Sausage, pork and beef, fresh, cooked (LK)	1.30	0.15	1.56	13.91	104.65	24.57	0.01	0.24	1.95
Sausage, pork, fresh, cooked (LK)	4.16	0.16	2.21	23.92	168.22	46.93	0.02	0.32	1.95
Sausage, turkey, fresh, cooked (LK)	4.99	0.35	4.57	35.35	234.27	48.02	0.02	0.65	2.66
Sausage, turkey, smoked (OZ)	4.80	0.33	4.32	33	253.09	44.83	0.02	0.60	2.49
Scallops, cooked (LG)	17.25	0.45	10.35	50.70	39.75	71.40	0.01	0.23	13.6
Sausage, Vienna, cooked (LK)	1.60	0.14	1.12	7.84	152.48	16.16	0	0.26	5.28
Shrimp, cooked, canned without salt (OZ)	11.06	0.88	9.54	38.84	63.50	51.60	0.05	0.44	18.14
Shrimp, cooked, canned with salt (OZ)	16.73	0.78	11.62	66.06	651.77	59.53	0.09	0.36	18.14
Squid, cooked (OZ)	11.91	0.25	12.19	61.80	16.44	91.85	0.60	0.57	22.71
Surimi (OZ)	2.55	0.07	12.19	79.95	244.94	31.75	0.01	0.09	12.76
Sushi or sashimi (raw tuna) (OZ)	2.27	0.29	14.17	72.01	11.06	71.44	0.03	0.17	29.37
Tuna, canned, oil pack, drained (CP)	20.80	2.22	49.60	497.60	566.40	331.20	0.11	1.44	124.8
Tuna, canned, oil pack, drained, no salt added (CP)	20.80	2.22	49.60	497.60	80	331.20	0.11	1.44	124.8
Tuna, canned, water pack, drained (CP)	19.20	5.12	46.40	297.60	569.60	502.40	0.02	0.70	165.76

FOOD	CALC (mg)	IRON (mg)	MAG (mg)	PHOS (mg)	SOD (mg)	POTA (mg)	COP (mg)	ZINC (mg)	SELE (µg)
Tuna, canned, water pack, drained, low sodium (CP)	19.20	5.12	46.40	297.60	324.80	502.40	0.02	0.70	165.76
Tuna, canned, water pack, drained, no salt (CP)	19.20	5.12	46.40	297.60	80	502.40	0.02	0.70	165.76
Turkey breast, processed (OZ)	2.55	0.19	5.95	60.67	112.55	70.31	0.01	0.43	4.04
Turkey ham (OZ)	2.83	0.78	4.54	54.15	282.37	92.14	0.03	0.83	14.46
Veal, breast (25% fat), cooked (OZ)	3.12	1.11	7.94	66.06	24.66	138.91	0.07	0.93	3.4
Veal, cutlet (10% fat), cooked (OZ)	3.69	0.26	7.37	63.22	23.53	99.51	0.04	0.95	3.4
Veal, rib roast (14% fat), cooked (OZ)	3.12	0.27	6.24	55.85	26.08	83.63	0.03	1.16	3.4
Veal, rump roast (6% fat), cooked (OZ)	7.65	0.33	7.65	64.07	25.80	100.93	0.04	1.22	3.4
MILK, DAIRY, AND RELATED PRODUCTS									
Buttermilk, 1% fat (CP)	285.18	0.12	26.83	218.54	257	370.68	0.02	1.03	2.52
Buttermilk, whole (CP)	273.60	0.24	31.20	211.20	230.40	369.60	0.07	0.98	2.47
Cheese, 17–26% fat (feta) (OZ)	139.62	0.18	5.45	95.60	316.41	17.52	0.01	0.82	3.12
Cheese, 22–28% fat (Camembert, Brie, Jarlsberg) (OZ)	109.88	0.09	5.66	98.26	238.62	52.90	0.01	0.67	3.12

Food									
Cheese, 25–30% fat (Edam, Gouda, Romano, provolone, Tilsit) (OZ)	207.24	0.12	8.44	151.84	273.58	53.21	0.01	1.06	3.12
Cheese, 26–31% fat (blue, Roquefort, Limburger, Liederkranz) (OZ)	149.57	0.09	6.50	109.83	395.57	72.66	0.01	0.75	3.12
Cheese, 28–32% fat (Muenster, brick, Monterey Jack, fontina, Cheshire) (OZ)	203.35	0.12	7.75	132.59	177.95	38.10	0.01	0.80	3.97
Cheese, 29–33% fat (process American) (OZ)	142.03	0.11	6.31	178.04	405.52	45.93	0.01	0.85	3.69
Cheese, 31–37% fat (cheddar, colby, Havarti) (OZ)	147.99	0.19	7.88	122.47	175.91	27.90	0.01	0.88	5.1
Cheese, imitation, low cholesterol, 19–26% fat (OZ)	136.36	0.14	6.01	106.03	395.48	41.67	0.01	0.57	3.52
Cheese, mozzarella, part skim milk, low moisture (OZ)	207.32	0.07	7.45	148.58	149.60	26.89	0.01	0.89	4.15
Cheese, Parmesan, fresh or dry (TB)	68.78	0.05	2.54	40.35	93.07	5.35	0	0.16	1
Cheese, ricotta, part skim milk (CP)	669.12	1.08	36.33	449.20	306.76	307.50	0.07	3.30	15.6
Cheese, ricotta, whole milk (CP)	509.22	0.93	27.80	388.93	206.89	257.32	0.05	2.85	17.24
Cheese foods and spreads, pasteurized processed, 20–26% fat (TB)	90.88	0.10	4.89	130.24	257.60	41.60	0.01	0.45	2.69
Cottage cheese, 1% fat (CP)	137.63	0.32	12.07	302.39	917.56	193.23	0.07	0.86	11.75
Cottage cheese, 2% fat (CP)	154.81	0.36	13.56	340.13	917.56	217.41	0.07	0.95	11.75
Cottage cheese, 2% fat, no salt added (CP)	155.36	0.36	13.61	341.33	45.36	218.18	0.07	0.95	11.79

FOOD	CALC (mg)	IRON (mg)	MAG (mg)	PHOS (mg)	SOD (mg)	POTA (mg)	COP (mg)	ZINC (mg)	SELE (μg)
Cottage cheese, 4% fat (CP)	126	0.29	11.05	276.78	850.08	177.03	0.06	0.78	10.92
Cottage cheese, 4% fat, no salt added (CP)	126	0.29	11.05	276.78	42	177.03	0.06	0.78	10.92
Cottage cheese, low fat (CP)	154.81	0.36	13.56	340.13	917.56	217.41	0.07	0.95	11.75
Cottage cheese, uncreamed (CP)	45.96	0.33	5.71	150.80	18.56	46.98	0.04	0.68	7.54
Cream, half and half (CP)	253.86	0.17	24.61	230.38	98.49	313.63	0.02	1.23	1.33
Cream, heavy whipping (CP)	153.75	0.07	16.73	148.51	89.49	179.45	0.02	0.55	0.48
Cream, light (CP)	230.88	0.10	20.76	191.76	95.04	292.08	0.02	0.65	0.48
Cream, whipping (CP)	165.87	0.07	17.28	146.03	81.98	231.35	0.02	0.60	0.48
Cream, whipping, unsweetened (TB)	5.20	0	0.54	4.58	2.57	7.26	0	0.02	0.01
Cream cheese, 35% fat (TB)	11.19	0.17	0.90	14.62	41.37	16.72	0	0.08	0.7
Cream cheese, light, 18% fat (TB)	19.83	0.10	0.94	18.73	81.66	15.84	0	0.07	0.76
Cream cheese, Neufchâtel (TB)	10.54	0.04	1.06	19.08	55.92	15.97	0	0.07	0.57
Ice cream, 7% fat (light), all flavors except chocolate or coffee (CP)	162.81	0.11	17.68	130.49	100.61	250	0.01	0.68	8.54
Ice cream, 7% fat (light), chocolate or coffee (CP)	151.22	0.62	26.83	131.71	98.17	280.48	0.09	0.62	8.54
Ice cream, 11% fat (average), all flavors except chocolate and coffee (CP)	168.96	0.12	18.48	138.60	105.60	262.68	0.03	0.91	9.24

Ice cream, 11% fat (average), chocolate or coffee (CP)	143.88	1.23	38.28	141.24	100.32	328.68	0.18	0.77	9.24
Ice cream, 16% fat (rich), all flavors except chocolate or coffee (CP)	173.16	0.07	16.28	140.60	82.88	235.32	0.03	0.59	10.36
Ice cream, 16% fat (rich), chocolate or coffee (CP)	173.16	0.07	16.28	140.60	82.88	235.32	0.03	0.59	10.36
Ice milk, hardened, 4% fat, all flavors except chocolate (CP)	183.48	0.13	19.80	143.88	112.20	278.52	0.01	0.58	9.24
Milk, 1% fat (CP)	300.12	0.12	33.72	234.73	123.22	380.88	0.02	0.95	9.44
Milk, 2% fat (CP)	296.70	0.12	33.35	232.04	121.76	376.74	0.02	0.95	7.27
Milk, canned, condensed, sweetened (CP)	867.51	0.58	78.49	775.10	388.62	1136.48	0.03	2.88	5.72
Milk, canned, evaporated skim, undiluted (CP)	741.12	0.74	69.12	498.94	294.40	848.64	0.05	2.30	3.2
Milk, canned, evaporated whole, undiluted (CP)	657.22	0.48	60.96	510.30	266.62	763.81	0.05	1.94	3.15
Milk, low fat (CP)	296.70	0.12	33.35	232.04	121.76	376.74	0.02	0.95	7.27
Milk, powdered, nonfat, instant (TS)	17.48	0	1.66	13.98	7.79	24.22	0	0.06	0.24
Milk, powdered, nonfat, regular (TS)	30.75	0.01	2.93	24.60	13.71	42.61	0	0.11	0.42
Milk, skim (CP)	302.33	0.10	27.83	247.20	126.17	405.72	0.02	0.98	11.64
Milk, whole (CP)	291.34	0.12	32.79	227.90	119.56	369.66	0.02	0.93	2.93
Sherbet (CP)	103.68	0.27	15.36	76.80	88.32	184.32	0.06	0.92	1.21
Sour cream, low fat (CP)	319.92	0.50	85.19	319.92	240.56	560.01	0	2.73	1.93

FOOD	CALC (mg)	IRON (mg)	MAG (mg)	PHOS (mg)	SOD (mg)	POTA (mg)	COP (mg)	ZINC (mg)	SELE (µg)
Whipped topping, aerosol, saturated vegetable fat (TB)	0.23	0	0.04	0.80	2.69	0.84	0	0	0
Whipped topping, frozen, saturated vegetable fat (TB)	0.30	0.01	0.08	0.36	1.19	0.85	0	0	0
Whipped topping, powdered, reduced calorie, with aspartame (TB)	3.26	0	0.70	4.64	6.58	8.08	0	0.01	0
Yogurt, 1% fat, all flavors (CP)	323.40	1.96	34.30	269.50	102.90	475.30	0.02	0.98	4.53
Yogurt, 1% fat, sweetened with aspartame, all flavors (CP)	248.48	0.27	27.07	206.09	108.22	392.51	0.12	0.83	10.71
Yogurt, 2–4% fat, all flavors (CP)	1.13	365.05	0.17	34.30	286.65	139.65	465.50	0.02	1.76
Yogurt, 2–4% fat, unflavored or plain (CP)	295.71	0.12	28.37	232.50	113.68	378.77	0.02	1.45	3.06
Yogurt, frozen, 1–2% fat, all flavors except chocolate (CP)	293.17	0.14	28.12	230.44	112.71	375.38	0.15	1.43	5.11
Yogurt, frozen, 1–2% fat, chocolate (CP)	288.11	0.87	53.27	259.82	109.30	440.50	0.37	1.74	6
Yogurt, low fat, all flavors except coffee (CP)	372.15	0.17	35.70	292.53	143.08	476.52	0.20	1.81	6.49
Yogurt, low fat, coffee flavor (CP)	370.39	0.20	36.87	291.97	142.34	488.70	0.20	1.81	6.52
Yogurt, low fat, unflavored or plain (CP)	447.37	0.20	42.75	351.57	171.99	572.81	0.02	2.18	3.80

Almonds, unsalted (CP)	377.72	5.20	420.32	738.40	15.62	10?.44	1.33	4.15	6.67
Brazil nuts, unsalted (CP)	246.40	4.76	315	840	2.80	8?0	2.48	6.43	2261
Cashews, salted (CP)	53.30	5.33	331.50	553.80	813.80	?9	2.82	6.17	26
Cashews, unsalted (CP)	53.30	5.33	331.50	553.80	22.10	?9	2.82	6.17	26
Chestnuts, unsalted (CP)	95.81	3.40	105.82	250.25	52.91	14?.98	0.93	0.50	2.57
Coconut, fresh (PC)	6.30	1.09	14.40	50.85	9	10?.20	0.19	0.49	6.3
Coconut, shredded, sweetened (TS)	0.29	0.04	0.97	2.08	5.08	?54	0.01	0.04	0.28
Coconut, shredded, unsweetened (TS)	0.43	0.06	1.50	3.44	0.62	?07	0.01	0.03	0.43
Filberts, hazelnuts, unsalted (CP)	253.80	4.41	384.75	421.20	4.05	6?0.75	2.04	3.24	4.32
Hickory nuts, unsalted (CP)	61	2.12	173	336	1	?36	0.74	4.31	8.1
Macadamia nuts, salted (CP)	60.30	2.41	156.78	268	348.40	4?0.86	0.40	1.47	NA
Peanut butter, no salt added, creamy or chunky (TS)	1.81	0.09	8.37	17.22	0.91	?.43	0.03	0.13	0.53
Peanut butter, with salt, creamy or chunky (TS)	1.81	0.09	8.37	17.22	25.48	?8.43	0.03	0.13	0.53
Peanuts, salted (CP)	126.72	2.64	266.40	744.48	623.52	?32.08	1.87	9.55	10.08
Peanuts, unsalted (CP)	126.72	2.64	266.40	744.48	8.64	?2.08	1.87	9.55	10.08
Pecans, salted (CP)	37.40	2.52	141.90	323.40	831.60	?94.90	1.32	6.05	12.87

FOOD	CALC (mg)	IRON (mg)	MAG (mg)	PHOS (mg)	SOD (mg)	POTA (mg)	COP (mg)	ZINC (mg)	SELE (µg)
Pecans, unsalted (CP)	38.88	2.30	138.24	314.28	1.08	423.36	1.27	5.91	12.64
Pine nuts, unsalted (CP)	9.60	3.67	280.80	42	86.40	753.60	1.24	5.14	NA
Pistachio nuts, salted (CP)	89.60	4.06	166.40	609.28	998.40	1241.60	1.55	1.74	576
Pumpkin seeds, salted (CP)	59.34	20.62	736.92	1617.36	793.50	1112.28	1.90	10.27	7.73
Pumpkin seeds, unsalted (CP)	59.34	20.62	736.92	1617.36	24.84	1112.28	1.90	10.27	7.73
Sesame seeds (TB)	10.48	0.62	27.76	62.08	3.20	32.56	0.12	0.82	0.06
Sunflower seeds, hulled, salted (CP)	167.04	9.75	509.76	1015.20	1123.20	992.16	2.52	7.29	87.84
Sunflower seeds, hulled, unsalted (CP)	167.04	9.75	509.76	1015.20	4.32	992.16	2.52	7.29	87.84
Tahini (sesame butter) (TS)	21.30	0.45	4.75	36.60	5.75	20.70	0.08	0.23	2.5
Walnuts, unsalted (CP)	94	2.44	169	317	10	502	1.39	2.73	7.4
VEGETABLES AND LEGUMES									
Artichokes, cooked, without salt (CP)	75.60	2.17	100.80	144.48	159.60	594.72	0.39	0.82	1.18
Arugula, raw (CP)	32	0.24	9.40	10.40	5.40	73.80	0.02	0.09	0.3
Asparagus, canned, drained solids, with salt (CP)	38.72	4.43	24.20	104.06	943.80	416.24	0.24	0.97	9.83
Asparagus, fresh or frozen, cooked without salt (CP)	41.40	1.15	23.40	99	7.20	392.40	0.31	1.01	10.75

Food									
Baked beans with franks, canned (CP)	137.19	4.06	77.95	261.93	1163.08	643.96	0.23	3.98	16.55
Bamboo shoots, canned, cooked, with salt (CP)	10.48	0.42	5.24	32.75	9.17	104.80	0.14	0.85	NA
Beans, kidney, dry, cooked or canned, without fat, without salt (CP)	49.56	5.20	79.65	251.34	3.54	713.31	0.42	1.89	3.65
Beans, kidney, dry, cooked or canned, without fat, with salt (CP)	50.48	5.26	80.71	253.57	425.76	719.74	0.42	1.91	3.72
Beans, lima, cooked, fresh or frozen, without salt (CP)	37.40	2.31	57.80	107.10	90.10	693.60	0.08	0.75	0.24
Beans, lima, dry, cooked or canned, without fat, without salt (CP)	31.96	4.49	80.84	208.68	3.76	955.04	0.43	1.79	4.55
Beans, lima, dry, cooked or canned, without fat, with salt (CP)	32.58	4.51	81.52	209.43	449.85	938.59	0.43	1.79	4.61
Beans, navy, dry, cooked or canned, without fat, without salt (CP)	127.40	4.51	107.38	285.74	1.82	669.76	0.53	1.93	8.41
Beans, navy, dry, cooked or canned, without fat, with salt (CP)	127.76	4.51	107.63	285.45	431.67	669.18	0.53	1.93	8.44
Beans, northern dry, cooked or canned, without fat, without salt (CP)	161.10	6.62	112.77	202.27	10.74	1004.19	0.52	2.47	7.8
Beans, northern dry, cooked or canned, without fat, with salt (CP)	161.10	6.62	112.77	202.27	433.18	1004.19	0.52	2.47	7.8
Beans, pinto, dry, cooked or canned, without fat, without salt (CP)	82.08	4.46	94.05	273.60	3.42	800.28	0.44	1.85	12.59

FOOD	CALC (mg)	IRON (mg)	MAG (mg)	PHOS (mg)	SOD (mg)	POTA (mg)	COP (mg)	ZINC (mg)	SELE (μg)
Beans, pinto, dry, cooked or canned, without fat, with salt (CP)	83.23	4.50	95.18	275.86	411.07	806.98	0.44	1.86	12.72
Beans, yellow, canned, drained solids, with salt (CP)	35.36	1.22	17.68	25.84	341.36	148.24	0.05	0.39	0
Beans, yellow, cooked, fresh or frozen, without salt (CP)	60.75	1.11	28.35	32.40	17.55	151.20	0.09	0.84	0
Beets, Harvard (CP)	30.58	3.30	33.81	33.61	313.09	277.96	0.12	0.41	16.81
Beets, pickled (CP)	39.48	1.84	49.18	69.29	398.98	564.41	0.15	0.66	36.17
Beets, red, canned, drained solids, with salt (CP)	25.50	3.09	28.90	28.90	231.20	251.60	0.10	0.36	1.53
Beets, red, cooked, fresh or frozen, without salt (CP)	27.20	1.34	39.10	64.60	130.90	518.50	0.12	0.59	1.53
Broccoli, cooked, fresh or frozen, without salt (CP)	93.84	1.12	36.80	101.20	44.16	331.20	0.07	0.55	1.51
Broccoli, raw (CP)	42.24	0.77	22	58.08	23.76	286	0.04	0.35	1.5
Brussels sprouts, cooked, fresh or frozen, without salt (CP)	37.20	1.15	37.20	83.70	35.65	503.75	0.11	0.56	3.49
Cabbage, Chinese (pak-choi), cooked, drained (CP)	158.10	1.77	18.70	49.30	57.80	630.70	0.03	0.29	3.48
Cabbage, Chinese (pak-choi), raw, shredded (CP)	73.50	0.56	13.30	25.90	45.50	176.40	0.01	0.13	1.54

Cabbage, Chinese (pe-tsai), cooked, drained (CP)	38.08	0.36	11.90	46.41	10.71	267.75	0.04	0.21	2.62
Cabbage, Chinese (pe-tsai), raw, shredded (CP)	58.52	0.24	9.88	22.04	6.84	180.88	0.03	0.17	1.67
Cabbage, cooked, without salt (CP)	46.50	0.25	12	22.50	12	145.50	0.01	0.13	1.86
Cabbage, raw (CP)	32.90	0.41	10.50	16.10	12.60	172.20	0.01	0.13	1.57
Carrot, raw (CP)	29.70	0.55	16.50	48.40	38.50	355.30	0.05	0.22	3.19
Carrot juice (CP)	59.04	1.13	34.44	103.32	71.34	718.32	0.12	0.44	6.57
Carrots, canned, drained solids, with salt (CP)	36.50	0.93	11.68	35.04	351.86	261.34	0.15	0.38	1.9
Carrots, fresh or frozen, cooked, without salt (CP)	48.36	0.97	20.28	46.80	102.96	354.12	0.20	0.47	1.28
Cauliflower, fresh or frozen, cooked, without salt (CP)	30.60	0.74	16.20	43.20	32.40	250.20	0.04	0.23	5.76
Cauliflower, raw (CP)	22	0.44	15	44	30	303	0.04	0.28	3.2
Celery, raw (CP)	48	0.48	13.20	30	104.40	344.40	0.04	0.16	1.32
Chard, Swiss, fresh or frozen, cooked, without salt (CP)	101.50	3.95	150.50	57.75	313.25	960.75	0.28	0.58	45.5
Chickpeas, dry, cooked or canned, without fat, without salt (CP)	80.36	4.74	78.72	275.52	11.48	477.24	0.57	2.51	6.4
Chickpeas, dry, cooked or canned, without fat, with salt (CP)	80.36	4.74	78.72	275.52	398.52	477.24	0.57	2.51	6.4

FOOD	CALC (mg)	IRON (mg)	MAG (mg)	PHOS (mg)	SOD (mg)	POTA (mg)	COP (mg)	ZINC (mg)	SELE (μg)
Corn, ear, cooked (MD)	1.54	0.47	24.64	79.31	13.09	191.73	0.04	0.37	1.17
Corn, whole kernel, drained solids, canned, with salt (CP)	8.20	1.41	32.80	106.60	529.72	319.80	0.10	0.64	0.66
Corn, whole kernel, fresh or frozen, without salt (CP)	3.28	0.49	29.52	77.08	8.20	227.96	0.05	0.57	1.97
Cucumber, raw (CP)	14.56	0.27	11.44	20.80	2.08	149.76	0.03	0.21	6.55
Eggplant, cooked, boiled, without salt, diced (CP)	5.76	0.34	12.48	21.12	2.88	238.08	0.11	0.14	6.43
Endive, raw (CP)	15.08	0.24	4.35	8.12	6.38	91.06	0.03	0.23	3.77
Fennel, bulb, raw (CP)	42.63	0.26	14.79	43.50	45.24	360.18	0.06	0.17	NA
Garlic, fresh (TS)	5.65	0.05	0.78	4.77	0.53	12.51	0.01	0.04	0.81
Ginger root, raw (CP)	17.28	0.48	41.28	25.92	12.48	398.40	0.22	0.33	NA
Green beans, canned, drained solids, with salt (CP)	35.36	1.22	17.68	25.84	341.36	148.24	0.05	0.39	1.22
Green beans, fresh or frozen, cooked, without salt (CP)	60.75	1.11	28.35	32.40	17.55	151.20	0.09	0.84	2.02
Greens, collard, fresh or frozen, cooked, without salt (CP)	29.44	0.20	8.96	10.24	20.48	167.68	0.04	0.14	2.94
Greens, turnip, fresh or frozen, cooked, without salt (CP)	197.28	1.15	31.68	41.76	41.76	292.32	0.36	0.20	1.41

Food								
Jicama, cooked, without salt (CP)	14.87	0.77	14.87	21.63	5.41	182.52	0.07	0.20	NA
Jicama, raw (CP)	19.50	0.78	20.80	23.40	7.80	227.50	0.05	0.43	0
Kohlrabi, fresh or frozen, cooked, without salt (CP)	41.25	0.66	31.35	74.25	34.65	561	0.21	0.51	NA
Kohlrabi, raw (CP)	33.60	0.56	26.60	64.40	28	490	0.18	0.04	NA
Lentils, dry, cooked or canned, without fat, without salt (CP)	37.62	6.59	71.28	356.40	3.96	730.62	0.49	2.51	7.39
Lentils, dry, cooked or canned, without fat, with salt (CP)	37.78	6.53	70.98	352.93	467.50	723.63	0.49	2.49	7.35
Lettuce (CP)	10.45	0.27	4.95	11	4.95	86.90	0.02	0.12	0.44
Mushrooms, canned, drained solids, with salt (CP)	17.16	1.23	23.40	102.96	663	201.24	0.36	1.12	8.42
Mushrooms, fresh or frozen, cooked, without salt (CP)	9.36	2.71	18.72	135.72	3.12	555.36	0.78	1.36	10.78
Mushrooms, raw, whole or sliced (CP)	3.50	0.87	7	72.80	2.80	259	0.34	0.51	7.7
Okra, fresh or frozen, cooked, without salt (CP)	176.64	1.23	93.84	84.64	5.52	430.56	0.18	1.14	0.74
Onions, fresh or frozen, cooked, without salt (CP)	46.20	0.50	23.10	73.50	6.30	348.60	0.15	0.44	6.51
Onions, raw (CP)	32	0.35	16	52.80	4.80	251.20	0.10	0.30	4.96
Parsley, fresh (TB)	5.17	0.23	1.87	2.17	2.10	20.77	0.01	0.04	0.02

FOOD	CALC (mg)	IRON (mg)	MAG (mg)	PHOS (mg)	SOD (mg)	POTA (mg)	COP (mg)	ZINC (mg)	SELE (µg)
Parsnips, fresh or frozen, cooked, without salt (CP)	57.72	0.90	45.24	107.64	15.60	572.52	0.22	0.41	11.54
Peas, blackeye, dry, cooked or canned, without fat, without salt (CP)	41.04	4.29	90.63	266.76	6.84	475.38	0.46	2.21	28.18
Peas, blackeye, dry, cooked or canned, without fat, with salt (CP)	41.04	4.29	90.63	266.76	410.40	475.38	0.46	2.21	28.18
Peas, blackeye, fresh, cooked (CP)	211.20	1.85	85.80	84.15	6.60	689.70	0.21	1.70	31.18
Peas, edible podded, fresh or frozen, cooked without salt (CP)	67.20	3.15	41.60	88	6.40	384	0.13	0.59	8.98
Peas, green, canned, drained solids, with salt (CP)	34	1.61	28.90	113.90	372.30	294.10	0.14	1.21	0.97
Peas, green, fresh or frozen, cooked, without salt (CP)	38.40	2.51	46.40	144	139.20	268.80	0.22	1.50	0.91
Peas, split, dry, cooked or canned, without fat, without salt (CP)	27.44	2.53	70.56	194.04	3.92	709.52	0.35	1.96	0.98
Peas, split, dry, cooked or canned, without fat, with salt (CP)	27.44	2.53	70.56	194.04	466.48	709.52	0.35	1.96	0.98
Peas and carrots, fresh or frozen, cooked, without salt (CP)	36.80	1.50	25.60	78.40	108.80	252.80	0.13	0.72	1.1
Pepper, chili, Mexican, canned (CP)	9.52	0.68	19.04	23.12	1595.28	254.32	0.14	0.23	2.72

Pepper, chili, fresh, cooked, without salt (CP)	23.26	1.55	32.30	56.30	9.04	416.16	0.22	0.38	2.72
Pepper, green, fresh or frozen, cooked, without salt (CP)	12.24	0.63	13.60	24.48	2.72	225.76	0.08	0.16	2.99
Pepper, green, raw (CP)	9	0.46	10	19	2	127	0.06	0.12	2.2
Pepper, red, fresh or frozen, cooked, without salt (CP)	12.24	0.63	13.60	24.48	2.72	225.76	0.08	0.16	2.99
Pepper, red, raw (CP)	9	0.46	10	19	2	127	0.06	0.12	2.2
Plantains, fresh, cooked, without salt (CP)	3.08	0.89	49.28	43.12	7.70	716.10	0.11	0.20	3.08
Potatoes, French fried (REG)	0.48	0.02	1.32	2.66	6.77	213.82	0.01	0.02	0.07
Potatoes, French fried, without salt (REG)	0.53	0.02	1.33	2.66	0.33	213.82	0.01	0.02	0.07
Potatoes, baked, without skin, without salt (MD)	4.65	0.33	23.25	46.50	4.65	362.63	0.20	0.27	1.05
Potatoes, baked, with skin, without salt (CP)	12.20	1.66	32.94	69.54	9.76	505.96	0.37	0.39	1.61
Potatoes, boiled, without skin, without salt (CP)	12.48	0.48	31.20	62.40	7.80	511.68	0.27	0.42	1.62
Potatoes, boiled, with skin, without salt (MD)	11.98	1.56	30.98	65.15	9.32	477.72	0.34	0.37	1.52
Pumpkin, canned, cooked (CP)	63.70	3.41	56.35	85.75	12.25	500.70	0.27	0.42	NA
Radicchio, raw (CP)	7.60	0.12	5.20	16	8.80	120.80	0.14	0.25	0.6
Radish, raw (CP)	24.36	0.34	10.44	20.88	27.84	269.12	0.05	0.35	2.32
Refried beans, canned (CP)	116.38	4.48	98.67	212.52	1072.72	994.29	1.04	3.47	13.81

FOOD	CALC (mg)	IRON (mg)	MAG (mg)	PHOS (mg)	SOD (mg)	POTA (mg)	COP (mg)	ZINC (mg)	SELE (µg)
Romaine, raw (CP)	10.80	0.33	1.80	13.50	2.40	87	0.01	0.07	NA
Rutabaga, fresh or frozen, cooked, without salt (CP)	81.60	0.90	39.10	95.20	34	554.20	0.07	0.59	0.17
Sauerkraut, cooked, canned, solids and liquid (CP)	70.80	3.47	30.68	47.20	1559.96	401.20	0.24	0.45	0.24
Scallion, cooked (CP)	131.40	0.96	43.80	67.89	8.76	529.98	0.13	0.92	5.04
Scallion, raw (CP)	72	1.48	20	37	16	276	0.08	0.39	2.3
Seaweed, kelp, raw (CP)	134.40	2.28	96.80	33.60	186.40	71.20	0.10	0.98	NA
Soybean curd (tofu) (OZ)	29.77	1.52	29.20	27.50	1.98	34.30	0.05	0.23	0.09
Soybeans, dry, cooked or canned, without salt (CP)	175.44	8.84	147.92	421.40	1.72	885.80	0.71	1.98	10.32
Soybeans, roasted (CP)	237.36	6.71	249.40	624.36	280.36	2528.40	1.43	5.40	27.02
Soy flour (CP)	175.10	5.41	364.65	419.90	11.05	2137.75	2.48	3.33	7.65
Spinach, canned, drained solids, with salt (CP)	271.78	4.92	109.14	94.16	419.44	479.36	0.39	0.98	2.55
Spinach, fresh or frozen, cooked, without salt (CP)	277.40	2.89	131.10	91.20	163.40	566.20	0.27	1.33	2.75
Spinach, raw (CP)	55.44	1.52	44.24	27.44	44.24	312.48	0.07	0.30	0.67
Sprouts, alfalfa, raw (CP)	10.56	0.32	8.91	23.10	1.98	26.07	0.05	0.30	NA

Sprouts, mung bean, canned, cooked, without salt (CP)	17.36	0.53	11.16	39.68	173.60	33.48	0.20	0.35	NA
Sprouts, soybean, raw (CP)	46.90	1.47	50.40	114.80	9.80	338.80	0.30	0.82	NA
Squash, summer, all varieties, fresh or frozen, cooked, without salt (CP)	48.60	0.65	43.20	70.20	1.80	345.60	0.18	0.70	0
Squash, winter, all varieties, fresh or frozen, cooked, without salt (CP)	34.30	0.81	19.60	49	2.45	406.70	0.22	0.64	3.18
Sweet potato, canned, syrup pack, drained solids, with salt (CP)	33.32	1.86	23.52	49	76.44	378.28	0.33	0.31	1.23
Sweet potatoes, candied (MD)	49.97	0.86	28.48	68.34	262.74	605.69	0.29	0.37	1.13
Sweet potatoes, canned, vacuum pack, drained solids, with salt (CP)	44	1.78	44	98	106	624	0.28	0.36	1.4
Sweet potatoes, fresh or frozen, cooked, without salt (CP)	71.40	1.15	51	140.25	25.50	1206.15	0.54	0.74	1.78
Tempeh, fresh or frozen (PTY)	210.92	5.13	158.76	467.21	13.61	832.36	1.52	4.11	13.61
Tomatillos, raw (CP)	9.24	1.19	26.40	51.48	1.32	353.76	0.11	0.29	5.28
Tomatoes, canned, no salt added (CP)	62.40	1.46	28.80	45.60	31.20	530.40	0.26	0.38	2.28
Tomatoes, canned, with salt (CP)	62.40	1.46	28.80	45.60	391.20	530.40	0.26	0.38	2.28
Tomatoes, fresh, cooked, without salt (CP)	14.40	1.34	33.60	74.40	26.40	669.60	0.22	0.26	2.28
Tomatoes, raw (CP)	9	0.81	19.80	43.20	16.20	399.60	0.13	0.16	2.34
Tomatoes, sun dried (CP)	59.40	2.99	104.76	192.24	1131.30	1850.58	0.77	1.07	8.73

FOOD	CALC (mg)	IRON (mg)	MAG (mg)	PHOS (mg)	SOD (mg)	POTA (mg)	COP (mg)	ZINC (mg)	SELE (µg)
Tomatoes, sun dried, oil pack, drained (CP)	51.70	2.61	89.10	152.90	292.60	1721.50	0.52	0.86	10.43
Tomato juice, no salt added (CP)	21.84	1.41	26.69	46.10	24.26	533.81	0.24	0.34	0
Tomato juice, salt added (CP)	21.84	1.41	26.69	46.10	875.93	533.81	0.24	0.34	0
Tomato paste, canned, no salt added (CP)	91.70	7.83	133.62	206.98	170.30	2441.84	1.55	2.10	13.83
Tomato paste, canned, with salt (CP)	91.70	7.83	133.62	206.98	2069.80	2441.84	1.55	2.10	13.83
Tomato sauce, canned, without fat, no salt added (CP)	34.30	1.89	46.55	78.40	73.50	908.95	0.49	0.61	2.74
Tomato sauce, canned, without fat, with salt (CP)	34.30	1.89	46.55	78.40	1482.25	908.95	0.49	0.61	2.74
Turnips, fresh or frozen, cooked, without salt (CP)	34.32	0.34	12.48	29.64	78	210.60	0.09	0.31	1.4
Vegetable juice, cocktail, no salt added (CP)	26.62	1.02	26.62	41.14	55.66	467.06	0.48	0.48	0.48
Vegetable juice, cocktail, salt added (CP)	26.62	1.02	26.62	41.14	883.30	467.06	0.48	0.48	0.48
Water chestnuts, cooked, canned (CP)	25.20	0.70	4.21	100.80	19.60	215.60	0.04	0.24	NA
Watercress, raw (CP)	40.80	0.07	7.14	20.40	13.94	112.20	0.03	0.04	NA
Zucchini, fresh or frozen, cooked, without salt (CP)	23.40	0.63	39.60	72	5.40	455.40	0.16	0.32	1.8
Zucchini, raw (CP)	19.50	0.55	28.60	41.60	3.90	322.40	0.08	0.26	3.9

Index

Beta-tocopherol, 186
Bioflavonoids, 51, 199–200
Biotin
  content of common foods,
    152
  deficiency, 153–154
  dietary requirements, 153
  functions, 152–153
  history, 151
  overview, 150–151
  sources, 153
  use and misuse, 154
Birth control pills, vitamins and,
    47, 146, 157, 176
Birth defects, 115, 117. *See also*
    Neural tube defects.
Blood pressure. *See*
    Hypertension.
Booher, L. E., 126
Boron, 266
Breast cancer, 95
Breast disease, fibrocystic, 192
Breast-feeding
  iron requirements, 248
  niacin requirements, 135
  RDAs for, 17
  riboflavin requirements, 127
  vitamin B_6 requirements,
    146
  vitamin B_{12} requirements,
    164
  vitamin C requirements,
    174–175
  vitamin supplements, 60, 67
Bugs Bunny Complete,
    273–274
Bugs Bunny Plus Iron,
    274–275
Bugs Bunny with Extra C,
    275–276

C

Cadmium, 206
Caffeine, 209

Calcium
  authorized health claims for
    foods, 37, 38
  cancer and, 216, 217–218
  content of common foods,
    226–227
  deficiency, 227–228
  dietary requirements, 225
  functions, 223–224
  hypertension and, 215, 216
  osteoporosis and, 103–104,
    221, 228
  sources, 224–225
  use and misuse, 228–229
  vitamin K and, 194
Calories, defined, 11
Caltrate 600, 276
Caltrate 600 + D, 276–277
Caltrate Plus, 277
Cancer
  antioxidants and, 78–79
  dietary habits and, 49
  free radicals and, 75, 78–79
  minerals and, 216–218
  phytochemicals and, 85–86
  vitamins and, 92–96, 177
Carbohydrates
  calories in, 11
  as essential nutrients, 12, 13
Carnitine, 51, 201
Carotenes, 41
Carotenoids, 41, 81, 85–86,
    107, 117
Carpal tunnel syndrome, 148
Castle, William, 161
Cataracts
  free radicals and, 75, 79
  phytochemicals and, 87
  vitamins and, 101
Centrum Advanced Formula
    (liquid), 279–280
Centrum Advanced Formula
    (tablets), 278–279

549

Lead, 206
Lecithin, 198
Life Extension (book), 71
Lind, James, 167, 168
Lipofuscin, 191
Lipoic acid, 51, 200
Low-density lipoprotein (LDL)
    cholesterol, 78, 87, 90,
    214
Lycopene, 85, 86, 107

M

Macrocytic anemia, 158, 160
Macrominerals, 205
Macrophages, 99
Magnesium
    content of common foods,
        233–234
    diabetes and, 218–219
    functions, 232–235
    hypertension and, 215, 216
    osteoporosis and, 221–222
Manganese, 75, 263
Median heights and weights, 22
Medications, vitamins and, 59,
    73. *See also* Antibiotics;
    Anticoagulants; Birth
    control pills.
Megavitamin therapy, 47, 48,
    69–73
Menaquinone. *See* Vitamin K.
Menopause, 26, 192, 221, 228
Menstruation, 26, 249
Mercury, 206
Metabolism, energy and, 11–12
Microminerals, 205
Minerals. *See also* Disease and
        minerals; Trace minerals;
        Water, minerals and.
    deficiency, 207–208
    defined, 13
    functions, 14, 77, 206–207
    history, 203–205
    individual profiles, 223–259

Minerals *(continued)*
    as inorganic elements,
        205–206
    labeling, 64–68
    RDAs for, 16–24
    toxicity, 208
Minoxidil, 115
Molybdenum, 265
Monosodium glutamate,
    sensitivity to, 148
Monounsaturated fats, 189
Myadec Professional
    Formula, 303–304

N

Natalins, 304–305
National Academy of Sciences,
    15, 20
National Cancer Institute, 260
National Center for Health
    Statistics, 53
National Health and Nutrition
    Examination Survey
    (NHANES), 17, 81
National Institutes of Health,
    87, 225
National Research Council, 206
Nationwide Food Consumption
    Survey, 146
Neural tube defects, 38,
    101–103, 158
Niacin
    blood cholesterol and, 47,
        131, 138, 139
    content in two daily diets,
        136–137
    deficiency, 135, 138
    dietary requirements, 135
    functions, 133
    history, 132–133
    manufacture in body, 43
    sources, 133–135
    use and misuse, 138–139
Niacin equivalent, defined, 133

552

Recipe Index